HEALTH AND DISEASE IN BYZANTINE CRETE (7TH–12TH CENTURIES AD)

Daily life and living conditions in the Byzantine world are relatively underexplored subjects, often neglected in comparison with more visible aspects of Byzantine culture, such as works of art. The book is among the few publications on Greek Byzantine populations and helps pioneer a new approach to the subject, opening a window on health status and dietary patterns through the lens of bioarchaeological research. Drawing on a diversity of disciplines (biology, chemistry, archaeology and history), the author focuses on the complex interaction between physiology, culture and the environment in Byzantine populations from Crete in the 7th to 12th centuries.

The systematic analysis and interpretation of the mortality profiles, the observed pathological conditions, and of the chemical data, all set in the cultural context of the era, brings new evidence to bear on the reconstruction of living conditions in Byzantine Crete. Individual chapters look at the demographic profiles and mortality patterns of adult and non-adult populations, and study dietary habits and breastfeeding and weaning patterns. In addition, this book provides an indispensable body of primary data for future research in these fields, and so furthers an interdisciplinary approach in tracing the health of the past populations.

Medicine in the Medieval Mediterranean

Medicine in the Medieval Mediterranean is a series devoted to all aspects of medicine in the Mediterranean area during the Middle Ages, from the 3rd/4th centuries to the 16th. Though with a focus on Greek medicine, diffused through the whole Mediterranean world and especially developed in Byzantium, it also includes the contributions of the cultures that were present or emerged in the area during the Middle Ages and after, and which interacted with Byzantium: the Latin West and early vernacular languages, the Syrian and Arabic worlds, Armenian, Georgian and Coptic groups, Jewish and Slavic cultures and Turkish peoples, particularly the Ottomans.

Medicine is understood in a broad sense: not only medical theory, but also the health conditions of people, nosology and epidemiology, diet and therapy, practice and teaching, doctors and hospitals, the economy of health, and the non-conventional forms of medicine from faith to magic, that is, all the spectrum of activities dealing with human health. The series includes texts and studies, bringing to light previously unknown, overlooked or poorly known documents interpreted with the most appropriate methods, and publishing the results of important new research.

Health and Disease in Byzantine Crete (7th–12th centuries AD)

CHRYSSI BOURBOU
Hellenic Ministry of Culture, Greece

Routledge
Taylor & Francis Group
LONDON AND NEW YORK

First published 2010 by Ashgate Publishing

Published 2016 by Routledge
2 Park Square, Milton Park, Abingdon, Oxon OX14 4RN
711 Third Avenue, New York, NY 10017, USA

Routledge is an imprint of the Taylor & Francis Group, an informa business

British Library Cataloguing in Publication Data
Bourbou, Chryssi.
Health and disease in Byzantine Crete (7th–12th centuries AD). – (Medicine in the medieval Mediterranean) 1. Medical archaeology – Greece – Crete. 2. Human remains (Archaeology) – Greece – Crete. 3. Medicine, Medieval – Greece – Crete. 4. Diseases – Greece – Crete – History – To 1500. 5. Diet – Greece – Crete – History – To 1500. 6. Byzantine Empire – Civilization – 527–1081. I. Title II. Series
306.4'61'094959–dc22

Library of Congress Cataloging-in-Publication Data
Bourbou, Chryssi.
Health and disease in Byzantine Crete (7th–12th centuries AD) / Chryssi Bourbou.
p. cm. — (Medicine in the medieval Mediterranean) Includes bibliographical references and index. ISBN 978-0-7546-6615-8 (hardcover : alk. paper)—ISBN 978-1-4094-1756-9 (ebook) 1. Human remains (Archaeology)—Greece—Crete. 2. Paleopathology—Greece—Crete. 3. Nutrition—Greece—Crete--History. 4. Diseases—Greece—Crete—History. 5. Cretans—Health and hygiene—History. 6. Human ecology—Greece—Crete. 7. Excavations (Archaeology)—Greece—Crete. 8. Crete (Greece)—Antiquities. I. Title.
DF221.C8B625 2010
610.939'18—dc22

2010028979

ISBN 13: 978-0-7546-6615-8 (hbk)

To Dionysis and my family with love

Contents

List of Figures

List of Tables

Foreword

Careful excavation and research on archaeological human skeletons provide insight into important aspects of the lives of our ancestors that is not accessible through any other source. Like our older living relatives, archaeological human burials have much to teach us through the information we can gain through analysis of data from these remains. However, there are challenges in achieving this objective. Increasingly archaeologists are recognizing the value of biological data in reconstructing the culture of past human societies. Similarly biological anthropologists recognize that data from human remains are affected by the culture represented by human skeletal samples. This reality has promoted cooperation and collaboration between an archaeologist excavating a site and the biological anthropologist analyzing the human burials that may be recovered from the site – ideally with active involvement of the biological anthropologist during excavation. This emphasis on the need to integrate cultural and biological data in the interpretation of skeletal data has led to the use of the term bioarchaeology to describe a research emphasis in which archaeology provides an important context for interpreting the data extracted from archaeological human remains. Dr Chryssi Bourbou's book provides a commendable example of this emphasis in which she provides the archaeological context for the skeletal remains which are the main focus of her book and utilizes this context in interpreting the results of her analysis.

The remarkable improvements I have witnessed during my lifetime in both the quality and quantity of data that can be obtained from comprehensive skeletal analysis highlights the fact that current scientific methods, if rigorously applied, provide the pathway to a more complete understanding of our past and our relationship to those who have lived before us. It also emphasizes the fact that new methods are likely to be developed in the future and that long-term storage and curation of archaeological skeletal samples is highly likely to provide a source of important new data in the future.

In the following pages, Bourbou has provided the reader with a careful analysis and interpretation of human remains dated to the Byzantine Period (seventh to twelfth centuries AD) and excavated from archaeological sites on the island of Crete in Greece. In her research she has demonstrated again the value of data obtained through the study of human remains. My late mentor and colleague, Dr J. Lawrence Angel, had done remarkable pioneer research on human skeletal biology in the eastern Mediterranean with an emphasis on Greece from the Neolithic Period through the Greek Classical Period. As Bourbou notes, Angel was one of the early scientists to attempt the linkage between the cultural and biological environment with the evidence of the human biological adjustment to this environment provided through analysis of the skeleton. Bourbou has applied more recent bioarchaeological methodology to highlight a phase in Greek history that has not received the attention from which earlier periods have benefited.

The analytical methods available today provide tools that I could not even imagine early in my career. Refinements in dating methods permit much greater accuracy in determining the archaeological age of human remains and radiocarbon dating using accelerator mass spectrometry requires much smaller samples than earlier dating methods. Furthermore we are much more aware of the factors that can distort dating methods. Mass spectrometry has also made possible analysis of stable isotopes that provide data for reconstructing some aspects of the diet in human archaeological skeletal samples. This research methodology is tangibly demonstrated in Bourbou's interpretation of stable isotope data in Chapter 4 indicating a dietary emphasis on wheat, oil and wine.

Our knowledge about the skeletal disorders that one encounters in the study of human remains has increased dramatically during the 40 years I have been conducting research on human skeletal paleopathology. Ongoing research continues to improve and provide data on the health of past human populations. One of the developments has been a heightened understanding of the skeletal manifestations of two of the metabolic disorders, scurvy and rickets. My own research on scurvy provided the observations needed to identify this disorder in sub-adult skeletons. However, it also raised questions about the pathological significance of porous lesions in the skull. The porous and sometimes hypertrophic lesions apparent in the orbits and skull vault of some sub-adult skulls had been attributed by Angel to one of the genetic anemias. Since Angel's 1966 paper in *Science*, in which he coined the term 'porotic hyperostosis' for the porous, hypertrophic lesions of the skull, the additional possibility of iron deficiency anemia was added to the list of diagnostic options associated with skull porosity. The term porotic hyperostosis, which should mean abnormal, porous bone formation, has become virtually synonymous with anemia including porous lesions not associated with new bone formation.

However, porous lesions of the skull and lesions in which there is porous hypertrophic bone formation can be caused by several disorders, including anemia, scurvy, rickets, infection and cancer. Anemia can only be identified anatomically if there is evidence of marrow hyperplasia associated with porotic hyperostosis. Angel knew this and assumed that everyone else using the term would as well. However, this has not been the case, with the result that the porous and porous hypertrophic lesions of the skull have been attributed, in most published reports, to anemia with virtually no attention being paid to the presence or absence of marrow hyperplasia. Bourbou is aware of the problem and in her research has wisely insisted on a multifactorial interpretation of these lesions. What is certainly true is that porotic and porotic hypertrophic lesions are indicative of a disorder and this has value as long as it is not attributed to a specific disorder without further evidence of pathogenesis such as the location of the lesions or the presence of marrow hyperplasia.

There are troublesome problems that remain to be dealt with in interpreting data from human skeletal samples. A vigorous scientific debate continues regarding the representativeness of archaeological skeletal samples relative to the living population from which the sample came. Clearly skeletal samples are not fully representative of the living population even in ideal situations. What is less clear is just how significant this limitation is. However, at the very least, bioarchaeologists need to be aware of the potential biases inherent in archaeological skeletal samples and avoid drawing conclusions that are not justified because of the limitations associated with the sample they are studying. For example, Bourbou notes that in Classical Greece children were not full members of society until the age of three and below that age may have been treated differently in the burial tradition. Many of the diseases that affect the skeleton can occur in infants and young children. If these are missing from the skeletal sample, disease prevalence will be distorted. Males and females may be buried in different areas of a cemetery. If the entire cemetery is not excavated this could result in a ratio between males and females that does not represent the living population.

Interpreting the significance of skeletal disease involves variables which current research has little ability to control. Although there are exceptions, the disorders one usually encounters in an archaeological burial are rarely the cause of death and may have had minimal morbidity. Skeletons with no evidence of disorder may represent very healthy people but it is also possible, for example, that they represent people with a poor immune response to infection and who die quickly before the skeleton can be involved.

Despite the limitations in interpreting the data recovered from archaeological human remains, there is much that we can learn from the analysis and Bourbou's book provides a helpful example of the insight available from rigorous analysis of skeletal samples. As we define more carefully the biases in skeletal samples and achieve greater understanding of the disorders that affect the skeleton, the quality and the interpretation of our data will improve. With growing experience in skeletal analysis it is probable that methods will be developed that will permit researchers to control for at least some of the limitations that currently exist.

Donald J. Ortner
Smithsonian Institution
National Museum of Natural History
March 2010

Acknowledgments

There are many people to thank, since without their help and support the publication of this book could never have happened. Friends and colleagues reviewed parts of the first draft, and their valuable comments and suggestions enhanced its format and content: Marie-Hélène Congourdeau (Centre d'Histoire et Civilisation de Byzance), Benjamin Fuller (Max Planck Institute), Sandra Garvie-Lok (University of Alberta), Cecily Hennesy (Christie's Education), Mary Lewis (University of Reading), Donald Ortner (Smithsonian Institution), Mike Richards (Max Planck Institute; University of British Columbia), Charlotte Roberts (University of Durham), Dionysios Stathakopoulos (King's College London), and Dimitris Tsougarakis (Ionian University). I am also grateful to many people who shared with me information on the various topics of my study, making substantial contributions of bibliographical references and data from their individual projects: Ilias Anagnostakis (National Institution of Research), Efrosyni Vika, Anastasia Fiolitaki (28th Ephorate of Byzantine Antiquities), Sherry Fox (Wiener Laboratory, American School of Classical Studies at Athens), Maria Kyrimi (13th Ephorate of Byzantine Antiquities), Alice-Mary Talbot (Dumbarton Oaks), Eirini Petroutsa, and Anastasia Papathanasiou (Ephorate of Speleology and Paleoanthropology). I especially thank Vassiliki Zygouri for entrusting me with data from her unpublished master's thesis.

Permission to examine the human skeletal material in this study was provided by Michalis Andrianakis (28th Ephorate of Byzantine Antiquities), Liana Starida (13th Ephorate of Byzantine Antiquities), and Petros Themelis (University of Crete; Society of Messenian Archaeological Studies). Generous financial support for the bioarchaeological and stable isotope analysis of the collections was granted by the Wiener Laboratory of the American School of Classical Studies at Athens, the Society of Messenian Archaeological Studies, the Ioannis Costopoulos Foundation, and the British School at Athens. Images and permission for their use were kindly provided by Petros Themelis and the Society of Messenian Archaeological Studies.

Images of pathological conditions for the collection from Eleutherna were made by Katerina Painesi, and all images have been skillfully reworked by Constantinos Andronis. Special thanks go to Constantinos Trompoukis (Faculty of Medicine, University of Crete) and Ilias Kosmidis for undertaking the radiographic analysis of the pathological specimens. I also warmly thank

Argyro Mamalaki and Vaso Mylona for access to the Library of the University of Crete, and Molly Richardson for her thorough and meticulous editing of the original manuscript. I am much obliged to John Smedley (Ashgate Publishing) for his guidance and for his patience in answering my questions on the format of the book.

I deeply thank Alain Touwaide (Institute for the Preservation of Medical Traditions, Smithsonian Institution) for inviting me to contribute to the series *Ancient Medicine in the Mediterranean World*, for which he serves as an editor, and for his continuous help and encouragement in the writing of this book. Dionysis, my family and my friends offered tremendous support, standing next to me during moments of stress and gently reminding me of the bright side of life.

Introduction

This book is about the analysis and interpretation of lifestyle and disease in Byzantine Crete through the study of human skeletal remains and the use of innovative techniques such as chemical analysis (stable isotopes) for the reconstruction of dietary, breastfeeding and weaning patterns. The interaction between humans and their environment is a millennia-long affair that has attracted increasing interest from archaeologists since the development of science-based multidisciplinary applications in the field. In the last decade, the term 'bioarchaeology' has been applied to the subfield that through a multidisciplinary approach focuses on the human biological component of the archaeological record and offers insights into the lifestyle, demography, disease patterns (palaeopathology) and diet of past populations.[1]

Major or minor, each adaptation to a continuously changing environment is potentially reflected in our bodies. Thus, without studying humans themselves we could only partially reconstruct life in the past. Bones and teeth, as well as mummified remains, serve as the primary source of evidence for anthropological and palaeopathological analysis, while iconography and documentary evidence supplement the study of diseases in the past. The methods most frequently applied to the study of human remains are macroscopic (visual) observation, radiology and computed tomography.[2] More sophisticated techniques are increasingly being employed, providing more accurate information, but also leading to higher costs and technical demands. The application of biomolecular techniques such as ancient DNA (aDNA) analysis[3] has proven particularly useful for recognizing diseases that only affect soft tissues, such as the Black

---

1 Larsen 1997; for the use of the term 'bioarchaeology' since its first application during the 1970s, see Buikstra 2006, xvii–xx.

2 For the use of palaeoradiology, see Chhem and Rülhi 2004; for examples of the application of computed tomography, see Chhem et al. 2004; Ryan and Milner 2006; Kuhn et al. 2007.

3 For the contribution of ancient DNA analysis to archaeology, see Brown 2000; for a thorough review on methods and applications, see Kaestle and Horsburgh 2002.

Death.[4] Research to date has concentrated mainly on tuberculosis[5] and leprosy,[6] although DNA from the causative organisms for diseases such as venereal syphilis,[7] malaria,[8] Spanish influenza[9] and typhoid fever[10] has also been extracted and amplified from archaeological material. Microscopic applications (for example, palaeohistology) have also presented exciting possibilities, providing detailed information to make or confirm specific diagnoses.[11] Also of increasing importance has been the application of chemical analysis (for example, stable isotope analysis) for looking at dietary patterns in order to better understand the quality and balance of foodstuffs and their effect on health[12] or migration patterns.[13]

Limitations (for example, not all pathological conditions produce lesions on dry bone) and pitfalls in bioarchaeology, as in every discipline, give rise to various problems inherent to the study of human remains recovered from archaeological contexts. In 1992, Wood et al. published a thought-provoking paper that brought these problems to the attention of researchers. Their observations were – and still are – shared by the majority of specialists working in bioarchaeology, skeletal biology and related disciplines, who recognize that from the soil to the laboratory, human remains are subject to a number of extrinsic and intrinsic factors that potentially complicate any attempt to reconstruct past lifestyle and disease patterns.[14] Much criticism has also stemmed from the argument that since the early 1980s, a lack of shared and combined research between archaeology and physical anthropology is noted. Goldstein pointed to the need for more science- and laboratory-oriented research on human remains, whereas today physical anthropologists ignore archaeological data, and bioarchaeology seems to be solely the study of human remains recovered from an archaeological context.[15] Although some of her arguments and concerns are valid and are

---

4 See, e.g., Drancourt et al. 1998, 2004, 2007; Wiechmann and Grupe 2005.

5 See, e.g., Taylor 1996; Taylor et al. 1999; Nerlich et al. 1997; Gernaey et al. 1999; Haas et al. 2000; Mays, Fysh and Taylor 2002.

6 Taylor et al. 2000.

7 Kolman et al. 1999.

8 Taylor, Rutland and Molleson 1997.

9 Reid et al. 1999.

10 Using aDNA, Papagrigorakis et al. 2006 have diagnosed typhoid fever as the cause of the Athenian plague.

11 Pfeiffer 2000; Bell and Piper 2000; Schultz 2001.

12 See, e.g., Müldner and Richards 2005, 2007a; Richards, Fuller and Molleson 2006.

13 Katzenberg 2000.

14 Roberts and Cox 2003, 16–17; Wright and Yoder 2003, 43–7.

15 Goldstein 2006, 376–9.

partially explained by the different trajectories the two disciplines have followed during the years, it must be always remembered that it is actually the educational background of the researcher that weighs most heavily upon the type of analysis applied. In other words, for an archaeologist specializing in the study of human remains the integration of archaeological, cultural and biological data is unquestionable in every attempt to reconstruct past lives, especially within historic contexts. Nevertheless, the 'bioarchaeological approach' is recognized as an important tool of investigation and, although still burdened with several complex unresolved issues, it remains our best option to understand fully the ways of life and death in the past.

During the last quarter of the nineteenth and the first half of the twentieth centuries, the educational background in medicine and biology of researchers involved in the study of human remains in Greece influenced their interests, which centered on exhaustive measurements and indices of variations between and within populations.[16] The physical anthropologist J. Lawrence Angel (1915–86) was the first to exhibit an interest in the skeletal biology of the Eastern Mediterranean, with Greece being the major focus throughout his life.[17] Angel belongs to the group of researchers who were responsible for shifting the research interests of palaeopathology from a static concern with the history of disease to questions concerning the epidemiology of diseases and their relation to other biocultural factors. Apart from his many reports on skeletal material from a variety of archaeological sites in Greece,[18] Angel had a keen interest in a number of areas of physical anthropology, such as palaeodemography,[19] palaeopathology (with publications on thalassaemia and its relationship to malaria in the Mediterranean area),[20] trauma[21] and occupationally related pathology.[22]

In the years that followed, bioarchaeology in Greece demonstrated a shift from hesitant and sporadic case studies to population-based analysis on a wider regional and temporal level. Most of these studies initially focused on prehistoric or classical populations.[23] Laskaris, in his survey of Byzantine cemeteries

---

16 For a thorough discussion of early studies of biological anthropology in Greece, see Roberts et al. 2005, 38–9, and for the current state of play, see Buikstra and Lagia 2009.

17 For the contribution of J. Lawrence Angel and Angel's corpus of publications, see Roberts et al. 2005, 4–5, and 51–8.

18 Perhaps one of his most important publications was on the population of Lerna, where he successfully combined biological and cultural data; see Angel 1971.

19 Angel, 1968, 1969.

20 Angel, 1964a, 1966, 1967, 1977, 1978.

21 Angel, 1974.

22 Angel, 1964b, 1982.

23 See, e.g., Papathanasiou 2001; Triantaphyllou 2001; Lagia, forthcoming.

and scattered burials throughout Greece, lists 561 sites, out of which only a very small number have received a thorough study of their recovered human skeletal remains.[24] This lack of skeletal studies for Byzantine populations can be explained to a great extent by the fact that very few systematic excavations have been carried out on Byzantine cemeteries and most of the material has been retrieved from rescue excavations, where it is at best viewed as a time- and money-consuming issue. Under these circumstances most Byzantine burial grounds are hastily excavated, and the material recovered is poorly stored and far less available for study and publication. In addition, human remains from Christian burials excavated within churches often end up in a communal grave after a brief ceremony by the local priest. In other European countries, such as the United Kingdom, specific guidelines are published for the treatment of human remains excavated in Christian burial grounds.[25] However, such protocols do not currently exist in Greece, highlighting the need for public awareness of the scientific value of human skeletal remains.

It is only in recent years that an increased interest has been expressed in the study of populations dating to Byzantine and post-Byzantine periods, or of specific segments of these populations such as non-adults.[26] Besides these population studies, researchers are increasingly using stable isotope analysis for detecting dietary, breastfeeding and weaning patterns, surveying as well the abundant documentary evidence against which the biological data can be projected and compared.[27] The present study focuses on the reconstruction of health status and dietary patterns of early (fourth to ninth centuries AD) and middle (tenth to thirteenth centuries AD) Byzantine populations from Crete.[28] Human skeletal collections from the early Byzantine period date mainly to the sixth–seventh centuries AD, and from the middle Byzantine period to

---

24 Laskaris 2000, 284–7.

25 Mays 2005.

26 Barnes, 2002; Bourbou 2001a, 2004; Tritsaroli 2006; Bourbou and Tsilipakou 2009.

27 Garvie-Lok 2001; Bourbou and Richards 2007; Bourbou 2008; Bourbou, Fuller and Richards 2008; Bourbou and Garvie-Lok 2009; Bourbou and Garvie-Lok forthcoming.

28 Besides publications on Byzantine populations from Crete, some work has been also conducted on populations from the mainland: Tritsaroli 2006, the Peloponnese: Bourbou 2004; Wesolowsky 1973, North Greece: Agelarakis and Agelarakis 1989; Bourbou 1996; Bourbou and Tsilipakou 2009; Georgakopoulou and Xirotiris 2009, Thasos: Buchet and Sodini 1984. For a thorough review of publications for early Byzantine populations in Greece, see Bourbou 2004, 31–9. Current research on Byzantine populations is being conducted by Dr P. Tritsaroli at the sites of Xironomi (Boeotia), Porto Rafti and Taxiarchis Kalyvion (Attica), P. Tritsaroli pers. comm. 2008, and by Dr S. Garvie-Lok at Isthmia and Kenchreai (the Peloponnese), S. Garvie-Lok pers. comm. 2008.

the eleventh–twelfth centuries AD. Little information has been available for Byzantine Crete, making the contribution of an interdisciplinary approach essential. Documentary and archaeological evidence gives sparse and scattered information, resulting in more questions than answers for the transitional and idiosyncratic character of the period in question.[29] The multiple and intensive stresses (including invasions and natural disasters such as earthquakes) suffered periodically throughout the Byzantine period highlight the need for caution in order to avoid simplistic generalizations about everyday life and the socio-economic and cultural activities of its populations. Nevertheless, in the past few years a growing interest can be noted in the rather neglected and largely unknown Byzantine Crete. The international conference *Creta Romana e Protobizantina* (Heraklion, 2000) represented a pioneering effort to bring together researchers from a variety of specializations in order to determine the effects of the complex phenomena observed during the gradual transformation from the ancient to the Byzantine world, and the resulting four-volume corpus of papers was published in 2004.[30] Added to these proceedings is the extensive publication of the results obtained from years of systematic excavation at the early Byzantine site of Eleutherna.[31] Piece by piece, the picture of Byzantine Crete is being roughly shaped and, although still much work remains to be done, a solid background exists upon which science-based research can be conducted.[32]

Since studies published on health in past populations vary in quality, data for inclusion in this book have been mainly derived from the work conducted by the author for the sites of Eleutherna, Kastella and Stylos. For comparison, published data for other Byzantine populations from Crete have been scrutinized and modified as appropriate in order to provide a more complete picture of the era in question; the publications that have proven helpful include those on the early Byzantine sites of Gortyn, Knossos and Kefali Pediados.[33] For the reconstruction of dietary patterns it was thought more useful to include all available data from sites outside Crete, in order to have a better idea of the Byzantine dietary profile and attitudes towards breastfeeding and weaning patterns.

---

29 Tsougarakis 1988.

30 Atti del Congresso Internazionale Creta Roman e Protobizantina, 2004.

31 Prof. P. Themelis, who supervised the field seasons from 1986 through 2003, acted as the editor of four distinctive volumes devoted to the meticulous study of the archaeological finds of Eleutherna: Themelis 2000, 2004; Bourbou 2004; Yangaki 2005.

32 It must be noted that the *International Conference on Cretological Studies*, which takes place every five years, and the *Conference on the Archaeological Work in Crete*, established in 2008 and expected to occur every two years, are the major forums for presenting archaeological projects conducted on the island.

33 Gortyn: Mallegni 1988; Knossos: Musgrave 1976; Kefali Pediados: Zygouri 2005.

The book begins with a presentation on the general context of Byzantine Crete, in order to contextualize the biological data and the methodology used for the anthropological and palaeopathological analysis (Chapter 1). The next two chapters discuss the results obtained from the study of the adult (Chapter 2) and non-adult (Chapter 3) segments of the populations, respectively. These chapters present the demographic profile and mortality patterns of the populations, as well as the observed pathological conditions.

There are a number of broad categories of disease that most palaeopathologists consider when studying past populations, some of which are more common than others. In this book the major disease categories (dental, joint and infectious diseases, hematopoietic and metabolic disorders, as well as traumatic incidents) are the areas focused on, but where evidence exists for rarer conditions (such as neoplastic and congenital) they are also included. Notably pathological conditions are better viewed in their biocultural context. Thus, for example, in terms of periodic crises and culturally influenced practices, it is impossible to ignore the impact of impoverished conditions on the development of specific pathological conditions.

Chapter 4 is devoted to stable isotope analysis applied to the study of dietary habits, as well as of breastfeeding and weaning patterns. The results obtained from such an analysis are viewed within the specific cultural context of the era: for example, it is essential to determine the likely $\delta^{13}C$ and $\delta^{15}N$ values of some of the items mentioned in the sources and known to be included in the Byzantine diet. Furthermore, fasting rules targeting some key animal products in the diet, or restrictions applied according to gender, should be considered when reconstructing Byzantine diets. Similarly, since attitudes towards breastfeeding and weaning patterns are cited in the written sources, isotopic data can ideally be projected and compared against documentary evidence. As the effects of weaning have been associated with the development of specific pathological conditions, special attention is given to metabolic and hematopoietic disorders. Finally, a synthesis of the obtained data is presented in the last chapter (Conclusions), where the integration of biological, chemical and cultural data provides a holistic picture of Cretan populations during the Byzantine era.

The diversity of fields that bioarchaeology draws from (for example, biology, chemistry, social sciences) reflects the fact that humans more than any other living organism experience a complex interaction between physiology, culture and the environment. The interpretation of this interaction – which usually affects human remains in multiple and not always clear ways – is the bioarchaeologist's primary task. Since the mid-1980s the changes seen in the field of bioarchaeology demonstrate an increasing sophistication, which permits us to share Larsen's enthusiasm when noting that:[34]

> Bioarchaeology is enjoying a period of robust growth.

The same spirit of vitality and innovation in bioarchaeology is shared among specialists working in Greece. The increasing number of publications has stimulated a series of events convened to highlight the burgeoning of bioarchaeological studies in Greece.[35] Currently, a number of institutions support and promote the study of human skeletal remains in Greece (university departments in Athens, Rhodes, Thessalonike, Thrace and Heraklion; the Ephorate of Speleology and Palaeoanthropology; the Wiener Laboratory of the American School of Classical Studies at Athens), offering a rich environment for fruitful work. Recognizing the significance of modern reference collections for research and teaching purposes, such a collection is currently housed at the Department of Animal and Human Physiology at the University of Athens.[36] The establishment of such a collection highlights the emergence of a clearly science-based discipline in Greece. It is also promising to see that archaeologists are incorporating into their research projects the study of human skeletal remains and encouraging the presence of a specialist in the field. They also understand the benefits of integrating the results of such an analysis into the general discussion of the funerary and cultural context, rather than including a separate appendix at the end of a cemetery report.

It is very important to emphasize the hope that bioarchaeological studies will further promote the interest of all related specialists in the education of the general public on the scientific value of human remains, a task that can be

---

34 Larsen 2006, 373.

35 In 2003 Dr L. Schepartz and Dr S. Fox organized a colloquium on *New Directions in the Skeletal Biology of Ancient Greece* at the 104th Annual Meeting of the Archaeological Institute of America; the following year, the author organized a session on *Studies of Bioarchaeology in Greece* at the 15th European Meeting of the Palaeopathology Association. The participants in these sessions, along with other scholars pursuing research on Greek skeletal populations, were invited to contribute to an edited volume; Schepartz, Fox and Bourbou 2009. Finally, in 2006 Greece hosted at Santorini the 16th European Meeting of the Palaeopathology Association, continuing a successful line of previous meetings in other European countries.

36 The first part of the collection was built between 1996 and 1997 at the Wiener Laboratory and consisted of 72 skeletons, see Pike 1997; currently the *Modern Reference Collection of the University of Athens* includes 225 specimens, see Eliopoulos, Lagia and Manolis 2007.

accomplished if bones take an actual place in museum halls.[37] A brief survey of how skeletal remains are displayed in museum exhibitions designed to teach people that archaeology discovers not only elaborate structures and precious artifacts but also the remains of the people who actually produced them, is limited to a handful of examples. While artifacts derived from funerary contexts are displayed and presented with much detail, the associated skeletal remains are usually absent. The Kerameikos Museum in Athens hosts only one funerary urn with cremated remains – and that is the only visual presence of human remains in a museum devoted exclusively to the finds retrieved from an extensive burial ground (Figure Intro. 1).

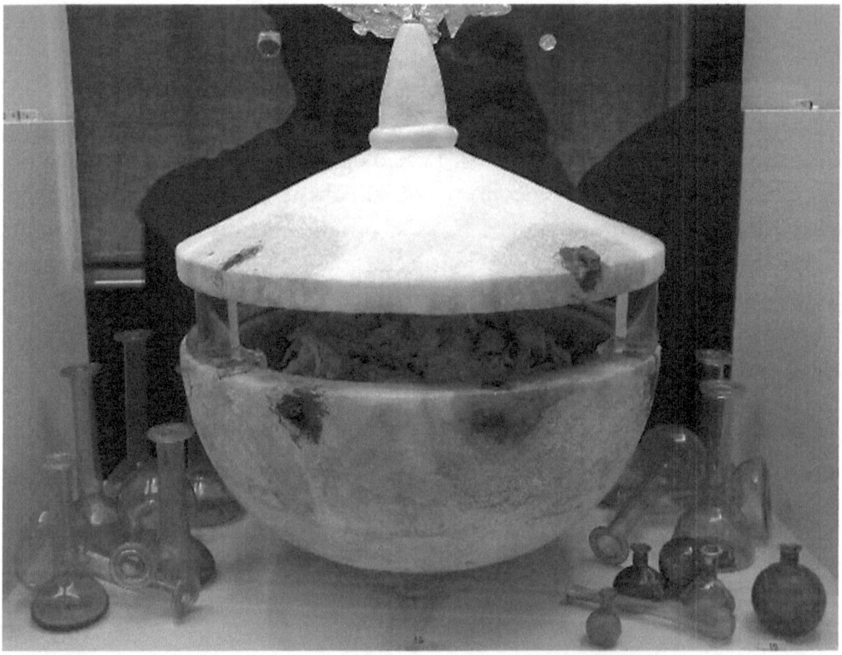

Figure Intro. 1 A funerary urn with cremated human bones. Kerameikos Museum, Athens (photo: C. Bourbou)

[37] At the Syntagma Metro Station in Athens, the exhibition of the finds recovered during construction work includes the display of a fourth century BC grave with its in situ skeleton. Feelings of passengers crossing the station daily varied from discomfort to curiosity, but no one passed by indifferent. Visitors are usually gathered around similar displays when they exist in Museum halls (for example, at the National Archaeological Museum in Athens). For a brief discussion on the display of human remains in museums, see Roberts 2009, 30–33.

In a more optimistic view, though, it must be highlighted that several temporary exhibitions have devoted a special section to the wealth of information we obtain from the study of human remains when observing pathological conditions and their treatment, diet or genetic affiliations (*Minoans and Mycenaeans: Flavors of their Times*, National Archaeological Museum of Athens, 1999), or have reconstructed burial environments including the skeletal remains (*Eleutherna: Polis, Acropolis, Necropolis*, Museum of Cycladic Art, Athens, 2005). A truly innovative way of displaying human remains has been admired by visitors at a recent exhibition (*Andritsa Cave – Fateful Refuge*, Byzantine and Christian Museum, 2005): bare bones were not exhibited; instead a sandy outline was carefully arranged to mimic the actual position of the skeleton as found within the burial context.

It is hoped that in the near future archaeologists and biological anthropologists will work together so that skeletons will come out of their closets, revealing secrets of their past lives. The bioarchaeological approach applied to Byzantine populations from Crete is expected to be such a stimulus for future analyses in Greece, especially for cases in which documentary and archaeological evidence is scarce and incomplete. The solid background of the discipline in Greece and the increasing interest in multidisciplinary applications to archaeological projects demonstrate a field where fruitful research is yet to be done.

Chapter 1
The Jigsaw Puzzle of Health in Context

The attainment of health is one of human life's many challenges, and the study of health and disease patterns in a population can potentially reflect many aspects of how a society functions. Health and disease as variables may affect the social, political and economic systems of a society and, in turn, those systems may influence disease load on a population. The relationship between humans, their environment and cultural context (the 'ecosystem') is interdependent. Thus, the etiology of a disease may be the result of a number of factors, both intrinsic (the immune system, age and sex) and extrinsic (subsistence, diet, population density, levels of hygiene, geographical location and climate). In the complex interrelationship of these intrinsic and extrinsic influences on health, none of them acts in isolation. Using the evidence of these variables for the reconstruction of health and disease patterns in the past can be particularly difficult, as critical information may need to be deduced from inadequate or incomplete data.[1]

The immune system is the key to protecting humans from disease. The ability of a person's immune system to resist disease depends on both the natural immune system, which is genetically inherited, and the adaptive immune system, which can change to protect the body against pathogens upon being exposed to them. A strong association exists between the immune status and diet, as a healthy balanced diet contributes to the normal development and effectiveness of a person's immune system. One's age and sex can also have an impact on a person's disease experience, often because of related changes in immune responses.[2]

What people do for a living, what they eat and where they live all affect their acquisition of diseases.[3] Social inequalities present in both past and modern populations define the quality of life and affect disease frequency in rich and poor; so, for example, high-status individuals have access to better diet, living conditions and medical treatment in comparison with their poorer counterparts. The type of settlement (rural or urban), its location (for example, in a marshy

---

1 For a thorough discussion, see, e.g., Roberts and Manchester 2005, 1–20; Roberts and Cox 2003, 2–12.

2 Armelagos 1998.

3 The impact of environmental and cultural factors on human health and disease has been a subject of extensive investigation; see, e.g., Salares 1991; Hope and Marshall 2000; Horden and Purcell 2000.

area) and local climatic conditions, especially weather extremes, influence the disease load on a population. The link between hot climates – which favor the survival of disease vectors – marshy areas and malaria provides a clear example of how climatic conditions, general topography and geology intertwine.[4] Agriculturally and pastorally based societies tend to develop specific health problems (for example, infectious and metabolic conditions, zoonotic diseases) as a result of sedentism, population density, poor sanitation and a limited food base. At the start of sedentism, people lack both effective sewage and clean water supplies, and accumulate domestic waste.[5] It takes only a single infected water-pump for an epidemic of cholera to spread, as was the case in nineteenth-century London.[6] Hygiene is not only environmental; although personal hygiene is culturally defined and influenced, individuals' effectiveness in cleaning their bodies, clothes, households and food affects the sanitary levels at which a population lives.

The factors briefly outlined above form the complex web that may affect an individual's predisposition to developing a disease. However, in the jigsaw puzzle of health, adaptation to a continuously changing environment also holds a fundamental role. Apart from their use of cultural mechanisms to adapt to their environment (such as medical practices), humans also deal with illness and potential disability through genetic adjustments to changes at a population level and through physiological adjustments to changes on the individual level.[7] Clearly, humans have demonstrated their ability to alter their environments in order to adapt to occurring changes. To what extent such alterations are beneficial or detrimental is uncertain, though, as changes carry with them new challenges and new risks that populations may or may not be able to deal with.

The present book aims to consider health and disease in Crete during the Byzantine period through a bioarchaeological approach, thereby contextualizing the biological evidence in the culture of the selected society. To this end, the present chapter provides an overview of the society's particular cultural conditions, all of which had the potential to affect the health status of the population: the history, archaeology, environment and natural phenomena, settlement patterns, economy and diet, general living conditions and social dynamics. Against this context, the derived biological data can then be projected, to yield a better understanding of

---

4 The geographical and meteorological location of particular sites has long been perceived to predispose populations to the development of specific diseases or to enhance the maintenance of good health. One of the most vivid examples of such notions is the Hippocratic treatise on *Airs, Waters and Places*; see Jouanna 1996; Nutton 2004, 72–86.

5 Cohen 1989.

6 Learmonth 1988.

7 McElroy and Townsend 1996.

the interacting human and environmental factors that predispose, enhance or buffer the development of specific pathological conditions.

Historical Outline

The history of Byzantine Crete is scantily documented in both the textual and archaeological record. The greater emphasis given to prehistoric and classical antiquities has resulted in a relative neglect of Byzantine sites, few of which have been properly excavated and investigated, and even fewer of which have been the subject of detailed publication.

The general turbulence in the Balkan Peninsula during the fifth and sixth centuries does not appear to have affected the peaceful life of the island. A possible invasion by the Vandals in the sixth century had no documented consequences. The Slavic raids had far less effect on Crete than in the rest of Byzantine Greece. The written sources mention only one Slavic raid on the island, occurring in AD 623; and even if Crete suffered other Slavic raids, it was apparently too remote to be a focus of Slavic invasion.[8] The hypothesis of a Slavic presence on Crete has been rejected, further, on the evidence of archaeological findings, including the bronze buckles discovered at Eleutherna that have now been firmly reclassified as Byzantine.[9]

The peaceful and uneventful life of the sixth and the first half of the seventh century, a period of great prosperity on Crete, underwent dramatic changes upon the appearance and rapid expansion of the Arabs. Raids started soon after the Arabs developed as a powerful naval force in the Mediterranean basin, and resulted in general instability in the region. The first known Arab raid was in AD 654, and during the course of the eighth century Crete had become the object of repeated Arab attacks, culminating in the gradual occupation of the island between AD 827 and 828.[10] Byzantine sources often provide vague and/or inaccurate accounts of this event, but some Arab sources preserve more reliable testimonies. The success of the Arab expedition is best explained as a consequence of the administrative and defensive organization of Crete at that time. Prior to the Arab invasion, and at the beginning of the conquest, Crete was an *archontia* governed by *archons* and thus lacked the more sophisticated organization of a *theme*, particularly on the military level.

---

8 Tsougarakis 1988, 22.

9 For a detailed discussion, see Poulou-Papadimitriou 2002; 2004b, 240–43.

10 Panagiotakis 1961-62; Tsougarakis 1988, 22–6, 30–41; Christides 1984; Makrypoulias 2000.

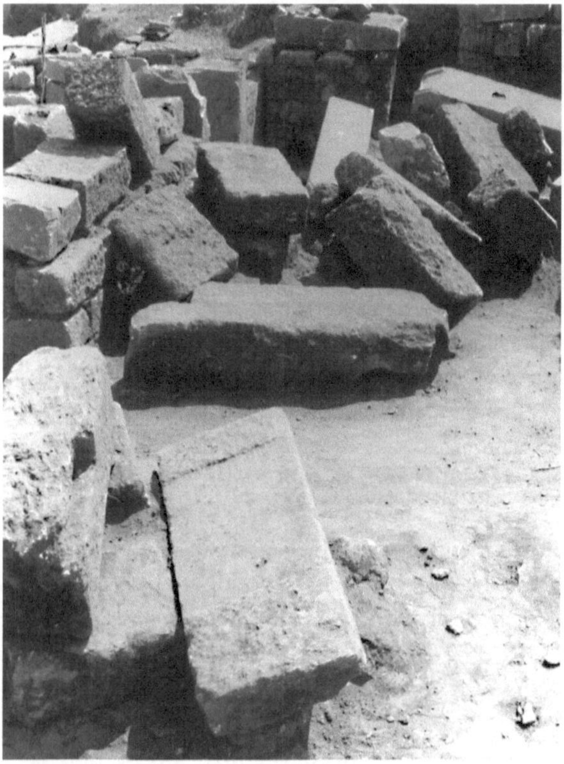

Figure 1.1 Ruins of buildings at Eleutherna (photo: courtesy of Prof. P. Themelis and the Society of Messenian Archaeological Studies)

The fifth century on Crete was marked by the presence of natural disasters, including earthquakes (Figure 1.1).[11] The seismic action persisted in the succeeding centuries, resulting in minor and major interruptions of everyday life.[12] These exceptional disasters added to the usual and constant hazards of rural life that included unpredictable droughts, infestations of locusts, hot dry summers and bleak winters. Written references to early Byzantine famines, shortages and epidemics, mainly of plague, sporadically include the island of Crete. The historian Procopius, for example, records a major outbreak of plague in AD 541 that originated in Egypt and quickly spread throughout the eastern

[11] Platakis 1950; Di Vita 1979/80; Pirazzoli 1986, 2004; Pirazzoli, Laborel and Stiros 1996.

[12] Di Vita 1997 refers to destruction of Gortyn by either one or possibly two major earthquakes.

Mediterranean, including Crete.[13] In the Vita of Andreas, Archbishop of Crete, is attested an epidemic (presumably an outbreak of plague), coinciding with famine and drought, to be dated probably shortly before AD 740.[14] The form of the episode is stereotypical – that of the holy man who prayed for the cessation of the crises, followed by ample rain that swept the disease away – but the core may be historic.[15] Frequent suffering in the Balkan area from epidemics and other crises, such as famine and shortages, is documented also in the written sources. Stathakopoulos, in his meticulous survey of crises in the later Roman and early Byzantine era, found that the Balkans experienced 13 crises of famine and shortages (eight during the sixth and five during the seventh century) and 11 epidemics (nine during the sixth and two during the seventh century).[16] Although it is difficult to assess patterns of range and duration of crop and food crises, Patlagean argues that a famine becomes catastrophic if these conditions persist over at least two consecutive annual cycles and if stocks have been exhausted.[17]

Readily apparent in the archaeological record is the abandonment of buildings and sites in Crete during the seventh century. At Eleutherna, for example, coinage dating to the end of the reign of Constans II (AD 661–668) or possibly to the first years of the reign of Constantine IV (AD 668–674) is considered the *terminus post quem* for the abandonment of the site.[18] Comparison of sites that are sufficiently documented by architectural and numismatic evidence, such as Eleutherna and Gortyn on Crete and other sites elsewhere in the Empire, attests a fairly undifferentiated continuity of social and economic life, even as populations at extramural and less protected sites, as at Eleutherna and Gortyn, moved for greater safety to mountainous and walled locations.[19]

The Byzantines tried numerous times to reconquer the island from the Arabs, and after a succession of failures, Nicephoros Phokas in AD 961 brought Crete back into the Byzantine domain.[20] His successful expedition is an historic

13 For outbreaks of plague in the sixth to the eighth centuries in the Byzantine Empire, see Congourdeau 1993a, 21–9; Stathakopoulos 2007a; Sarris 2007.

14 *Vita Andreae Cretensis* (ed. Papadopoulos-Kerameus 1898); 177–8; Detorakis 1969-70, 93; 1970-71, 119–20; Stathakopoulos 2004, 367.

15 Stathakopoulos 2002.

16 Stathakopoulos 2004, 23–34, tables 2.4 and 2.5.

17 Patlagean 1977, 82. For a thorough review of the social response to these crises, see Stathakopoulos 2004, 56–87, esp. pp. 81–5.

18 Sidiropoulos 2000; Themelis 2004, 62.

19 Di Vita 2000, 29; Themelis 2004, 69. See also the relevant discussion based on the pottery finds in Yangaki 2005, 311–13.

20 Tsougarakis 1988, 41–58.

event about which a great deal is known, with reasonable certainty, from both Byzantine and Arab sources.[21] Following the re-establishment of Byzantine rule on Crete and the subsequent incorporation of the long-isolated island into the ecclesiastical and administrative framework of the Empire, we have almost no contemporary information concerning the social and economic conditions on the island for more than a century. It is only from later sources and indirect indications that we gain an impression of this period as one of quiet and creativity, characterized by a noted increase in monetary circulation, agricultural production and stock-raising. During this period, and increasingly during the Comnenian period (AD 1081–1185), Crete ensured its safety and strengthened its ties with the imperial capital. This direct and unquestionable influence of Constantinople is strongly evidenced in contemporary art, including architectural features and wall-paintings as, for example, in the church of Zoodochos Pigi in Alikianos, southwest of Chania, dating to the fourth decade of the eleventh century.[22] The revolt of Karykis during the second half of the eleventh century, which failed even to win the support of the population, is the only upheaval known to have occured until the capture of the island first by the Genoese (in AD 1204) and later by the Venetians (in AD 1210/1211).[23]

Christianity: The New Religion

Although the exact date of the Christianization of the island is not known, the Church of Crete is traditionally said to have been founded by Saint Paul, who then handed over the organization of the Christian communities to his disciple Titos. Information on the internal organization of the Church is extracted mainly from the Conciliar Acts and the Notitiae Episcopatuum of the Eastern Church.[24] By the second century AD a thriving Christian community had been established in Gortyn, and others must have existed in various towns throughout the island. The fate of the Church during the Arab occupation is obscured by the lack of relevant information in the sources. Some concessions would have been granted to the Church, but judging from the situation in other regions (for example, in Cyprus and Palestine) we can assume the presence of some kind of ecclesiastical and monastic organization.

---

21 For an account of the expedition, see Tsougarakis 1988, 58–74.

22 Andrianakis 2008, 261.

23 Tsougarakis 1988, 74–88.

24 Tsougarakis 1988, 197. For the organization of the Church on Crete, see Tsougarakis 1988, 197–248.

The most obvious modification of both the urban and rural environment was the construction of religious buildings, especially basilicas, during the fifth century and into the second half of the sixth century.[25] The great number of basilicas built in the latter period may be connected to the victories of Justinian against the Vandals and Ostrogoths and also to the island's importance as a crossroads of commerce.[26] The introduction of Christianity to the island inevitably brought new ideological and religious concepts into the society. Facilitated by the *Pax Romana* and supported by monastic activity in the east, Christianity spread throughout Greece.[27] The success of Christianity, however, did not result in the elimination of the pagan world-view, which was deeply rooted in the everyday life of most people, and its persistence is especially apparent in the area of burial rituals.[28] Due to the teaching of the new religion about the resurrection of the body, the practice of cremation went into decline, in favor of inhumation, as early as the second century, and was eventually abandoned in the fourth. Reflecting aspects of religious and social change and new ideological conceptions of death and the afterlife, burial practices in this instance responded to the Christian conception of death as *koimesis* rather than *thanatos*.[29] These changes are clearly represented in contemporary Christian texts and symbols, epitaphs and grave goods, which become fewer and less valuable in conformity with the simple and humble Christian life.[30]

Settlement Patterns and Byzantine Houses

The investigation of settlement patterns in Byzantine Crete relies mainly on the reports of geographers and travelers, hagiographical texts and archaeological evidence (namely the basilicas, defensive constructions, pottery and numismatic finds). The relevant literary evidence is scant, in many cases laconic and not

---

25 For the role of the Church in early Byzantine topography and life, see Saradi 2006, 385–432.

26 Sanders 1982; Rendini 1985.

27 Cameron 1993; Brown 1998.

28 On pagan monuments in the Christian city, see Saradi 2006, 355–84.

29 Kyriakakis 1974; Abrahamse 1984; Emmanouilidis 1989; Kourkoutidou-Nikolaidou 1997; Dennis 2001; Velkovska 2001; Alexakis 2001; Saradi 2006, 432–9. For the relevance of current Greek funerary practices to understanding Byzantine customs, see Danforth 1982; Alexiou 2002.

30 For a survey of Byzantine cemeteries and other funerary constructions throughout Greece and for useful comments on the typology of the graves and accompanying goods, see Laskaris 2000.

always reliable, while the archaeological evidence enables us to recognize a larger number of settlements.[31] The works of early geographers and Renaissance travelers, although offering interesting information on economy, trade and customs, are of limited value in respect to the geography and topography of the island. For example, the sixth-century *Hieroclis Synecdemos*, which despite its omissions probably lists settlements active at that time, and the description of the island by Cristoforo Buondelmonti in the fifteenth century, are among the few accounts that distinguish the status of settlements.[32] Especially in the case of the earliest works, the focus on 'cities' overlooks other kinds of settlements.[33] The same incomplete picture is characteristic of the relevant hagiographical texts, with the possible exception of the autobiographical work of Ioannis Xenos from the end of the tenth and beginning of the eleventh century.[34] Although economic prosperity is evident in the archaeological evidence after AD 961 and well into the twelfth century, contemporary written sources refer more often to villages than to settlements of urban character, providing only sporadic references to Chandax (Heraklion). This change in focus undoubtedly reveals two historical trends: first, a disinterest in resettling the urban centers, and secondly, a 'ruralization' of the island. Evidently, the contribution of rural settlements to the economic growth played an important role in their survival throughout the period of Arab occupation.

The documentary and archaeological evidence attests a succession of distinctive settlement patterns. The fifth through the seventh centuries present thriving settlements primarily agricultural in character but containing a considerable urban environment, as, for example, at Gortyn. Between the seventh and ninth centuries, amid a notable lack of large-scale activities, the population appears to be organized in small rural communities, a tendency that continued into the next centuries. The Arab occupation contributed to the decay of the already declining urban centers, and the re-establishment of Byzantine rule after AD 961 did not restore the necessary economic and social conditions for an urban revival. Until the twelfth century, when urban expansion can again be detected, Chandax remained the only recognizably urban settlement, in contrast to settlements that were little more than oversized villages.

The role of rural households (farms) in the economic and social life of the island is obscured by the poverty of the architectural testimony. Evidence of

---

31 For a review of settlement patterns in the light of documentary and archaeological evidence, see Tsougarakis 1988, 91–153, and 1991, 591–4, 596–9.

32 *Hieroclis Synecdemos* (ed. Honigmann 1930); *C. Buondelmonti* (ed. van Spitael 1981).

33 Saradi 2006, 96–100.

34 *Vita of Saint Ioannis Xeni* (ed. Tomadakis 1948).

rural structures rarely comes to light. A recent rescue excavation at the site of Kefala, near Vryses in northwestern Crete, has revealed evidence of a wide range of activities carried out at one rural household.[35] Located near the river Almyros and along a road artery leading to Cydonia (Chania) that had been well known since Roman times, the farm structure consisted of five rooms. Four of the rooms served as storage areas, as indicated by the presence of pithoi bases on the floor and built-in benches, and the fifth room is characterized as a workshop of uncertain type. The open space to the west of the excavated area has been identified as a courtyard, and finds from the site include a circular construction, most probably a silo, and two hearths. On the evidence of coins and pottery, the building dates to the sixth or early seventh century AD. Although we cannot infer much about the contribution of this particular farmhouse to the surrounding economy, a considerable number of farmhouses and rural settlements may have existed in the fertile plains around urban centers like Cydonia and Gortyn.[36] Such farmhouses might have acted as intermediary points for the sale of products in the closest urban center, thereby contributing to the economic growth of the island as early as the sixth and seventh centuries AD.

We can expect that extensive documentation on individual houses within these various types of settlements could tell us much about the communities that inhabited them.[37] The limits of our present data on Byzantine houses, however, allow us to draw few conclusions of more than local significance.[38] Evidence for

---

[35] Fiolitaki 2010.

[36] Tsougarakis 1991, 593.

[37] Few studies have dealt satisfactorily with the topic of Byzantine housing. Early studies by de Beylié 1902 and Gerland 1915 did not draw on the archaeological evidence and included many inaccuracies; the substantial research presented by Orlandos 1937, which remains fundamental, was limited to the houses of Mistra; and the studies by Koukoules 1936, 1951, 249–317 relied exclusively on documentary sources. More recent and substantial contributions to our understanding of Byzantine architecture include Scranton 1957 on the Byzantine levels at Corinth; Bouras 1982-83 and Sigalos 2004a, critical overviews of houses from the tenth to the fifteenth century; Sigalos 2004b, 71–78, survey of houses in post-Roman Greece; Ellis 2004, an analysis of the typology of early Byzantine houses; Grünbart and Stathakopoulos 2002, 314–19, an overview of houses and households; and Sodini 2004, a thorough discussion of findings in the Mediterranean.

[38] Bouras 1982-83, 1. Discovery of a variety of items in addition to architectural remains could provide substantial information on aspects of everyday life: ceramic, glass and metal vessels (on kitchenware and storageware, see, e.g., Bakirtzis 2003; Papanikola-Bakirtzi 2005; on glass vessels, see, e.g., Stern 2001; Volanakis 2002; keys, locks and padlocks (on the technology used for the safety of houses, see, e.g., Vikan 1982); ceramic and metal lamps (on the lighting equipment, see, e.g., Petridis 1986; Oikonomou 1988). See also examples in Tsakalos 2005, 22–5, and Papanikola-Bakirtzi 2002, 272–7, 282–303.

early Byzantine houses is particularly scanty. The early Byzantine settlement at Eleutherna includes houses built hastily of material reused from earlier structures. The densely occupied neighborhoods of this era, located probably south of the basilica, remain unexcavated (Figure 1.2).[39] At Gortyn, in the area between the temple of Apollo Pythios to the west and the Praetorium to the east, a residential quarter of peasants and artisans was constructed, probably after an earthquake in the mid-fifth century. The houses, which were two storied, had small rooms and a court opening onto the street. Successive reconstructions of these houses were carried out until the demise of the city around AD 670.[40]

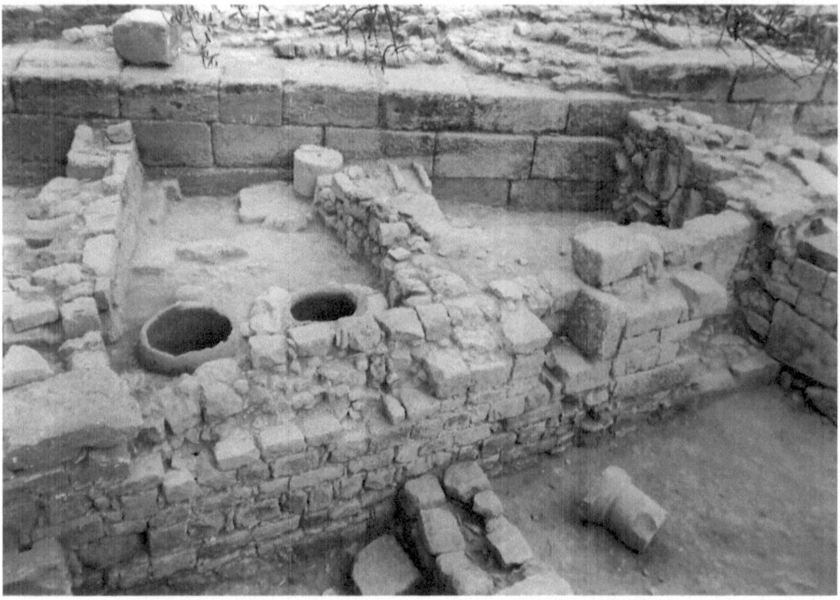

Figure 1.2 Room of an early Byzantine house at Eleutherna with storage pithoi (photo: courtesy of Prof. P. Themelis and the Society of Messenian Archaeological Studies)

The study of middle Byzantine houses provides a more complete picture of a contemporary household.[41] In the tradition of antiquity, the courtyard was the focal point of the house in respect to communication between rooms and as the setting for domestic activities such as cooking, household production and small-scale manufacturing. The location of kitchens remains unclear, as hearths within

[39] Themelis 2002, 105–8, and 2004, 64–5; see also Greco et al. 1998 for the late Roman/early Byzantine (fifth to seventh centuries AD) house complex at Itanos, Crete.

[40] Di Vita 2000, pl. LXI; Giorgi 2002; Zanini 2003, 2004.

[41] Sigalos 2004a, 55–65; Rheidt 1991; Rosser and Donovan 1983.

rooms have not been identified.[42] Although we cannot reject the possibility that particular areas within rooms or even specific rooms were reserved for cooking, it seems more likely that cooking took place in the courtyard. Storage rooms are more easily recognized, particularly on the evidence of pithoi sunk into or resting on the surface of floors. In addition to such courtyard houses, 'single-space' houses were also very common in Byzantine Greece. These structures took one of two forms: either a single room used for all household activities or two or more rooms arranged in a line or in an L-shaped plan, in which a spatial distribution of activities was probably expected. For either type of single-space house, 'a multifunctional space hypothesis' can be assumed, where the main living area served as the space for the activities of the family during the day and for resting during the night.[43] Built-in benches discovered in some rooms could have been used for seating and sleeping, and in the absence of these structures the floor could have been used, covered by the relevant sleeping equipment.[44] The only known example of a Byzantine house on Crete dating from the twelfth to the thirteenth centuries is the house excavated at the site of Pyrgi (Hagia Anna) at Eleutherna.[45] The one-story house with a courtyard consisted of three areas, set in a row, and was divided into at least six or seven smaller rooms. Area A served as the main room, area B most probably served as storage space and area C was the kitchen.

The practice of using the rooms of a house for multiple functions recommends the keeping of basic standards of personal hygiene and household cleanliness. By the Byzantine period, standards of personal hygiene were changed from those of antiquity, the ancient custom of visiting public baths having been replaced by less frequent personal washing at home. For clothes-washing, the Byzantines retained the ancient use of various kinds of earth, plant substances and wood ash, and perhaps also nitron, one of the most widespread cleaning agents of antiquity, which would foam when combined with ammonia or vinegar.[46] The extent to which thorough cleaning was possible has not been determined. Certainly in the context of densely occupied houses or settlements and close contact with animals,

---

42 Only in the case of Neon Syllaton at Veroia has a hearth been possibly identified, see Pazaras and Tsanana 1990, 359, fig. 4.

43 Sigalos 2004a, 60.

44 Oikonomides 1990, 209–10. On the basis of eleventh to fifteenth-century documentary evidence on household contents of the middle class, Oikonomides provides information on several categories of furnishings, including chests, sleeping equipment, kitchenware and storage vessels; see also Koukoules 1949, 60–116.

45 Kalpaxis 2008, 14 and note 6, proposes a typological correspondence with Pergamon house type d 1 or d 2.

46 Forbes 1995, 174–82; Rautman 2006, 49.

the ill effects of poor sanitation would have resulted in a faster and more efficient transmission of disease.[47] Although there have been references in the sources to dug cesspits, construction of clay pipes from house to house and central pipes within an extended drainage system, specific sanitary facilities have not been located in houses.[48]

Economy and Society

Estimating the extent of farming and herding activity on Byzantine Crete relies on the evidence of the geographical location, climate and geomorphology; natural disasters and invasions; and also on specific historical factors such as the economic policy of the Byzantine Empire, since, for example, the size of a tax burden could affect the abandonment of fields.[49] Some aspects of the economic activity already known from the Roman period likely continued through the Byzantine period.[50]

Crete is described in the sources as a very fertile and intensively cultivated island with orchards, fruit gardens and vineyards.[51] Agriculture formed the basis of the economy and products were sufficient for both local consumption and considerable exports.[52] Grain production, in particular wheat, was the dominant agricultural activity of the population, rising well above local requirements to allow for exports and donations to various institutions.[53] Wine production, although very few references to it exist in Byzantine sources, was second in

[47] Russell 1986, 144 noted that the subdivision of the areas within households to accommodate larger numbers of inhabitants was a typical phenomenon of declining standards of everyday life.

[48] Koukoules 1951, 307–13; Karpozilos 1989; Sigalos 2004a, 59. Pits have been found, for example at Corinth (see Scranton 1957), but their function has not been securely determined. A pit and open pipes for rainwater have been found at Eleutherna; see Themelis 2004, 64.

[49] See, e.g., Laiou 2003 on the factors affecting the price of land during the tenth century.

[50] For a general discussion of the Byzantine economy, see Morrisson and Sodini 2002; Lefort 2002; Dagron 2002.

[51] In addition, *Kitâb al-Dja'rafiyya* (ed. Hadj-Sadok 1968), 70, 87, refers to a wide range of medicinal and aromatic herbs that grew in the island, such as resin, laurel and epithyme. Hazelnuts, rhubarb and pomegranates were also known to be cultivated.

[52] For means of agricultural production, see Bryer 2002; on the early Byzantine agricultural tools from Eleutherna, see Brokalakis 2004.

[53] Tsougarakis 1988, 282–3.

importance.[54] The production of olive oil seems to have been more limited, making imports necessary.[55] The cultivation of flax and cotton must have been known during the Byzantine era. Breeding-stock of sheep, goats and cattle was also herded as a resource for wool, rawhide and dairy products.[56] One of the best-known products of Crete was cheese, highly appraised in a number of Arabic sources, which was produced especially in the White Mountains area of the west and was exported in large quantities.[57] Also well reputed was Cretan honey, and apiculture was common.[58] Fishing must have been a subsidiary activity, especially for the coastal populations.[59] Arabic sources note that tuna, in particular, was caught in large quantities during their migration period toward Spain and Crete in early May.[60] It is reasonable to assume that freshwater fish were also consumed, especially in areas near rivers and springs. The discovery of 63 fishing-net weights made of lead during the excavation at the early Byzantine site of Argyroupolis reinforces this hypothesis. The site is located some 7 kilometers from the coast and much closer to the river Mouselas, where it is probable that most of the local fishing took place.[61] Finally, trade in ores and minerals (mainly copper and iron),

54 *Vita of Saint Ioannis Xeni* (ed. Tomadakis 1948), 59–60.

55 Olive oil and walnuts are the only two agricultural products known to have been imported into Crete. It was only in the seventeenth century that Venice made the cultivation of olive trees compulsory in all her colonies; see Tsougarakis 1988. *Kitâb al-Dja'rafiyya* (ed. Hadj-Sadok 1968), 52–4, refers to some kind of oil extracted from turnips and oil derived from sesame seeds.

56 *Vita of Saint Ioannis Xeni* (ed. Tomadakis 1948), 60.

57 See, e.g., *Edrisi* (tr. Amadée Jaupert 1836-40) II, 126; *Aboulféda* (tr. Reinaud and MacGuckin de Slane 1848), 276; *Kitâb al-Dja'rafiyya* (ed. M. Hadj-Sadok), 54 and §358, where Cretan cheese is attested to have been exported to Egypt.

58 *Aboulféda* (tr. Reinaud and MacGuckin de Slane 1848), 276; *Vita of Saint Ioannis Xeni* (ed. Tomadakis 1948), 59. Archaeological remains of beehives have been found at the early Byzantine sites of Eleutherna, see Yangaki 2005, 162–3; Gortyn, see Albertocchi and Perna 2001, 533–5; Panormo, see Kalokyris 1955, 325; Hagia Galini, see Vogt 1991–93; Knossos, see Frend and Johnston 1967; Hayes 2001, 440–41; and Vafes, A. Fiolitaki, pers. comm. 2008. Yangaki 2005, 163 notes that sherds from beehives found at Eleutherna account for 1 to 5%, a percentage that remains steady between the fourth and seventh centuries, suggesting a continuous local production of honey during the early Byzantine period.

59 To what extent marine resources formed a basic supplement to the everyday diet is still under investigation; see Chapter 4.

60 *Kitâb al-Dja'rafiyya* (ed. Hadj-Sadok 1968), 17, 40, 61. In the fourth poem of Ptochoprodromos, however, tuna is considered to be of low quality; see *Ptochoprodromos* (tr. and ed. Eideneier 1991), IV 109, 115, 237, 296.

61 A. Fiolitaki pers. comm. 2008. The river Mouselas was known to be navigable in antiquity, as excavations undertaken by the 25th Ephorate of Prehistoric and Classical Antiquities revealed anchorages alongside the river.

timber, glass and salt was also conducted, although its relation to the economy was clearly subsidiary.[62]

The rich and prosperous island of Crete could provide a potentially well-balanced diet for those who had access to basic and seasonal foodstuffs. In urban areas a greater variety of food was available to those who could afford to buy it, while in rural areas working peasants could at least have seasonally supplemented their diets with their own produce of fruit, vegetables, eggs, milk and cheese.[63] However, the vulnerability of the rural population to shortages that resulted from adverse weather and disease should not be underestimated. Byzantine Crete had an important advantage of near self-sufficiency, and production not only met local demand but was adequate to allow exports, limiting imports largely to products of the specialized kind. Thus, from an economic point of view, basic needs could be fulfilled when no real crises emerged; but when calamities loomed, impoverished conditions would have had a significant effect on living standards.

Little information exists on the social structure of Byzantine Crete and thus our discussion is largely based on the general patterns seen in other parts of the Empire.[64] The scattered surviving evidence demonstrates that during the fifth to the seventh centuries cultivated lands belonged to free small-holder peasants, but we do not know the extent to which prominent families may have subsequently achieved dominance. One's experience of daily life was primarily shaped in the family. The Byzantine period saw family turn sharply inward, separating the public male world more clearly from the enclosed, largely domestic sphere of women and children.[65] Our necessarily generalized picture of the role of men and women in the Byzantine society of Crete reveals, to some extent, the different expectations that the society had of men and women, and thus tells us much about the society.[66] In Byzantium, early marriage was the norm, and Byzantine legislation permitted the betrothal of a girl after the age of seven, a figure later

62 See Tsougarakis 1988, 270–78. The copper mines in the area of Kantanos are the only mining area where a Byzantine presence is certain, although other sites, such as Argyroupolis-Lappa where lead and silver were exploited, may also have been mining centers. Timber is likely to have been an abundant raw resource, although evidence of dense forests is attested in no Byzantine documentary sources; much later, *C. Buondelmonti* (ed. van Spitael 1981), 115, 116, 118 refers to massive cypress forests on the southwest coast. Salt-pans (at, for example, Souda Bay, Elounda and Spinalonga) produced salt of good quality, as attested in the *Vita of Saint Niconis Metanoeite* (ed. Lambros 1906), 154.

63 For a thorough discussion of the Byzantine diet as attested in the sources and the derived isotopic data, see Chapter 4.

64 Tsougarakis 1988, 290–301.

65 For a discussion of Byzantine childhood, see Chapter 3.

66 Barber 1997.

raised to 12. The minimum age for marriage was 12, a practice that had much to do with concerns about ensuring both the virginity of the bride and the birth of children as soon as physically possible.[67] In the course of his lifetime a man would belong to a succession of social units: household, school, professional guild and church or monastery. Prominent roles for men were available in occupations linked with civil, military or ecclesiastical services, and men could play an active role in numerous professions, the cultivation of the land and the tending of livestock.[68] Women were excluded from the priesthood and the Church hierarchy, yet found a special place in female monasteries.[69] Women's daily routine included household activities, but for most women the central biological event in their lives was childbirth.[70] Caring for the children and being responsible for their primary education were major preoccupations, in which the variety of childhood experiences often accorded with social status.[71] Women worked in the family gardens and orchards, helped with the tending of livestock and were involved in household manufacture such as spinning and weaving. All these activities could subject them to a number of hazards and to an even higher mortality risk during pregnancy and childbirth. However, the role of women – influenced by two stereotyped female figures, the Virgin Mary (representing virginity and motherhood) and Eve (representing the sexual temptress) – was crucial to the perpetuation of the family line, and was of particular importance at the critical passages of life, namely marriage, birth and death.

Byzantine Medicine

Life in the past was difficult in both urban and rural settings. Farming, for example, was the dangerous occupation it has always been, and agricultural workers risked injury from equipment, large animals and falls. Risks from

---

67 Talbot 1997, 121.

68 The professions of doctor, tailor and horse doctor are attested for Crete; see Bandy 1970, 47, 70–71, 126–7.

69 For the role of women in Byzantine society, Kislinger 1989; Laiou 1981, 1982, 1985, 1992, 1999, 2000; Garland 1988, 2006; Beaucamp 1992; Herrin 1993; Nikolaou 1993, 2005; Talbot 1997; Kazhdan 1998; Kalavrezou 2003; Walker 2003; Connor 2004; professional life, Bourdara 1989; Margarou 2000; religious life, Talbot 1994, 2001; Beaucamp 2000; Constantinou 2005; political life, Beaucamp 1990; Garland 1999; Herrin 2001.

70 Women who could not conceive were considered very unfortunate and often turned to the use of various substances and magico-religious practices; see Talbot 1997, 123–4; Fulghum-Heintz 2003, 278.

71 For the role of children in Byzantine society, see Chapter 3.

even minor wounds, which can easily become infected and lead to permanent disability or even death, were significantly greater in the pre-antibiotic era. Although references in the literary sources point to a wide range of medicinal herbs that grew on the island, and we know of the presence of a physician from a probably funerary inscription dating to the fifth century,[72] we have no detailed accounts of medical practice in Byzantine Crete.

Until recent decades, medical historians, in general, viewed Byzantine medicine as summarized by Scarborough:[73]

> [Byzantine] medicine is one of stagnation, plagiarism of the great medical figures of classical antiquity and a somber boredom that seemingly awaited the Italian Renaissance.

However, Byzantine medicine is better viewed within the social matrix of the population it was developed to serve. Both the non-medical sources and contemporary art reveal a general awareness of medicine and medical practice in Byzantium, and shed light on the lively interaction of Greek medical history, notions of magic and astrology, traditions of folk medicine, the development of hospitals and the sophisticated medical knowledge practiced by skillful physicians in the upper strata of the Empire.[74]

Byzantine doctors successfully reworked, recombined and reorganized earlier traditions with new observations. Their ongoing activity in these pursuits is evident in the major medical works of Oribasius (c. AD 325–400), Aetius of Amida (*fl.* under Justinian [AD 527–565]), Alexander of Tralles (c. AD 525–605), Paul of Aegina (*fl.* c. AD 640, in Alexandria), Theophanes 'Nonnus' (*fl.* AD 912–59), Symeon Seth (*fl.* under Michael VII Ducas [AD 1071–78]) and many others. In these works, the influence of Greek and Roman medical tradition is constantly present, but the authors introduce useful comments and notes based on fresh observations, test modified or new applications of therapeutic measurements and attempt diagnosis on the basis of careful examination. In the manufacture of drugs, as well, some parts of the Greco-Roman tradition remain, but novelty in the use of herbs and herbals, medicinal minerals and

---

72 Bandy 1970, 47 no. 18 (found at Hagioi Deka, south of Gortyn).

73 Scarborough 1984a, ix; for accounts of Byzantine medicine, see, e.g., Garrison 1921; Temkin 1962; Singer and Underwood 1962; Majno 1975.

74 See, e.g., Keenan 1941, 1944; Magoulias 1964; Constantelos 1966-67; Duffy 1984; Vikan 1973, 1984; Kessler 1971; Weitzmann 1977; Eftychiadis 1983; Nutton 1984; Bennett 2000. On hospitals, see Horden 2004, 77–99; 2005, 361–89; Crislip 2005, 100–142.

animal products indicates that the theory of drug-action has shifted and that the substances used in pharmacology have been augmented in number and kind.[75]

The specialized treatise of Paul of Aegina on sophisticated surgical operations and the practical handbook of Alexander of Tralles on therapy for the working physician indicate the presence of an active scientific community concerned for the treatment and welfare of its patients and provide information about the medical man as both practitioner and teacher.[76] In a society that balanced concern for health and for salvation, the Byzantine physician is shown to support the application of charms, amulets and folk remedies.[77] Such use of superstition and magic in medical practice reveals that the Byzantine physician was well aware of notions and attitudes tightly woven into the matrix of Byzantine society, from the lower to the upper classes. Alexander of Tralles' response to this balance is quite bold: he openly associates himself with such practices at the risk of losing his intellectual respectability. Writing in a relatively clear language, he provides a vivid example of a caring physician, practicing his profession in such a way as to meet the needs of the society to which he belongs.[78] Kazhdan, studying the image of the medical doctor in the tenth to the twelfth centuries, argues that decline in the social standing of those in the medical profession began most probably after the seventh century.[79] From the numerous references to failing and incompetent doctors at the end of the tenth century, in which they are accused of daring to match the healing power of the saint, it is probably safe to deduce that physicians had become too influential to remain unchallenged. This anti-medical movement weakened during the eleventh century, and by the twelfth century physicians and the medical profession were highly respected.

The environmental and cultural characteristics of Byzantine Crete that have been sketched here indicate in general the living conditions in which the biological profile of its populations can be properly investigated. With this context in mind, the adaptive and functional meaning of the biological data provided by the human skeletal remains can be better situated in the cultural and natural environment in which they occurred. What was really happening in Byzantine Crete is the question we are called to answer, and by approaching the question at the point where historical, archaeological and biological analysis

75 Scarborough 1984b, 2002.

76 *Paul of Aegina* (ed. Heiberg 1921 and 1924; tr. Adams 1834); *Alexander of Tralles* (ed. and tr. Puschmann 1878–79); for the latter see also Guardasole 2004a, 2004b, 2004c, 2006.

77 See, e.g., Vikan 1984; Maguire 1995; Russell 1995; Vakaloudi 2001.

78 For a thorough review, see Duffy 1984.

79 Kazhdan 1984.

meet, we can provide groundwork for evaluating a population's adaptation to its continuously changing environment.[80]

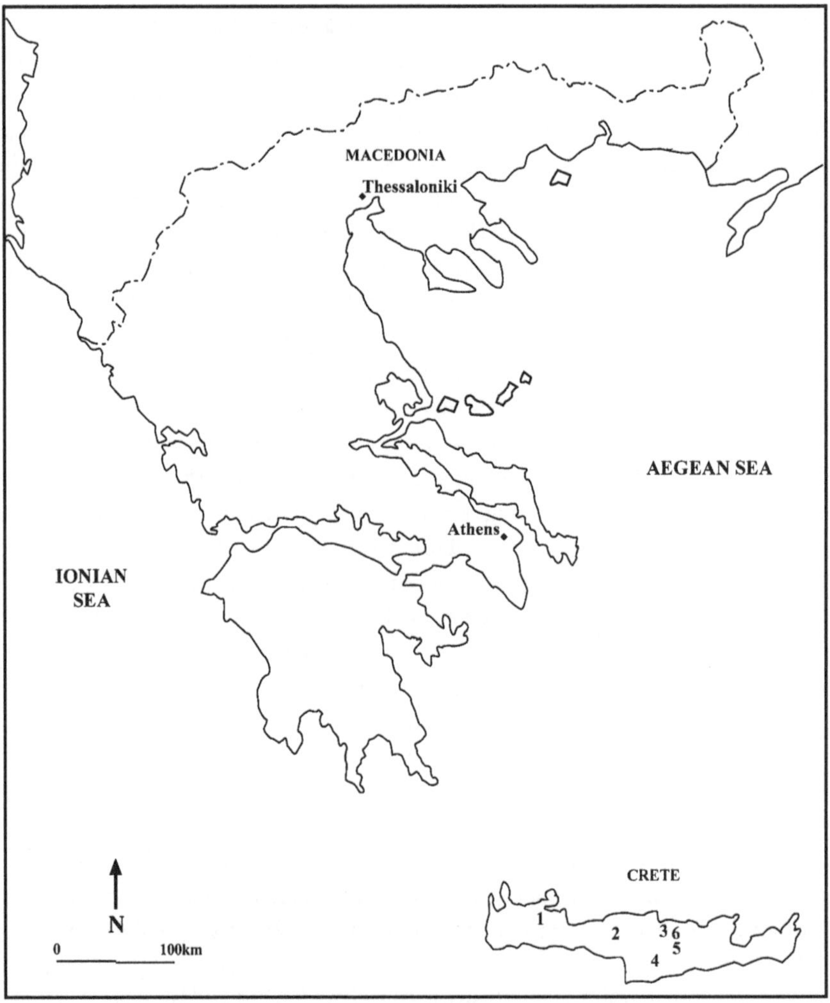

Figure 1.3 Map of the sites
Key: 1=Stylos; 2=Eleutherna; 3=Kastella; 4=Gortyn; 5=Kefali; 6=Knossos

[80] For application of this approach to early Byzantine populations throughout Greece, see, e.g., Bourbou 2004; Bourbou and Tsilipakou 2009. The transitional and idiosyncratic character of the period resulted in the use of differential adaptation patterns by the population under strenuous conditions; see, e.g., Bourbou 2004, 81–2 for the cases of early Byzantine Eleutherna and Messene.

Materials and Methods

Data to date published on the health of Byzantine populations from Crete is limited and varies in quality from study to study, reflecting in these respects the history of the development of bioarchaeological studies in Greece. Inadequate levels of detail and undefined methods of analysis have obscured the basis for many of the reported conclusions. The material under discussion here includes human skeletal collections studied by the author at Eleutherna, Stylos and Kastella and by other researchers at Gortyn, Kefali and Knossos, sites in the western and central parts of the island (Figure 1.3).[81] The total number of individuals is 445; 271 (60.8%) are adults and 174 (39.1%) are non-adults (Table 1.1). Of the total, 341 individuals (207 adults and 134 non-adults) represent the early Byzantine sites, and 104 individuals (64 adults and 40 non-adults) the middle Byzantine sites (Table 1.2).

Table 1.1 Demographic data for the skeletal series

Site	Date	Adult (%)	Non-adult (%)	Total	Reference
Eleutherna	Sixth to seventh centuries AD	100 (66.2%)	51 (33.7%)	151	Bourbou 2004
Gortyn	Sixth to seventh centuries AD	29 (54.7%)	24 (45.2%)	53	Mallegni 1988
Kastella	Eleventh to twelfth centuries AD	35 (59.3%)	24 (40.6%)	59	Bourbou 2006a, 2009; Bourbou and Richards 2007
Kefali	Sixth to seventh centuries AD	49 (55%)	40 (44.9%)	89	Zygouri 2005
Knossos	Sixth to seventh centuries AD	29 (60.4%)	19 (40.4%)	48	Musgrave 1976
Stylos	Eleventh to twelfth centuries AD	29 (64.4%)	16 (35.5%)	45	Bourbou 2003a, 2009
Total		*271 (60.8%)*	*174 (39.1%)*	*445*	

81 Eleutherna: Bourbou 2004; Gortyn: Mallegni 1988; Kastella: Bourbou 2006a, 2009; Bourbou and Richards 2007; Kefali: Zygouri 2005; Knossos: Musgrave 1976; Stylos: Bourbou 2003a, 2009.

Table 1.2 Demographic data for the skeletal series by time period

Early Byzantine period						
Sites	Adult	M	F	I	Non-adult	Total
Eleutherna	100	52	21	27	51	151
Gortyn	29	18	11	0	24	53
Kefali	49	18	11	20	40	89
Knossos	29	9	12	8	19	48
Total	*207*	*97*	*55*	*55*	*134*	*341*
Middle Byzantine period						
Kastella	35	15	8	12	24	59
Stylos	29	9	11	9	16	45
Total	*64*	*24*	*19*	*21*	*40*	*104*

M=Male, F=Female, I=Indeterminate

The collections of Eleutherna, Gortyn and Stylos are derived from the excavation of a cemetery of an associated ecclesiastical monument. Around the early Byzantine basilica at Eleutherna, 50 burials have been excavated. Most of them were tiled or cist graves, usually including multiple burials (Figure 1.4).[82] Although there is strong evidence that the cemetery was initially used for the burial of the clergy, it was soon used by the community at large. Accompanying goods are of great variety, including glass and ceramic vessels and jewels.

At Gortyn, in central Crete, in the area just southeast of the basilica of Hagios Titos, a densely packed necropolis was found in the ruins of a small late Antique bath complex. It was probably constructed during the last quarter of the fourth century and, after its destruction in the sixth century, it was again used until the second half of the seventh century. Almost all family tombs had been opened and reused more than once.[83] The village of Stylos, some 20 kilometers from Chania, is well known for its springs and for the river Koiliaris.[84] During excavations at the site in the 1980s and 1990s at the church of Hagios Ioannis Theologos, a large number of burials came to light (Figure 1.5).[85] Only a small part of the human skeletal collection, dating to the eleventh- to the twelfth-century phase

[82] On the basilica, see Themelis 2004, 46–63, and discussion in Andrianakis 2006, 51–2; on the burials, Yangaki 2004a; on the pottery, Vogt 2000; Poulou-Papadimitriou 2004a, Yangaki 2005; on the golden amulets, Yangaki 2004b; on the buckles, Poulou-Papadimitriou 2004b; on the inscriptions, Tzifopoulos 2000; on the coins, Sidiropoulos 2000.

[83] Di Vita 1988, 91–141.

[84] Spanakis 1993, 743.

[85] For the site of Stylos, only general information exists; M. Andrianakis pers. comm. 2009; Lassithiotakis 1969, 465–8.

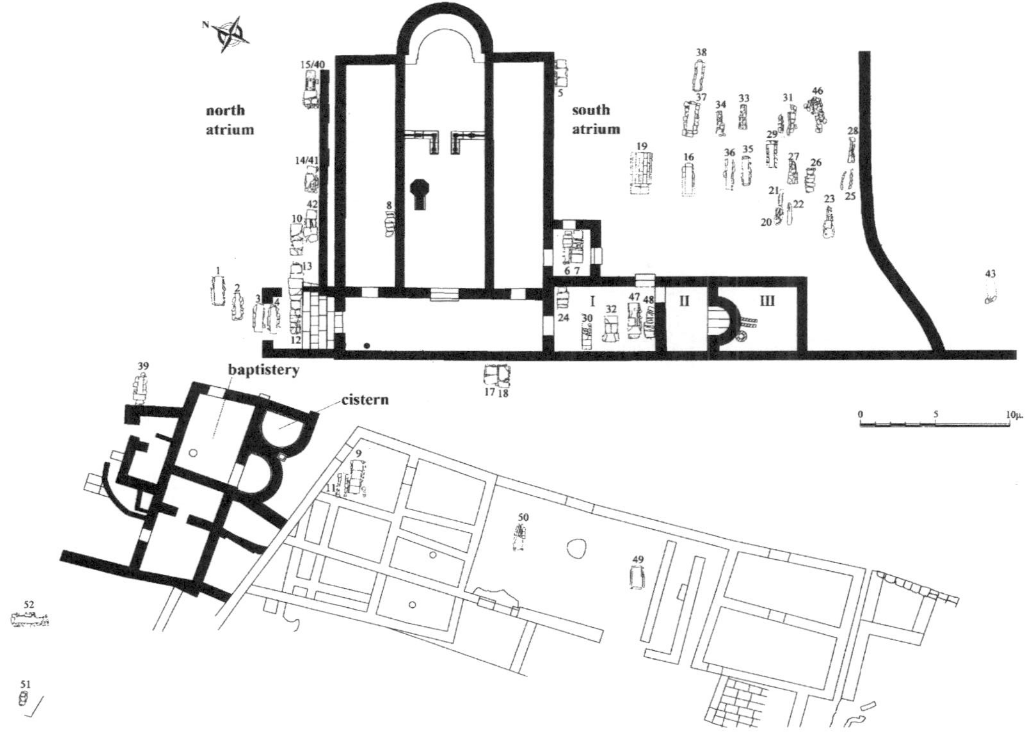

Figure 1.4 Cemetery plan of the basilica at Eleutherna (photo: courtesy of Prof. P. Themelis and the Society of Messenian Archaeological Studies)

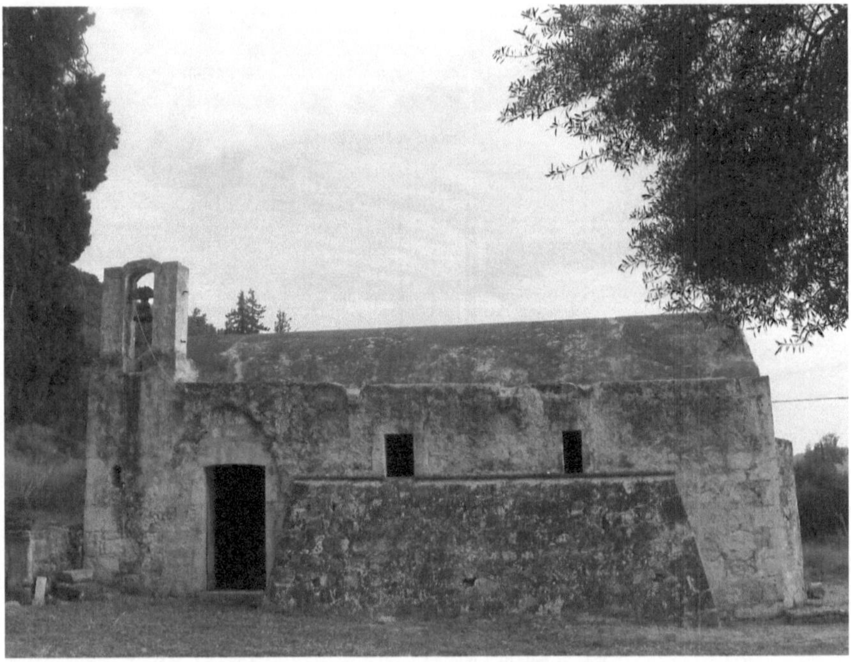

Figure 1.5 The church of Hagios Ioannis Theologos at Stylos (photo: C. Bourbou)

of the church, is available for study. The majority of the graves is cist or tiled. Secondary burials are frequent at the site, accounting in many cases for the disarticulation of the remains. Both adults and non-adults are represented, and the accompanying goods include jewels.

The skeletal collections of Knossos, Kastella and Kefali have not yet been associated with any ecclesiastical monument or specific settlement in the area. A built tomb (ossuary) was found on the road to Knossos, near the present-day Venizeleion Hospital in Heraklion, during excavations for the construction of a road; its chronology is based on the typology of the few clay vessels recovered among the generally poor accompanying goods. The excavators argue that this was a family tomb in use over a long period.[86] At Kastella in Heraklion, a middle Byzantine cemetery was discovered in 2003 during restoration work at the Venetian church of Saint Peter (Figure 1.6).

86 Catling and Smyth 1976. As the ossuary contained only commingled remains, Musgrave 1976 estimated the Minimum Number of Individuals (MNI).

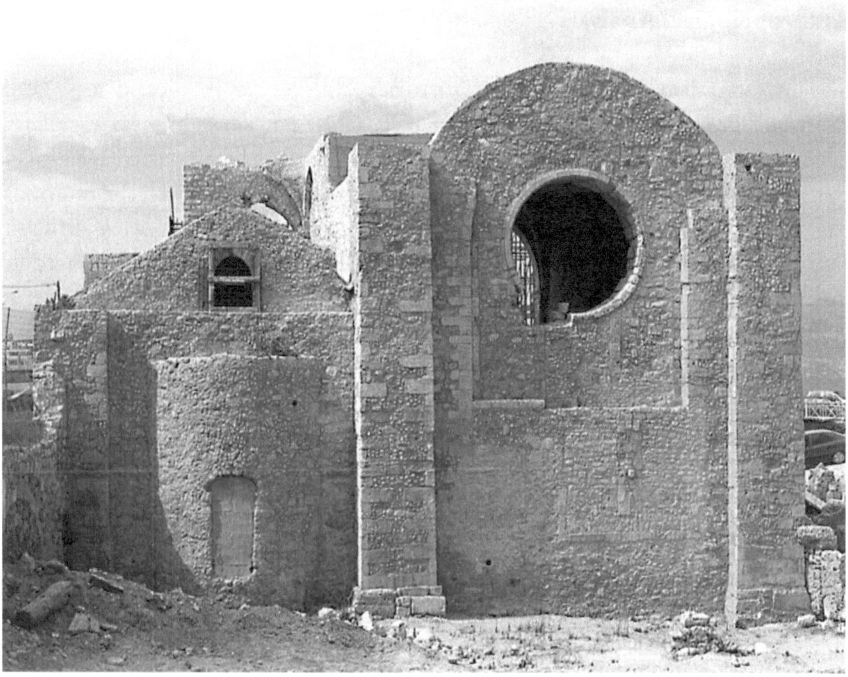

Figure 1.6 The Venetian church of Saint Peter in Heraklion (photo: C. Bourbou)

A total of 32 excavated burials containing single and multiple inhumations was exposed. The typology of the relatively few accompanying goods (mainly pottery and bronze jewellery) allowed for the dating of these burials to the eleventh century. In the history of the continuous occupation of the modern city of Heraklion, the discovery of this middle Byzantine cemetery is considered as the 'missing chronological link' for understanding the urban life of the city during that era.[87] Finally, in the area of Kastelli Pediados evidence has been found for continuous occupation from prehistoric to late Byzantine times.[88] In 2002, close to the top of the hillsite 'Kefali', an early Byzantine cemetery was discovered.[89]

87 Borboudakis 1968; Starida 2003; Poulou-Papadimitriou 2008.

88 Rethemiotakis 1992, 1997.

89 The excavation is not yet published. Available information on the architectural type of the graves and placement of the deceased is given in Zygouri 2005.

Anthropological Analysis

The investigation of demographic histories, differences in diet, disease and mortuary practices depends heavily on accurate age-at-death and sex estimates of human skeletal remains. The derived data used here often presented age ranges that varied considerably among the different studies and for which the methods of analysis were not always stated, making comparative analysis a difficult task. The construction of specific age categories for both adult and non-adult individuals resolved the problem presented by the various age-range systems (Tables 1.3 and 1.4). Regarding immature individuals, throughout this book the term 'non-adults' as suggested by Lewis is used,[90] including all children recovered from the sites up to the age of 17 years. Additional definitions have been used here to differentiate between the physiological periods in a child's life.

Table 1.3 Adult age categories

Age range	Definition
18–30 years	Young adult
31–40 years	Middle adult
41–50 years	Mature adult
51 years and over	Old adult

Table 1.4 Non-adult age categories

Age range	Definition
Embryo	The first 8 weeks (2 months) of intrauterine life
Fetus	From week 9 to birth
Perinatal	Around birth, from 24 weeks gestation to 7 postnatal days
Neonatal	Birth to 27 postnatal days
Infant	Birth to 1 year
Child	1–14.6 years
Adolescent	14.6–17.0 years

Adapted from Scheuer and Black 2004, 468; Lewis 2007, 2

[90] Lewis 2007, 1–2. Note that the terms applied in this study provide a biological basis for discussion and comparative analysis, rather than indication of the cultural symbolisms attributed to the Byzantine child; see Chapter 3.

The methodology for age estimation applied to the collections of Eleutherna, Kastella, Kefali and Stylos followed the criteria cited in Buikstra and Ubelaker.[91] For the documentation of age changes in adult individuals of Eleutherna, Kastella and Stylos different methods have been combined, primarily documentation of morphological changes in the pubic symphysis[92] and the auricular surfaces of the ilium,[93] dental wear[94] and cranial suture closure.[95] Age estimation of non-adult individuals was based on standards for dental eruption and development,[96] measurement of long-bone length and epiphyseal union.[97] In differentiating young adults from older individuals, special attention was given to several late-fusing skeletal elements such as the medial clavicle and the iliac crest of the ilium.

In respect to sex determination, if non-adult skeletons had been sexed in previous research, the determination was not accepted as valid; there are at present no widely agreed upon standards for diagnosing sex in immature remains. Although some advances have been made in the criteria used to sex non-adults from dry bone, the methodology needs further refinement and application to larger samples.[98] Sex in adult individuals was determined using dimorphic aspects of the pelvis and skull.[99] The pelvis is the most reliable indicator of sex in the human skeleton and, although rarely preserved intact, it was preferred to the skull. Emphasis was given to specific anatomical features such as the subpubic region (ventral arc, subpubic concavity, ischiopubic ramus ridge), the presence of a preauricular sulcus and the form of the greater sciatic notch.[100]

The estimation of stature for the collections of Eleutherna, Kastella, Stylos and Kefali followed the formulae suggested by Trotter.[101] The maximum length of only intact long bones (preferably left side bones) for each skeleton was separately estimated and then averaged.

---

91 Buikstra and Ubelaker 1994; for age changes in the pelvis, see Meindl and Lovejoy 1989; and for a full discussion on ageing adult individuals, see Cox 2000.

92 Todd 1920, 1921; Katz and Suchey 1986; Brooks and Suchey 1990.

93 Lovejoy et al. 1985.

94 Brothwell 1981.

95 Meindl and Lovejoy 1985.

96 Ubelaker 1989; Scheuer and Black 2000.

97 Brothwell 1981; Ubelaker 1989; Scheuer and Black 2000; for a thorough review of non-adult ageing methods, see Lewis 2007, 38–47.

98 Lewis 2007, 47–55; Wilson, MacLeod and Humphrey 2008.

99 Determination of sex based on the cranial features is a challenging process, as cranial morphology provides a reliable basis of sex determination for only some populations.

100 The ischiopubic ramus ridge and the greater sciatic notch, considered to be the least reliable indicators, were used with appropriate caution.

101 Trotter 1970.

Paleopathological Analysis

In this book the major and most commonly attested disease categories (dental, joint and infectious diseases, hematopoietic and metabolic disorders, as well as traumatic incidents) are the pathological conditions focused on, but where evidence exists for other conditions they are also presented. For the collections of Eleutherna, Kastella and Stylos the description of pathological conditions (macroscopically and radiographically examined), stated in terms such as side/location on the skeletal element and type of lesion, followed the protocols suggested by Buikstra and Ubelaker.[102] Differential diagnosis of diseases was generally based on specialized textbooks, such as those by Aufderheide and Rodríguez-Martín, and Ortner.[103] More specifically, the criteria that have been followed for the recording of diseases are those given by Lukacs for dental diseases;[104] by Rogers et al., and Rogers and Waldron for degenerative joint disorders;[105] and by Ortner and Ericksen, Ortner, Kimmerle and Diez, and Ortner et al. for scorbutic cases;[106] cases of scurvy were re-evaluated in respect to the pathognomonic features currently suggested by Ortner, and by Brickley and Ives.[107] Recording of fractures, which formed the main body of traumatic incidents, followed a specific protocol adopted by Lovell.[108] Each skull bone (frontal, parietal, temporal, occipital, zygomatic, nasal, maxilla and mandible) was scrutinized for fractures and was distinguished by side, with the exception of the nasal bones, which were counted as one bone only. In the postcranial skeleton, the presence of fracture was determined for the long bones (clavicle, humerus, ulna, radius, metacarpals, femur, tibia, fibula, metatarsals), the thorax and the vertebral column. Each long bone was identified as present (90% present), incomplete (50–90% present), fragmentary (<50% present) or absent.[109] Both incomplete and complete long bones with fractures formed the observable corpus. For each long-bone lesion the following information was documented: side and position of bone (proximal, middle and distal diaphyses, proximal and distal epiphyses) as well as type of fracture. Long-bone fracture description included length, apposition (shift), rotation and angulation (alignment). Also assessed were aspects of fracture healing, such as duration of

102 Buikstra and Ubelaker 1994.

103 Aufderheide and Rodríguez-Martín 1998; Ortner 2003.

104 Lukacs 1989.

105 Rogers et al. 1987; Rogers and Waldron 1995.

106 Ortner and Ericksen 1997; Ortner, Kimmerle and Diez 1999; Ortner et al. 2001.

107 Ortner 2003; Brickley and Ives 2006, 2008.

108 Lovell 1997.

109 Judd and Roberts 1999.

healing (for example, the presence of complete or partial callus formation) and complications during healing.

The research data that were consulted for this study often provided only partial description of the observed lesions with reference to clinical diagnostic criteria, methodology, differential diagnosis, prevalence rates or supporting illustrations. This lack was especially apparent in the data reported for degenerative joint disease, in which prevalence rates were rarely provided. An inconsistency was also noted in 'labeling' conditions that reflect osteoarthritis, as a wide range of terms like 'arthropathy', 'arthritis' and 'osteophytosis' was applied. In general, reference to the real prevalence rates of pathological conditions according to skeletal elements or individuals was a frequent piece of vital missing information. This obstacle was possible to overcome when an inventory of bones and teeth was included in the study. If such an inventory was present, an effort was made to estimate both the number of individuals affected by a pathological condition (crude prevalence rate) and the number of skeletal elements affected (true prevalence rate). The frequencies of the pathological conditions observed in the skeletal remains from the studied sites are presented in tables that include the total number of adult/non-adult individuals; total males, females and non-sexed adults; crude prevalence rates; and true prevalence rates if total teeth/parts of bone observed are provided. In the text, crude prevalence rates are stated as a percentage of the total number of individuals considered and are graphically represented (by site/age and sex distribution/time period). The observed pathological conditions are illustrated in figures.

The bioarchaeological approach employed here for overcoming the limitations of problematic information provides, in the first instance, a window onto health in Byzantine Crete. For the future, it suggests a model for a possible standardization of methodology and improved data quality that will provide greater insight into the reconstruction of health and disease patterns from archaeological populations.

Chapter 2

In Search of *Homo Byzantinus*

The focus in the Byzantine sources, written and visual, tends to lie on emperors, generals, the clergy and the aristocracy, of whom a great deal is known. But the 'average Byzantine' is an elusive figure that remains at the periphery of written texts and visual depictions. Investigating the concepts of gender and identity in Byzantine culture can meet many obstacles. In much early research, in fact, *Homo byzantinus* was identified as *vir byzantinus* (the Byzantine male), sustaining the idea that men were the 'natural' embodiment of Byzantine society. *Femina byzantina* (the Byzantine female) had to wait many years to leave the shadowy world to which she had been consigned.[1] The study of human skeletal remains of Byzantine populations is expected to shed more light on aspects of everyday Byzantine life and enable us to better understand what it was to be a Byzantine.

The present chapter is focused on the frequency of diseases in the adult segment of the population. The information provided, which is based on generally accepted clinical notions of disease, is discussed in light of the interaction of environmental and other influences on health status.

Table 2.1 Demographic data for the adult sample

Site	M	F	I	Total no. of individuals
Eleutherna	52	21	27	100
Gortyn[2]	18	11	0	29
Kastella	15	8	12	35
Kefali	18	11	20	49
Knossos[3]	9	12	8	29
Stylos	9	11	9	29
Total	*121*	*74*	*76*	*271*

M=Male, F=Female, I=Indeterminate[23]

[1] See Kazhdan and Constable 1982, and discussion in Barber 1997 and Bjørnholt and James 2007.

[2] According to Mallegni 1988, table 1, the total number of female individuals is 16; these five additional female individuals are not included in the table as they range from 'adolescent' to 18 years old.

[3] Minimum Number of Individuals and sex determination are modified after Musgrave 1976, tables 1 and 3.

Physical Anthropology

The adult sample includes 271 individuals, representing 60.8% of the total number of individuals under study. Sex determination was possible for 195 adults (43.9%), 121 males (62%) and 74 females (34.9%), while the sex of 75 individuals (10.1%) remained unknown (Table 2.1). Table 2.2 presents a summary of the data obtained from the life tables.[4] Minor and major variations were observed among the populations; for example, we note that the population of Gortyn experienced the lowest crude mortality rate (34.93 individuals), and the population of Stylos the highest (43.48 individuals). Similarly, the population of Gortyn presented the highest life expectancy at birth (28.63 years) and at age 15 (24.22 years), and Stylos the lowest at birth (23.00 years) and at age 15 (16.03 years). The data obtained is presented graphically in Figure 2.1. A cluster of deaths is observed in the most productive age categories, from 15 to 34 years, numbering 162 individuals (36.4%); at Eleutherna, for example, almost one-third of the population (58 individuals) died within this age range.[5] In the entire sample, 40 individuals (8.9%) are aged over 45 years; the populations of Gortyn and Eleutherna (12 and 11 individuals, respectively) included the majority of mature and old adult people.

Table 2.2 Summary of the data obtained from the life tables

Site	Crude mortality rate[1]	Life expectancy at birth	Life expectancy at 15 years
Eleutherna	40.13	24.92	17.97
Gortyn	34.93	28.63	24.22
Kastella	39.14	25.55	18.22
Kefali	37.20	26.88	17.21
Stylos	43.48	23.00	16.03

[1] Number of individuals dying in a year for a population of 1,000 individuals

Previous studies on early Byzantine populations indicate a mean age at death of around 40–45 years for males and 30–35 years for females.[6] These figures do not change considerably during the middle Byzantine period (Figure 2.2). The lower average age at death for females can be explained primarily in terms of the risks associated with complications during pregnancy and childbirth.

4 Life tables have been prepared for all samples with the exception of the Knossos sample, as it included only commingled remains.

5 As argued in Chapter 1, a fundamental reason for promoting teenage marriages may have been the desire to maximize the number of births.

6 Bourbou 2004, table 17. For the Roman imperial era, Angel and Bisel 1985, table 5 report that average age at death was 38.8 years for males and 34.2 years for females.

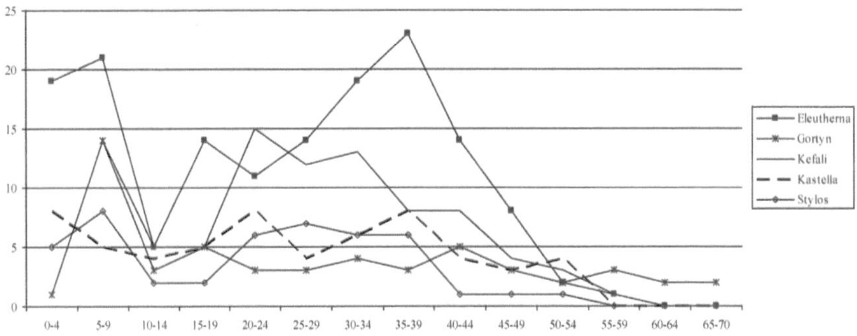

Figure 2.1 Mortality curve of the populations

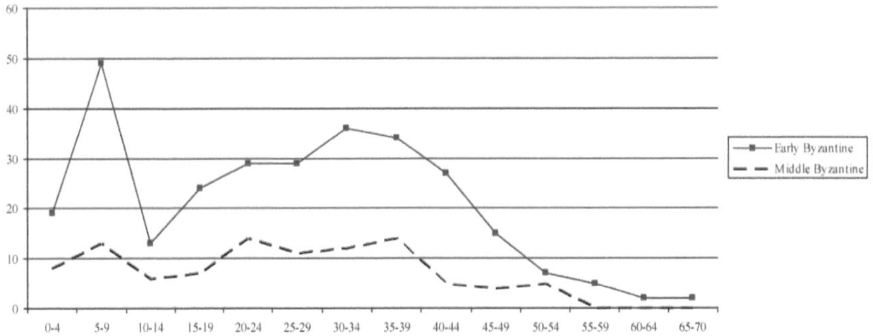

Figure 2.2 Mortality curve of the populations by time period

Possible causes include premature death due to miscarriages, complications of delivery and infection or hemorrhages during the postpartum period.[7] Based on the fact that most childbirths took place at home with the help of untrained, albeit experienced midwives, death at childbirth or shortly afterward was probably a common occurrence.[8] While women are undoubtedly put at risk by

[7] Talbot 1997, 125.

[8] Lascaratos, Lazaris and Kreatsas 2002 review a well-documented example of the difficulties confronted by physicians during the complicated labor of Eudoxia, wife of the emperor Arcadius (AD 395–408). However, evidence suggests that women also received treatment in hospitals, where beds were specifically reserved for new mothers. Talbot 1997, 124–5 and Fulghum-Heintz 2003, 280 note that the hospital in early Byzantine Alexandria had beds designated for new mothers and that the Pantokrator monastery in Constantinople (twelfth century AD) included a 12-bed female ward.

childbearing, males, in general, have a lower resistance to environmental stress and a less effective immune response than females.[9] Coupled with the hazards presented in the performance of various activities, males were also exposed to a number of risks that had the potential to put them under temporary or permanent disability, or even to cause their death.

Finally, data on average height in Byzantine Crete, although restricted by the limited number of intact long bones preserved, is estimated for males to have been between 1.61 and 1.78 cm, and for females between 1.46 and 1.62 cm (Table 2.3). These data compare with data from other Byzantine sites in Greece, apart from minor variations.[10]

Table 2.3 Mean adult height in Byzantine Crete

Site	Total no. of individuals	No. of males/ Males used for estimation	Mean height (cm)	No. of females/ Females used for estimation	Mean height (cm)
Eleutherna	100	52/16	1.69	21/7	1.60
Gortyn	29	18/11	1.73	11/3	1.60
Kastella	35	15/2	1.61	8/2	1.54
Kefali	49	18/8	~1.65	11/2	~1.48
Knossos	28	9/16[1]	1.61–1.78	12/8[1]	1.46–1.62
Stylos	29	9/3	1.66	11/0	–

[1] Number of long bones measured

Paleopathology

The distribution of the observed pathological conditions in our sample is graphically represented in Figure 2.3. Various pathological conditions that are attested include diseases of the dentition, degenerative joint diseases, hematopoietic diseases, infectious diseases, traumatic incidents, circulatory disorders, congenital abnormalities and tumors of bone. Figure 2.4 presents the distribution of pathological conditions attested in the early and middle

9 Armelagos 1998.

10 For example, at Messene the average height is 1.70 cm for males and 1.52 cm for females, see Bourbou 2004; at Corinth ('Lerna Hollow'), 1.63–1.73 cm for males and 1.50–1.62 cm for females, see Wesolowsky 1973; Abdera (Polystylon), 1.68 cm for males and 1.56 cm for females, see Agelarakis and Agelarakis 1989; at Aliki II (Thasos), 1.62 cm for males and 1.50 cm for females, see Buchet and Sodini 1984.

Byzantine periods on Crete. All pathological conditions are analyzed and discussed in detail below.

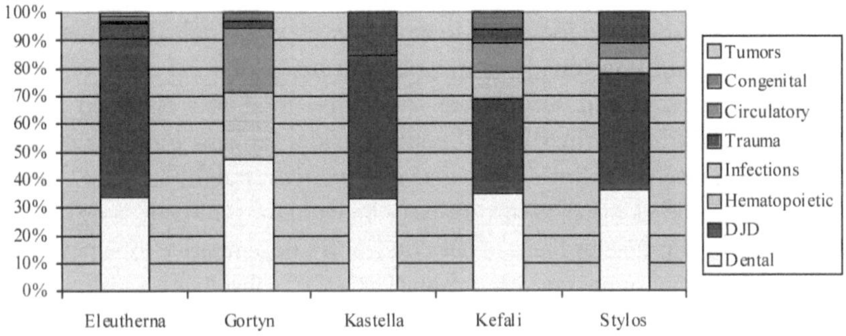

DJD=Degenerative Joint Disease

Figure 2.3 Distribution of pathological conditions by site (individuals affected)

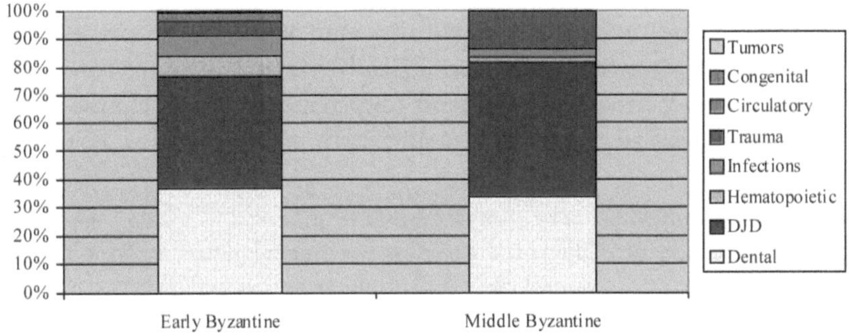

DJD=Degenerative Joint Disease

Figure 2.4 Distribution of pathological conditions by time period (individuals affected)

Diseases of the Dentition

Teeth tend to survive better than bones in the burial environment; thus dental diseases are perhaps the most commonly reported pathological conditions in any skeletal sample. Evidence of dental diseases yields valuable clues about diet (type of food consumed), nutrition (adequacy of food with regard to physiological needs) and subsistence (how that food was obtained and/or produced). In addition, the study of teeth provides information on individual health status as well as cultural influences and intercultural differences.[11] Dental diseases are classified either as infectious (when a pathogenic microorganism is responsible for the development of the condition), degenerative (due to the loss of a conspicuous amount of tooth or bone surface or substance), developmental (diseases occurring during the formation of dental tissues or during the developing interrelationship between teeth and jaws) or genetic.[12] Being able to identify the etiological pathway leading to a given dental pathology, for example, whether caries, calculus or attrition is primarily responsible for ante-mortem tooth loss – although not an easy task – is extremely useful in dietary reconstruction. However, despite a substantial bibliography on dental pathology, a full understanding of the diseases of the dentition and their implications awaits further analysis.[13]

For the purposes of this study, dental caries, ante-mortem tooth loss, abscesses, calculus (plaque or tartar accumulation) and enamel defects are considered, being the data most frequently and most consistently recorded.[14] In the sample of 271 individuals, 116 people (42.8%) suffered from dental diseases, 83 of them

---

11 Cultural influences: for example, the cases of dental mutilation applied for ornamental effect in pre-Columbian America. Intercultural differences: for example, populations with varying economies have revealed important relationships between diet and the development of specific dental pathologies.

12 Lukacs 1989, 264. For a thorough review of the dental diseases most likely to be encountered and diagnosed in archaeologically recovered human skeletal remains, see Hillson 1986, 283–314; 1996, 231–94; Aufderheide and Rodríguez-Martín 1998, 398–9, 400–407; Ortner 2003, 589–606.

13 See, e.g., Hillson 1986, 1996.

14 Data on attrition and periodontal disease are much more inconsistent and are therefore excluded from the overall discussion. The available data can be summarized as follows: Mallegni 1988 associates the most frequent pathology (ante-mortem tooth loss) in Gortyn with attrition, the latter being attributed to the quality of food consumed; Bourbou 2004, table Ia, refers to only one affected mandible with periodontal disease and ten mandibles and two maxillae exhibiting heavy attrition; finally, Zygouri 2005 reports that, of 156 teeth studied, 37 (23.7%) and 12 (7.6%) presented periodontal disease and attrition, respectively.

males (42.5%) and 26 females (13.3%) of 195 sexed adults. Absolute frequency rate is 31.9% or 597 affected teeth/tooth sockets of 1,870 (Figure 2.5). Dental diseases are attested more frequently for males than females, and although all age categories are affected, a cluster is noted for middle-aged adults (Figure 2.6).

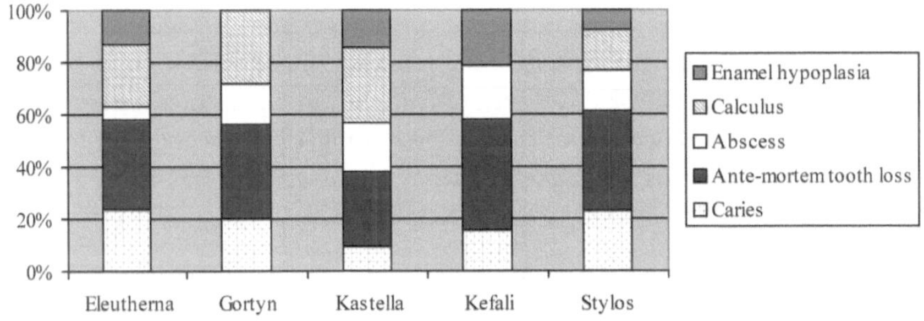

Figure 2.5 Distribution of dental pathologies by site (individuals affected)

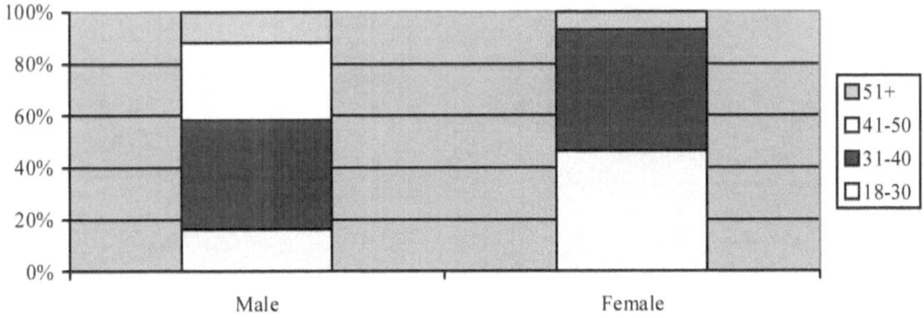

Figure 2.6 Distribution of dental disease by sex and age (individuals affected).

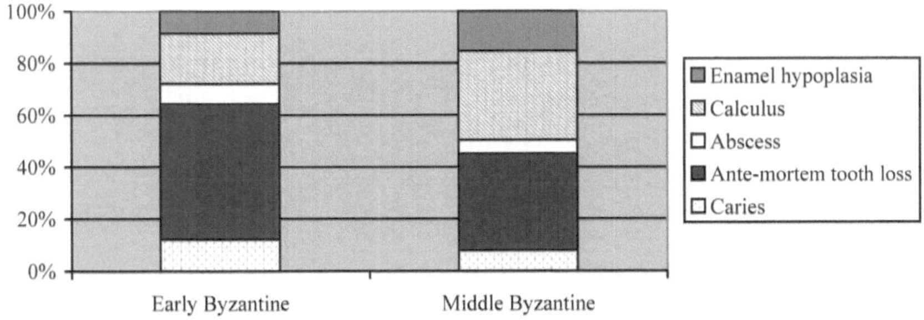

Figure 2.7 Distribution of dental pathologies by time period (individuals affected)

In comparison between time periods, 81 people (39.1%) and 35 people (54.6%) are attested for the early and middle Byzantine period, respectively. Absolute frequency rate is 27.9% or 409 affected teeth/tooth sockets of 1,461 for the early Byzantine sites, and 45.9% or 188 affected teeth/tooth sockets of 409 for the middle Byzantine sites (Figure 2.7).

The presence of food sugars in association with acidogenic bacteria produces demineralization of enamel and dentine, resulting in the formation of cavities (dental caries)[15] – Figure 2.8. Caries are recorded in all six sites, affecting 22 people, with a prevalence rate of 8.1%, representing 18 males and four females of 195 sexed individuals. Absolute frequency rate is 4.5% or 65 of 1,415 teeth, with a range of 2.1% (Gortyn) to 8.3% (Kefali) (Table 2.4).

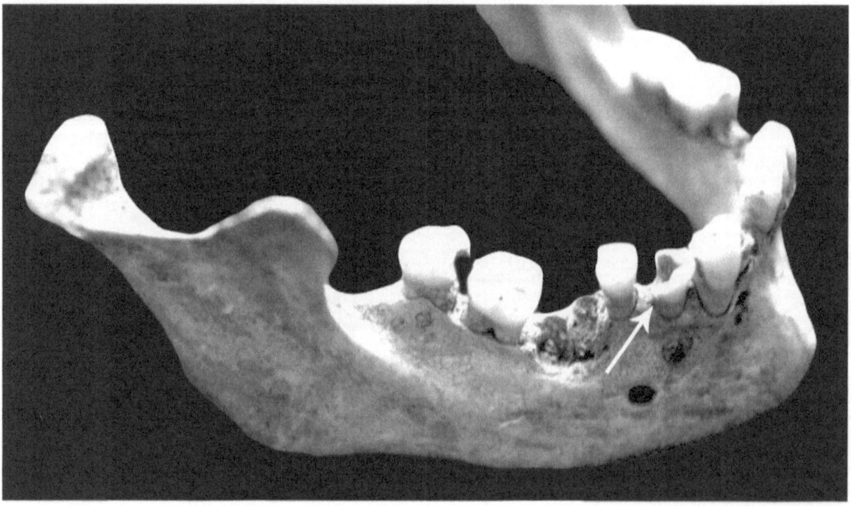

Figure 2.8 Kastella: Skeleton 014, carious lesion (arrow) on mandibular tooth (photo: C. Bourbou)

15 Lukacs 1989, 265.

Table 2.4 Dental caries in the adult sample (individuals and/or teeth affected)

Site	Total no.	Affected	M	F	CPR%	Total no. of teeth	Teeth affected	TPR%
Eleutherna	100	9	8	1	9.0	618	18	2.9
Gortyn	29	5	4	1	17.2	232	5	2.1
Kastella	35	2	2	0	5.7	267	9	3.3
Kefali	49	3	1	2	6.1	156	13	8.3
Knossos	29	-	-	-	-	-	14	-
Stylos	29	3	3	0	10.3	142	6	4.2
Total	*271*	*22*	*18*	*4*	*8.1*	*1,415*	*65*	*4.5*

M=Male, F=Female

Lukacs describes three distinctive pathways as primary causal factors contributing to the development of ante-mortem tooth loss: caries, calculus and attrition.[16] With the exception of Knossos, for which no precise relevant data are provided, ante-mortem tooth loss is observed in the rest of the sites (Figure 2.9). The pathology is seen in 41 people (16.9%), representing 27 males and 10 females of 195 sexed

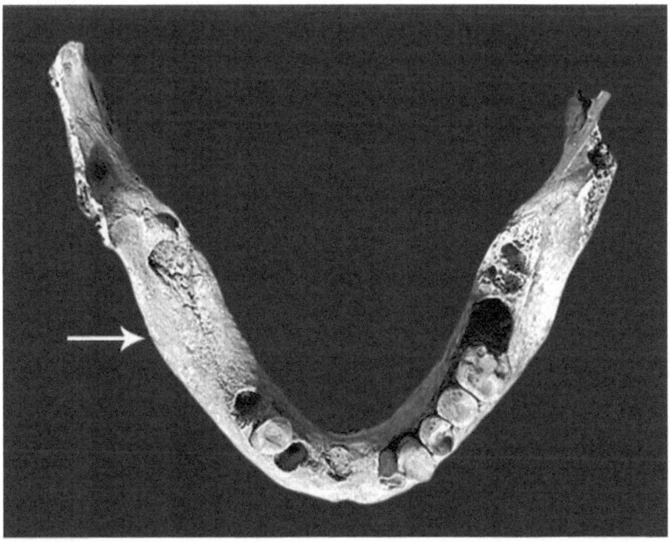

Figure 2.9 Eleutherna: Skeleton 011a, ante-mortem tooth loss (arrow) of mandibular teeth (photo: K. Painesi. Courtesy of Prof. P. Themelis and the Society of Messenian Archaeological Studies)

[16] Lukacs 1989, 265. Besides these primary causal factors, abscess and periodontal disease also cause ante-mortem tooth loss.

individuals. Absolute frequency rates for five sites are 20.0% or 283 of 1,415 teeth/tooth sockets with a range of 12.7% (Kastella) to 42.9% (Kefali) (Table 2.5).

Table 2.5 Ante-mortem tooth loss in the adult sample (individuals and/or teeth/tooth sockets affected)

Site	Total no.	Affected	M	F	I	CPR%	Total no. of teeth/ sockets	Total no. of teeth/ sockets affected	TPR%
Eleutherna	100	13	9	3	1	13.0	618	104	16.8
Gortyn	29	9	6	3	0	31.0	232	42	18.1
Kastella	35	6	4	2	0	17.1	267	34	12.7
Kefali	49	8	4	2	2	16.3	156	67	42.9
Stylos	29	5	4	0	1	17.2	142	36	25.3
Total	*242*	*41*	*27*	*10*	*4*	*16.9*	*1,415*	*283*	*20.0*

M=Male, F=Female, I=Indeterminate

Exposure of the pulp chamber through severe attrition or extensive carious decay produces an inflamed pulp which can result in an infected periapical tissue and osteitis. In archaeological bones such periapical abscess is recognizable if the spreading pathological process has destroyed the external bony surface of the jaw.[17] Dental abscess is recorded in all six sites, with a frequency rate of 5.9% (16 individuals), representing 13 males and three females of 195 sexed individuals. Absolute frequency rate is 2.2% or 42 of 1,870 teeth/tooth sockets, with a range of 0.3% (Eleutherna) to 12.1% (Kefali) (Table 2.6).

Table 2.6 Dental abscess in the adult sample (individuals and/or teeth/tooth sockets affected)

Site	Total no.	Affected	M	F	CPR%	Total no. of teeth/ sockets	Total no. of teeth/sockets affected	TPR%
Eleutherna	100	2	2	0	2.0	618	2	0.3
Gortyn	29	4	3	1	13.7	232	7	3.0
Kastella	35	4	3	1	11.4	267	8	2.9
Kefali	49	4	3	1	8.1	156	19	12.1
Knossos	29	-	-	-	-	455	4	0.8
Stylos	29	2	2	0	6.8	142	2	1.4
Total	*271*	*16*	*13*	*3*	*5.9*	*1,870*	*42*	*2.2*

M=Male, F=Female

[17] Lukacs 1989, 271. Because only visually diagnosed cases are reported in archaeological bone, the application of radiographic analysis is essential in order to assess the real abscess frequency.

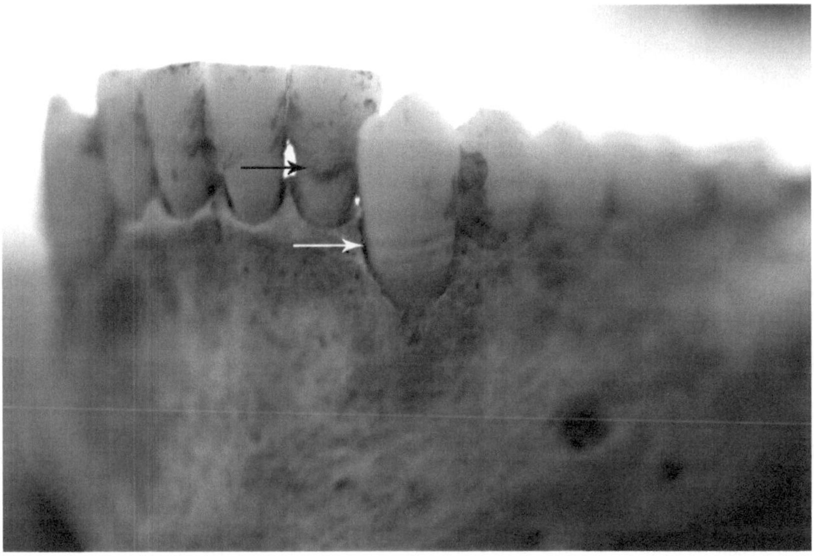

Figure 2.10 Kastella: Skeleton 021, calculus (black arrow) and enamel hypoplasia (white arrow) on mandibular teeth (photo: C. Bourbou)

Dental calculus is the mineralization of bacterial plaque[18] (Figure 2.10). Calculus is recorded in four sites, affecting 24 people (11.2%), 16 being males and six females of 195 sexed individuals. Absolute frequency rate is 12.0% or 143 of 1,183 teeth/tooth sockets, with a range of 4.5% (Eleutherna) to 32.6% (Kefali) (Table 2.7).

Table 2.7 Dental calculus in the adult sample (individuals and/or teeth affected)

Site	Total no.	Affected	M	F	I	CPR%	Total no. of teeth	Teeth affected	TPR%
Eleutherna	100	9	5	2	2	9.0	618	28	4.5
Kastella	35	7	5	2	0	20.0	267	51	19.1
Kefali	49	6	4	2	0	12.2	156	51	32.6
Stylos	29	2	2	0	0	6.8	142	13	9.1
Total	*213*	*24*	*16*	*6*	*2*	*11.2*	*1,183*	*143*	*12.0*

M=Male, F=Female, I=Indeterminate

18 Lukacs 1989, 267.

Enamel hypoplasia consists of sharply defined, linear, horizontal grooves or pits on the enamel surface of the tooth crown (see Figure 2.10). Although the classical linear lesion of enamel hypoplasia is not difficult to diagnose in archaeological teeth, atypical lesions may mimic enamel hypoplasia lines, and the anterior teeth, which are the most useful in the evaluation of the condition, are frequently lost, especially during excavation and post-excavation procedures. Enamel hypoplasia is reported in four sites for 13 individuals (6.1%), affecting nine males and three females of 195 sexed individuals. Absolute frequency rate is 5.4% or 64 of 1,183 teeth, with a range of 1.2% (Eleutherna) to 17.3% (Kefali) (Table 2.8).

Table 2.8 Enamel hypoplasia in the adult sample (individuals and/or teeth affected)

Site	Total no.	Affected	M	F	I	CPR%	Total no. of teeth	Teeth affected	TPR%
Eleutherna	100	5	4	1	0	5.0	618	8	1.2
Kastella	35	3	2	1	0	8.5	267	26	9.7
Kefali	49	4	3	1	0	8.1	156	27	17.3
Stylos	29	1	0	0	1	3.4	142	3	2.1
Total	*213*	*13*	*9*	*3*	*1*	*6.1*	*1,183*	*64*	*5.4*

M=Male, F=Female, I=Indeterminate

Teeth-cleaning appears not to have been a common activity of the Byzantine population of Crete, and the composition and consistency of foods consumed primarily determined the development of dental diseases. The quality of food consumed (sweetening agents, hard plant tissues or coarsely ground flour containing tiny stone particles from the mill-stones used for its production) affected the extent of abrasion on the teeth and pathological conditions in the oral cavity. For example, caries usually develop in the mouth in an acidic environment, while calculus usually develops in an alkaline environment, which is indicative of a more protein-rich diet. Most research suggests that the basic diet in early and middle Byzantine Crete was low in carbohydrates but rich in plant tissues and fluorides, conditions that contribute to good general oral hygiene.[19] In the samples from all six sites, ante-mortem tooth loss is the most striking of the dental diseases, and edentulous jaws have also been recovered. Two male individuals in Eleutherna had lost all their mandibular teeth ante-mortem. In the majority of cases, the smooth, completely healed dental sockets suggest that ante-mortem tooth loss must have taken place long before death occurred. The

19 See, e.g., Mallegni 1988, 46; Bourbou 2004, 71.

analysis of dental data in the samples revealed that male individuals suffered disproportionately from dental pathologies, suggesting possible differential access to food products depending on sex, but the isotopic evidence did not reveal substantial differences.[20]

Cases of enamel hypoplasia merit special attention, for paleopathologists have often interpreted individuals with hypoplasia to have been more stressed and correspondingly less well adapted than those without hypoplasia. Traditionally, enamel hypoplasia has been associated with non-fatal stress episodes, such as metabolic insults or malnutrition, although in most cases it has been impossible to associate the presence of the condition with specific etiological circumstances. Because hypoplasia is an indicator of stress, cases of enamel hypoplasia in the archaeological record are associated with hardship and are therefore important factors in elucidating the past human condition. For example, in the Eleutherna sample, an association can be made between hypoplasia, stress periods and longevity, since the mean age at death of individuals with hypoplasia is 36.8 years – appreciably lower than the mean age at death for the population overall, which is 40 to 45 years.[21]

Degenerative Joint Diseases of the Appendicular Skeleton

Diseases occurring in joints and their potential hardships (pain and disability) play an important role in any attempt to reconstruct lifestyles of past populations. The various joint diseases are typically accompanied by characteristic changes (osteophytes, erosion of the joint and especially eburnation and/or porosity of subchondral bone), enabling the researcher to classify the specific type, although in many cases, especially in fragmentary skeletons, a detailed classification is not possible.[22]

Despite the generally poor preservation of joint surfaces, degenerative diseases are among the most commonly observed pathological conditions at four of the six studied sites. At Gortyn, no degenerative lesions are reported, and at Knossos, osteoarthritis of carpal bones is summarily reported with no additional information. The report of degenerative joint diseases in the Kefali sample lacks detailed information and classification of the various types. We note here that for the Kefali sample, a case of ankylosing spondylitis has been diagnosed, but

20 See Chapter 4.

21 See the discussion in Goodman 1991; Bourbou 2004, 71–2.

22 See Rogers et al. 1987, 179–83; Rogers and Waldron 1995, 1–7.

has only been briefly described and documented as the sacro-iliac joints are not affected.

Osteoarthritis

Osteoarthritis affects synovial joints and its frequency increases with age; a predilection for the vertebral column, hands, hips, knees, the acromioclavicular joint, the first metatarsophalangeal and carpometacarpal joint is noted, and in modern populations females are usually more commonly affected than males. The typical set of diagnostic criteria for osteoarthritis on dry bone include the presence of osteophytes, areas of porosity or pitting, alteration of the bony contour of the joint and the most unequivocal marker of the condition, eburnation.[23]

Much of the work on osteoarthritis in the 1960s and 1970s considered the condition to be ideal for reconstructing past lifestyles, since its cause was largely interpreted as the result of repetitive mechanical load on specific joints; that is, the continuous use of specific muscles and joints in daily and repetitive activities.[24] Identification of osteoarthritis was used, in addition, to answer questions regarding possible links between subsistence economy and prevalence/patterning of the condition, and to track differences in activity patterns between males and females and among groups engaged in specific activities related to food production and trade.[25] Interest in osteoarthritis in anthropological studies declined in the late 1990s and although the condition continued to be incorporated in general skeletal studies, the inherent complexities of the disease process were often overlooked. Weiss and Jurmain provide a useful review of the relevant medical and anthropological research.[26] In the interest of affording better diagnoses and interpretation of osteoarthritis in past populations, and promoting a systematic evaluation of osteoarthritis as part of a more complete bioarchaeological investigation, Weiss and Jurmain emphasize the multifactorial etiology of the condition, considering genetic, anatomical, body mass index and mechanical influences on the development of the condition.[27]

---

23 Rogers et al. 1987, 185–6; Rogers and Waldron 1995, 43–5; Rogers 2000, 166.

24 See, e.g., Wells 1962, 1963, 1972; Angel 1966, 1971; Ortner 1968; Jurmain 1978; Merbs 1983; Bennike 1987; Waldron 1992.

25 See, e.g., Cohen and Armelagos 1984; Bridges 1992; Lovell and Dublenko 1999; Slaus 2000; Klaus, Larsen and Tam 2009.

26 Weiss and Jurmain 2007.

27 Weiss and Jurmain 2007, 439–44.

Table 2.9 Osteoarthritis of the appendicular skeleton in the adult sample (individuals affected)

Site	Total no.	One joint affected				Two joints affected				Three or more joints affected			
		M	F	I	CPR%	M	F	I	CPR%	M	F	I	CPR%
Eleutherna	100	6	0	3	9.0	0	1	0	1.0	3	0	0	3.0
Kastella	35	1	1	0	5.7	2	0	0	5.7	2	2	0	11.4
Kefali	49	0	0	1	2.0	2	0	0	4.0	1	1	0	4.0
Stylos	29	0	0	1	3.4	0	1	0	3.4	1	0	0	3.4
Total	*213*	*7*	*1*	*5*	*6.1*	*4*	*2*	*0*	*2.8*	*7*	*3*	*0*	*4.6*

M=Male, F=Female, I=Indeterminate

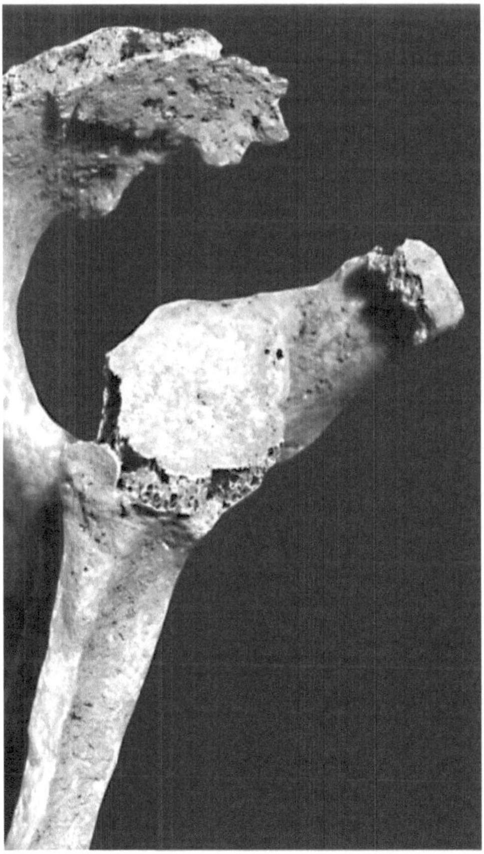

Figure 2.11 Eleutherna: Skeleton 011a, osteoarthritis of the acromioclavicular joint (photo: K. Painesi. Courtesy of Prof. P. Themelis and the Society of Messenian Archaeological Studies)

The distribution of osteoarthritis in the appendicular skeleton (Figures 2.11 and 2.12) is presented in Table 2.9. Twenty-nine individuals (10.7%) exhibited osteoarthritic lesions in one or multiple joints, 18 being males (9.0%) and six females (3.0%) of 195 sexed adults (Figure 2.13). Absolute frequency for the upper limbs is 2.7 % or 33 affected joints of the 1,193 examined, with a range of 0.6% (Eleutherna, sternoclavicular) to 9.0% (Kastella, hand) (Table 2.10).

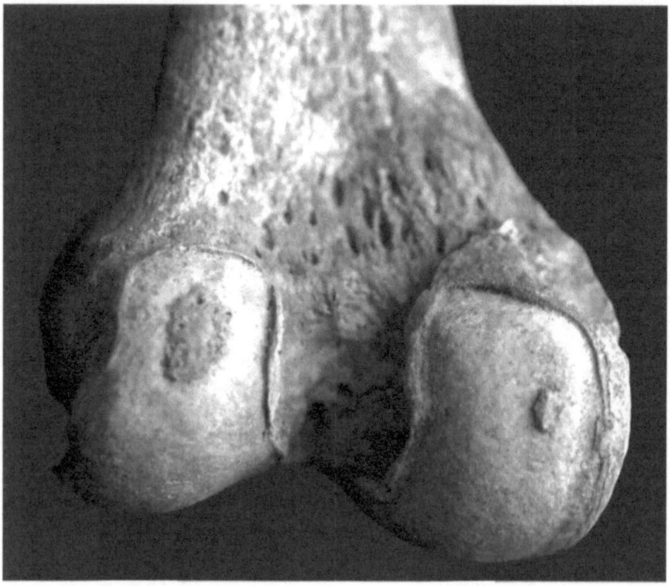

Figure 2.12 Kastella: Skeleton 004, osteoarthritis of the knee joint (photo: C. Bourbou)

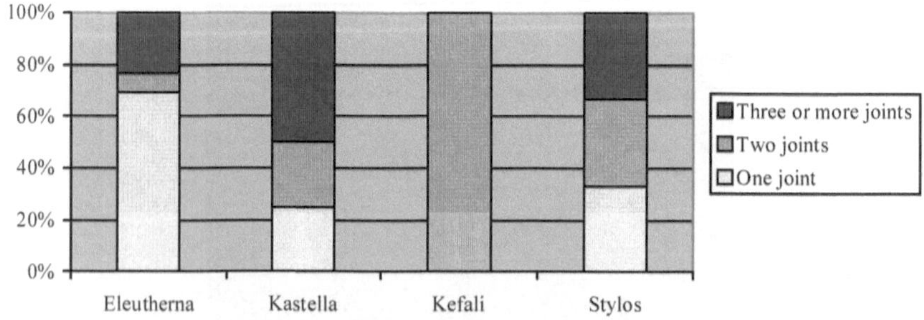

Figure 2.13 Distribution of osteoarthritis in the appendicular skeleton by site (individuals affected)

Absolute frequency for the lower limbs is 4.3 % or 21 affected joints of the 481 examined, with a range of 1.6% (Eleutherna, foot) to 19.5% (Kastella, knee) (Table 2.11). The majority of osteoarthritic lesions were observed on the upper limbs, and males are more frequently affected than females (Figure 2.14). When comparing between time periods, 18 people (8.7%) and 11 people (17.1%) are attested for the early and middle Byzantine period, respectively (Figure 2.15).

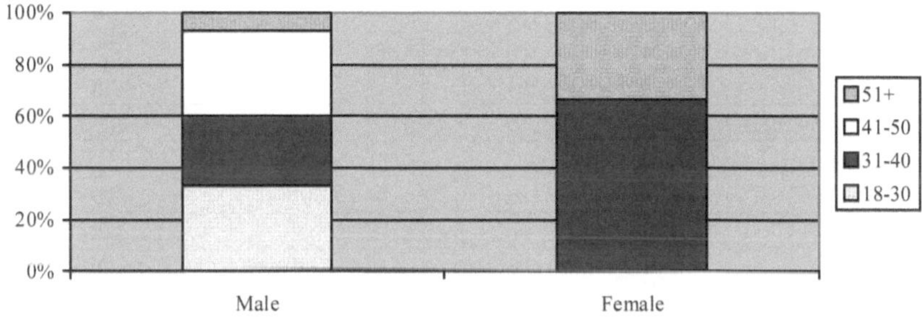

Only individuals of known sex and age are represented

Figure 2.14 Distribution of osteoarthritis in the appendicular skeleton by sex and age (individuals affected)

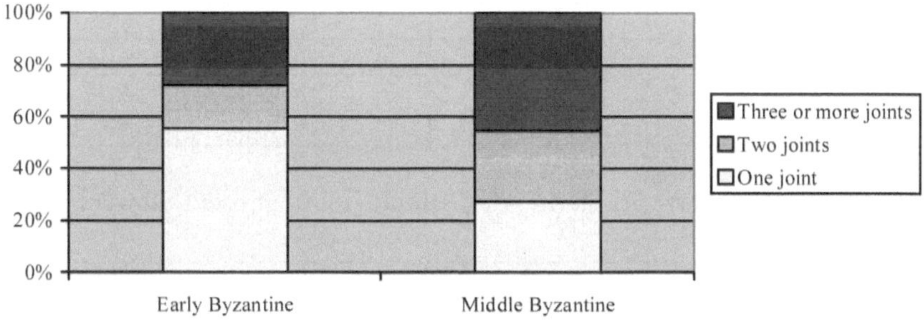

Figure 2.15 Distribution of osteoarthritis by time period (individuals affected)

Table 2.10 Osteoarthritis in the adult sample (joints affected): upper body

Site	Total joints	Joints affected	TPR%
Sternoclavicular			
Eleutherna	156	1	0.6
Kastella	24	1	4.1
Total (sternoclavicular)	*180*	*2*	*1.1*
Acromioclavicular			
Eleutherna	136	2	1.4
Kastella	45	4	8.8
Stylos	26	1	3.8
Total (acromioclavicular)	*207*	*7*	*3.3*
Glenohumeral			
Eleutherna	101	1	0.9
Kastella	41	2	4.8
Stylos	24	2	8.3
Total (glenohumeral)	*166*	*5*	*3.0*
Elbow			
Eleutherna	230	2	0.8
Kastella	48	3	6.2
Total (elbow)	*278*	*5*	*1.7*
Wrist			
Eleutherna	162	2	1.2
Hand			
Eleutherna	156	8	5.1
Kastella	44	4	9.0
Total (hand)	*200*	*12*	*6.0*
Total	*1,193*	*33*	*2.7*

Table 2.11 Osteoarthritis in the adult sample (joints affected): lower body

Site	Total joints	Joints affected	TPR%
Sacro-iliac			
Kastella	29	1	3.4
Knee			
Kastella	46	9	19.5
Foot			
Eleutherna	354	6	1.6
Kastella	35	4	11.4
Stylos	17	1	5.8
Total (foot)	*406*	*11*	*2.7*
Total	*481*	*21*	*4.3*

Degenerative Joint Diseases of the Spine

The vertebral column is also frequently affected by various degenerative conditions, mainly osteoarthritis, spondylosis and intervertebral disc displacement (Schmorl's nodes and discal prolapse). Spondylosis is a very common condition and an entity separate from osteoarthritis.[28] It affects the apophyseal (facet) joints of the vertebrae, and the most obvious manifestations include marginal osteophytes and coarse pitting of the vertebral bodies, usually manifested in mid-to-lower cervical, upper thoracic and lower regions of the spine.[29] One hundred and nine individuals (40.2%) exhibited one or multiple degenerative conditions in the vertebral column, in which the multiple conditions included coexistence of, for example, osteoarthritis and spondylosis (Figure 2.16). 68 are males (34.8%) and 23 are females (11.7%) of 195 sexed individuals (Figure 2.17). Absolute frequency is 35.9% or 400 affected vertebrae of 1,113 examined. When comparing between time periods, 71 people (34.3%) and 39 people (60.9%) are attested for the early and middle Byzantine period, respectively. Absolute frequency rate is 29.5% or 232 affected vertebrae of 786 for the early Byzantine sites, and 51.3% or 168 affected vertebrae of 327 for the middle Byzantine sites (Figure 2.18).

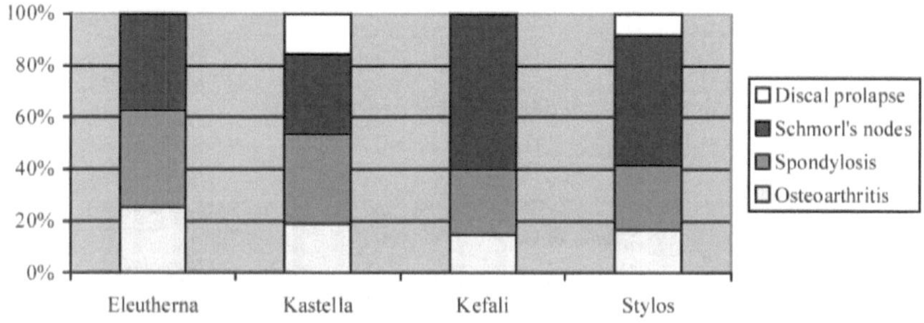

Figure 2.16 Distribution of degenerative disease of the spine by site (individuals affected)

[28] Spondylosis affects the vertebral bodies and osteoarthritis affects the synovial joints of the vertebrae.

[29] Rogers 2000, 169–70.

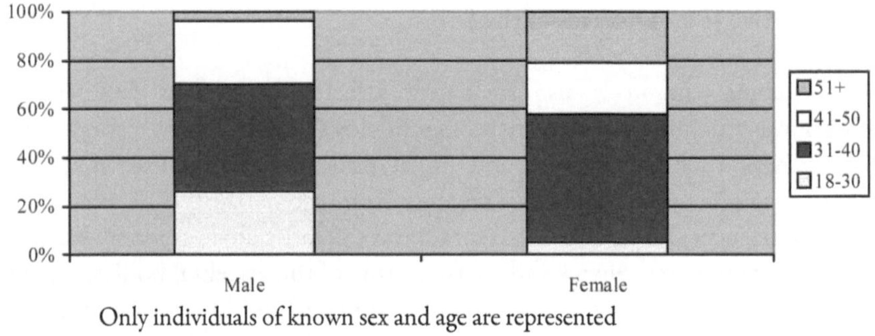

Figure 2.17 Distribution of degenerative disease of the spine by sex and age (individuals affected).

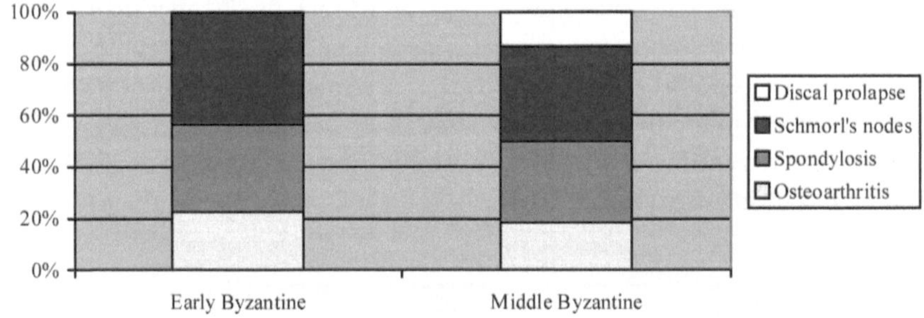

Figure 2.18 Distribution of degenerative disease of the spine by time period (individuals affected)

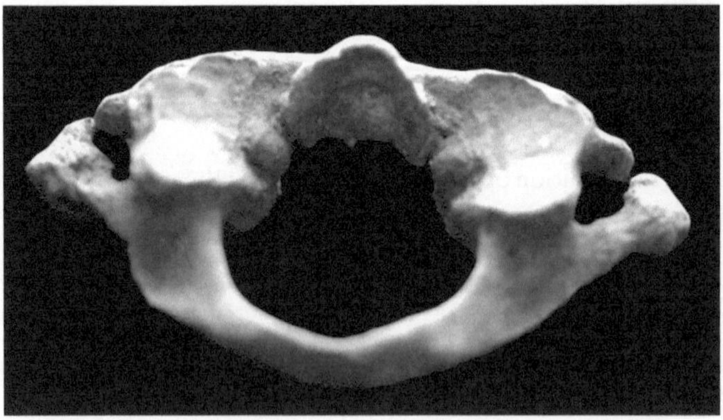

Figure 2.19 Kastella: Skeleton 011a, osteoarthritis of the first cervical vertebra (photo: C. Bourbou)

Osteoarthritis of the spine (Figure 2.19) is seen in 23 individuals (8.4%). Fifteen are males (7.6%) and six females (3.0%) of 195 sexed adults. Absolute frequency rate for spinal osteoarthritis is 7.1% or 80 affected vertebrae of 1,113 observed, with a range of 2.2% (Kefali) to 22.1% (Kastella) (Table 2.12). Spondylosis (Figure 2.20) is seen in 36 individuals (13.2%). Twenty-one are males (10.7%) and 10 are females (5.1%) of 195 sexed adults. Absolute frequency rate is 11.2% or 125 affected vertebrae of 1,113 observed, with a range of 2.2% (Stylos) to 37.5% (Kastella) (Table 2.13).

Table 2.12 Osteoarthritis of the spine in the adult sample (individuals and/or vertebrae affected)

Site	Total no.	Affected	M	F	I	CPR%	Total no.of vertebrae	Vertebrae affected	TPR%
Eleutherna	100	13	7	5	1	13.0	566	33	5.8
Kastella	35	5	4	1	0	14.2	104	23	22.1
Kefali	49	3	2	0	1	6.1	220	5	2.2
Stylos	29	2	2	0	0	6.9	223	19	8.5
Total	*213*	*23*	*15*	*6*	*2*	*10.8*	*1,113*	*80*	*7.1*

M=Male, F=Female, I=Indeterminate

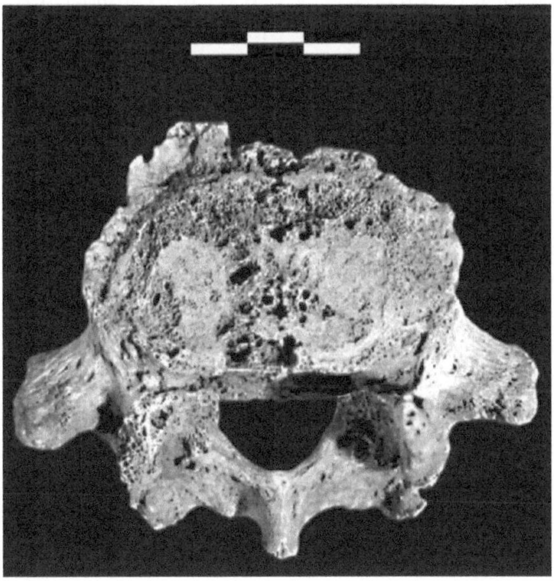

Figure 2.20 Eleutherna: Skeleton 007, spondylosis of the fifth lumbar vertebra (photo: K. Painesi. Courtesy of Prof. P. Themelis and the Society of Messenian Archaeological Studies)

Table 2.13 Spondylosis in the adult sample (individuals and/or vertebrae affected)

Site	Total no.	Affected	M	F	I	CPR%	Total no. of vertebrae	Vertebrae affected	TPR%
Eleutherna	100	19	12	5	2	19.0	566	59	10.4
Kastella	35	9	5	4	0	25.7	104	39	37.5
Kefali	49	5	3	1	1	10.2	220	22	10.0
Stylos	29	3	1	0	2	10.3	223	5	2.2
Total	*213*	*36*	*21*	*10*	*5*	*16.9*	*1,113*	*125*	*11.2*

M=Male, F=Female, I=Indeterminate

Intervertebral Disc Displacement

The intervertebral disc is a load-bearing structure that lies between the bodies of adjoining vertebrae in the spinal column. Each disc consists of an outer fibrous ring (annulus fibrosus) and an inner soft core (nucleus pulposus), both characterized by a high water content.[30] The precise amount of pressure within the disc is influenced by an individual's position and activity, and becomes elevated in the presence of abnormally increased externally applied loads, resulting in a prolapsed nucleus. Displacement of the nucleus from its confined space can result in various diseases of the spine; for example, anterior displacement can lead to spondylolysis deformans, while superior and inferior displacement is associated with cartilaginous node formation.

These cartilaginous nodes, usually termed 'Schmorl's nodes', consist of prolapsed intervertebral disc material that enters the vertebral body in a position either superior or inferior to the disc.[31] On dry bone they present as a smooth-walled cavitation seen on the inferior or superior surface of the affected vertebral body. Cartilaginous nodes are present in various disease processes, such as Scheuermann's disease (juvenile kyphosis), osteoporosis, infection and neoplasm, while traumatic incidents and senescent processes can also result from their formation. Idiopathic cartilaginous nodes, or those without obvious cause, are also encountered.[32] The predilection of Schmorl's nodes for the lower thoracic and lumbar regions is to be attributed to the anatomy and biomechanics of the lower spine, which typically result in a greater amount of loading on the lumbar vertebrae than on the cervical.[33] The presence of these nodes has been

---

30 Resnick 1995, 1419.

31 Schmorl and Junghanns 1959, 133.

32 Hansson and Ross 1983; Resnick 1995, 1420–21; Wagner et al. 2000.

33 Argoff and Wheeler 1998.

used as an indicator of differentiated activity patterns between males and females and among social groups.[34] In addition, the specific displacement of disc material designated as discal prolapse (protrusion), in which the nucleus pulposus has been displaced through some of the fibers of the annulus fibrosus but remains confined by the intact outermost fibers, has been observed in some of the archaeological samples under study here.[35] These conditions involving intervertebral disc displacement can provide crucial information about diseases of the disc as well as related neurological structures in a given population.

Schmorl's nodes (Figure 2.21) are seen in 45 individuals (16.6%); 28 individuals (14.3%) are males and seven (3.5%) are females of 195 sexed adults. Absolute frequency rate for Schmorl's nodes is 15.0% or 168 affected vertebrae of 1,113 observed, with a range of 10.4% (Eleutherna) to 28.8% (Kastella)

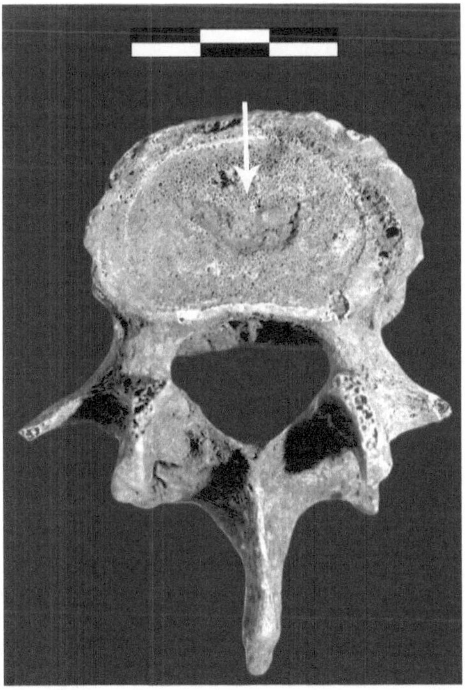

Figure 2.21 Eleutherna: Skeleton 002b, Schmorl's node (arrow) on the twelfth thoracic vertebra (photo: K. Painesi. Courtesy of Prof. P. Themelis and the Society of Messenian Archaeological Studies)

---

[34] See, e.g., Parrington and Roberts 1987; Robb et al. 2001.

[35] Following Resnick 1995, 1424 for the terminology.

(Table 2.14). Discal prolapse (Figure 2.22) is observed in the samples from Kastella and Stylos, including five individuals (1.8%). Four are males (2.0%) of 195 sexed adults. Absolute frequency rate for discal prolapse is 8.2% or 27 affected vertebrae of 327 (Table 2.15).

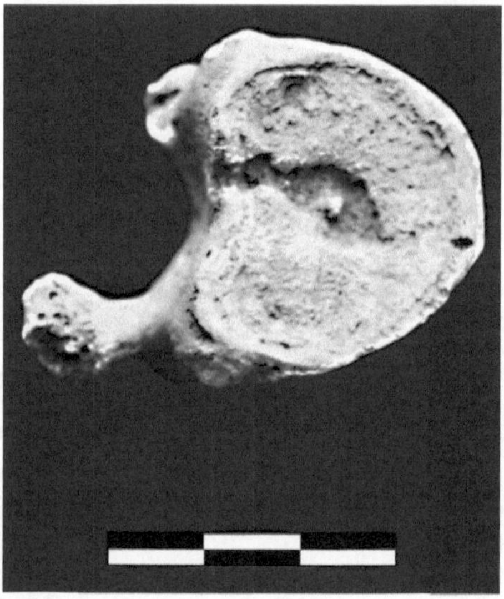

Figure 2.22 Kastella: Skeleton 002, discal prolapse on the twelfth thoracic vertebra (photo: C. Bourbou)

Table 2.14 Schmorl's nodes in the adult sample (individuals and/or vertebrae affected)

Site	Total no.	Affected	M	F	I	CPR%	Total no. of vertebrae	Vertebrae affected	TPR%
Eleutherna	100	19	13	3	3	19.0	566	59	10.4
Kastella	35	8	5	2	1	22.8	104	30	28.8
Kefali	49	12	8	1	3	20.4	220	54	24.5
Stylos	29	6	2	1	3	24.1	223	25	11.2
Total	*213*	*45*	*28*	*7*	*10*	*21.1*	*1,113*	*168*	*15.0*

M=Male, F=Female, I=Indeterminate

Table 2.15 Discal prolapse in the adult sample (individuals and/or vertebrae affected)

Site	Total no.	Affected	M	F	I	CPR%	Total no. of vertebrae	Vertebrae affected	TPR%
Kastella	35	4	4	0	0	11.4	104	9	8.6
Stylos	29	1	0	0	1	3.4	223	18	8.0
Total	*64*	*5*	*4*	*0*	*1*	*7.8*	*327*	*27*	*8.2*

M=Male, F=Female, I=Indeterminate

Osteoarthritis is the second most frequently encountered pathological condition in the skeletal sample, next to dental diseases. Although osteoarthritis is a multifactorial condition, the primary contributing factors are age and mechanical stress. The presence of degenerative changes in major joints and in the vertebral column is associated with the wear and tear occasioned by everyday activities and is distinguished from traumatic arthritis, which is caused by disruption of the biomechanical functioning of a joint. Even in cases where the articular cartilage is entirely missing as a result of severe osteoarthritis, the presence of eburnation and/or porosity is a reliable indication that the joint was still in use when death occurred.[36]

Schmorl's nodes are frequently observed in archaeological populations, occurring cross-culturally and throughout various time periods, geographical locations and overall activity patterns.[37] Faccia and Williams, in a clinical study that investigated the relationship between Schmorl's nodes and pain, have provided information that is also useful in the analysis of skeletal populations.[38] The results indicated that Schmorl's nodes in the central part of the vertebral body are significantly associated with patients' reporting of pain, and that the presence of osteophytes in the affected vertebral region may increase the possibility that an individual will report pain. On the basis of that evidence, Schmorl's nodes can be expected to have adversely affected the quality of life in past populations as well. Schmorl's nodes can occur idiopathically and can be associated with specific pathological conditions, but are most commonly the result of degenerative changes associated with ordinary stress on the vertebral column.[39] Due to the non-specific nature of these indicators, etiological determinations of specific activities are not attempted here.

36 Rogers and Waldron 1995.

37 See, e.g., Kramar, Lagier and Baud 1990; Coughlan and Holst 2000; Knüsel 2000; Knüsel and Boylston 2000; Robb et al. 2001.

38 Faccia and Williams 2008.

39 Schmorl and Junghanns 1959.

What is clear from the skeletal data is that males, particularly of younger age groups, suffered more than females from degenerative joint disease. Although sex differences may be a consequence of hormones, body size and anatomy, rather than of activity, the observed pattern may be suggestive of a more strenuous lifestyle for male individuals, for whom an early onset of work is also indicated.

Hematopoietic Disorders

The general term 'anemia' includes various red blood cell abnormalities that affect the normal exchange of oxygen in the circulatory system. Anemias such as sickle cell anemia and thalassemia are the result of genetic abnormalities that affect the synthesis of hemoglobin, while other types of anemia are caused by abnormalities in hemoglobin production or retention. Iron is an important constituent of hemoglobin, and anemia can also be caused by inadequate intake of iron. Abnormal blood loss through bleeding, due to a variety of causes such as infection of the gastrointestinal tract, can also lead to the development of anemia. Diagnosis of anemia on dry bone, regardless of the specific cause of the condition, requires evidence of marrow hyperplasia. Not all anemias affect the skeleton and the association between the severity of anemia and the extent of bone involvement is still poorly understood.[40]

Cribra orbitalia and porotic hyperostosis

Cribra orbitalia refers to porous lesions on the orbital roof, and porotic hyperostosis refers to porous lesions on the cranial vault. Both lesions can result from marrow hyperplasia, which can cause a thinning of the outer table of the skull, a widening of the inner diploë (spongy bone) and a characteristic 'hair-on-end' appearance of the trabecular structure detectable on radiographs. Cribra orbitalia and porotic hyperostosis have a morphological resemblance, but it is not yet clear whether they share the same etiology.[41] A variety of etiologies has been suggested for the interpretation of these porous lesions, including orbital hemangioma or chronic eye infection in leprous individuals, trachoma, genetic

---

40 For a thorough discussion of anemias, see Ortner 2003, 363–70. Lagia, Eliopoulos and Manolis 2007 discuss macroscopic and radiological characteristics associated with thalassemia, based on observation of the skeletal remains of a 14-year-old that are housed in the *Modern Reference Collection of the University of Athens.*

41 For the suggestion of an etiological relationship between the two, see, e.g., Stuart-Macadam 1989; Salvadei, Ricci and Manzi 2001; Facchini et al. 2004; no such relationship is argued in, e.g., Wiggins 1991; Ribot and Roberts 1996; Lewis and Roberts 1997.

anemias, dietary deficiency (mainly iron-deficiency anemia), parasitic infestation and infection.[42] Although cribra orbitalia and porotic hyperostosis should be viewed as descriptive rather than diagnostic terms, and despite evidence that various conditions (infections, metabolic disorders) can produce similar lesions, it is widely accepted by paleopathologists that porotic hyperostosis and cribra orbitalia are osseous responses to iron-deficiency anemia, and these lesions have become almost synonymous with iron-deficiency anemia in the bioarchaeological literature. Walker et al. have argued, however, that iron-deficiency anemia does not provide a reasonable physiological explanation for the marrow hypertrophy that produces porotic hyperostosis and cribra orbitalia. They suggest, instead, that a vitamin B12-deficient diet is much more likely to be the key nutritional component in the set of interacting variables responsible for porotic hyperostosis and many cases of cribra orbitalia.[43]

Table 2.16 Cribra orbitalia and porotic hyperostosis in the adult sample (individuals affected)

Site	Total no.	Affected with cribra orbitalia	M	F	CPR%	Affected with porotic hyperostosis	M	F	CPR%
Gortyn	29	9	5	4	31.0	0	0	0	0
Kefali	49	5	4	1	10.2	2	2	0	4.0
Stylos	29	1	0	1	3.4	1	0	1	3.4
Total	*107*	*15*	*9*	*6*	*14.0*	*3*	*2*	*1*	*3.0*

M=Male, F=Female

Cribra orbitalia is observed in 15 individuals (5.5%), affecting nine males (4.6%) and six females (3.0%) of 195 sexed adults. Porotic hyperostosis is observed in three individuals (1.1%), two being males (1.0%) and one female (0.5%) of the 195 sexed adults (Table 2.16) and (Figure 2.23). Absolute frequency rate for cribra orbitalia is 76.0% or 28 affected orbits of 37 observed, with the maximum prevalence (75.0%) at Kefali. Absolute frequency rate for porotic hyperostosis is 6.3%, or nine affected cranial bones of 141 observed, with the maximum prevalence (8.8%) at Kefali (Table 2.17). The majority of the cases include male individuals (Figure 2.24). Fourteen individuals (6.7%) are reported for the early Byzantine sites, and only one individual (1.5%) from the middle Byzantine site of Stylos (Figure 2.25).

[42] Møller-Christensen and Sadison 1963; Duggan and Wells 1964; Angel 1964a, 1966, 1971; El-Najjar 1977a, 1977b; El-Najjar et al. 1979; Cohen and Armelagos 1984; Gilbert and Mielke 1985; Walker 1986; Blom et al. 2005.

[43] Walker et al. 2009.

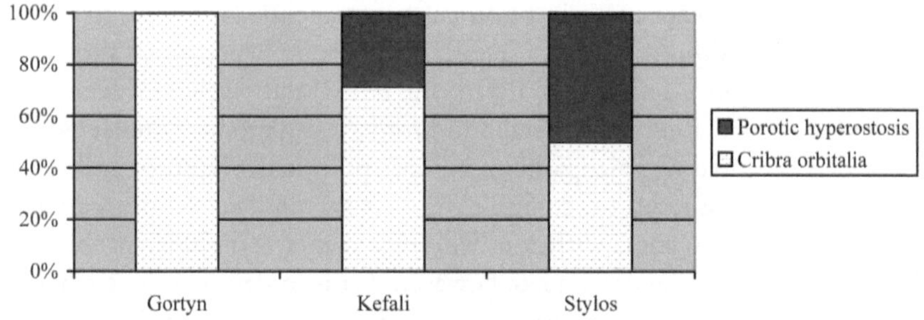

Figure 2.23 Distribution of hematopoietic disorders by site (individuals affected)

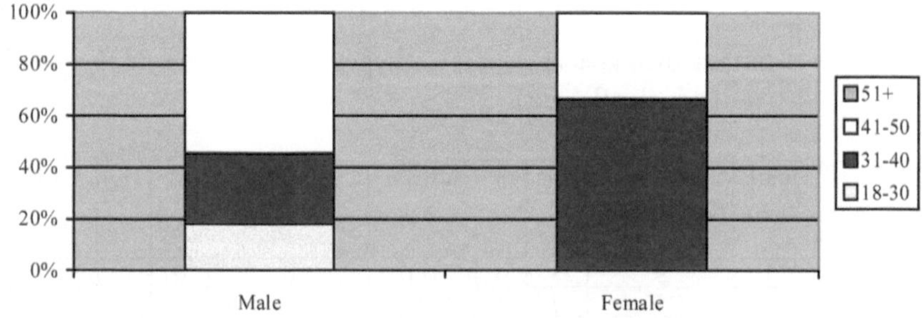

Only individuals of known sex and age are represented

Figure 2.24 Distribution of hematopoietic disorders by sex and age (individuals affected)

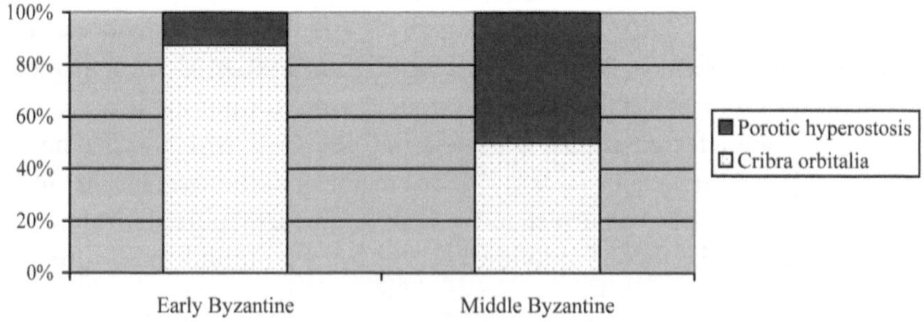

Figure 2.25 Distribution of hematopoietic disorders by time period (individuals affected)

Table 2.17 Cribra orbitalia and porotic hyperostosis in the adult sample (bones affected)

Site	Total cranial bones	Cranial bones affected	TPR%
Orbits			
Gortyn	-	18	-
Kefali	12	9	75.0
Stylos	25	1	4.0
Total (orbits)	*37*	*28*	*76.0*
Frontal			
Kefali	34	3	8.8
Parietal			
Kefali	40	3	7.5
Stylos	25	2	8.0
Total (parietal)	*65*	*5*	*8.0*
Temporal			
Kefali	42	1	2.3
Total	*178*	*37*	*21.0*

Angel's hypothesis that cribra orbitalia and porotic hyperostosis reflect thalassemia genotypes as a response to endemic malaria has influenced the diagnosis of these lesions on human skeletal remains from Greece.[44] Mallegni, for example, suggested thalassemia minor as a probable cause of the porotic lesions observed in Gortyn, adducing the marshy location of the site in the Messara plain, where a high incidence of malaria has been noted.[45] However, most recorded cases of porotic lesions fail to provide convincing evidence of genetic anemias, due to the absence of additional skeletal lesions associated with these disorders. Hapiot, having more recently investigated the impact of malaria in the ancient Aegean, from the Paleolithic to Geometric periods, concluded that the connection between malaria and the presence of porotic hyperostosis was not absolute in all surveyed sites.[46]

Current research on the subject has profited from the introduction of histological and DNA analysis, which enhances the differentiation between true cases of iron-deficiency anemia.[47] Histological analysis has been applied to investigation of the biogeographical profile of porotic hyperostosis in prehistoric

44 Angel 1964a, 1966, 1967, 1984; see also Keenleyside and Panayotova 2006; Walker et al. 2009, 112–13.

45 Mallegni 1988, 386.

46 Hapiot 2002, 2003.

47 For the application of DNA analysis to differential diagnosis see Filon et al. 1995; Faerman 1999; Faerman et al. 2000. For the application of histological analysis, see Schultz 2001; Wapler, Crubézy and Schultz 2004. The histological image indicative of iron-deficiency anemia presents gracile trabeculae, orientated in a perpendicular hair-on-end pattern extending from the diploic space.

Greece, including samples from Mesolithic, Neolithic and Bronze Age sites presenting differing environmental conditions.[48] Tentative results suggest that porotic hyperostosis exposes a broad range of morphotype variants in prehistoric Greece and that a significant relation exists between the prevalence of the lesions and the ecological settings, such as extreme environments. Still, the association of the pathology with nutritional and social shifts during the Neolithic period cannot be detected, and a combination of factors is expected to account for the prevalence of the pathology in certain sites.

The most appropriate model for paleoepidemiological studies of cribra orbitalia and porotic hyperostosis would seem to be a multifactorial etiology, although in each environmental/population niche certain specific synergistic factors would predominate. Reconsidering the etiology of porotic hyperostosis and cribra orbitalia has important implications for current interpretations of malnutrition and infectious disease in past populations. Distinction should be made, for example, between porotic hyperostosis resulting from marrow hyperplasia and porotic hyperostosis caused by superficial inflammatory conditions such as infection or scurvy. A more precise system of classification, enabling standardization between data on these lesions, would allow more scientifically valid comparison and would increase our understanding of the mechanisms responsible for their occurrence.[49]

Infectious Diseases

Infectious conditions of varying degree are very commonly found in skeletons from archaeological sites, since infection has played a significant role in human health for millennia. Perhaps more than any other category of disease, the causes and effects of infections offer skeletal biologists insight into the interaction of disease, diet, ecology, social structure, settlement patterns, plant and animal domestication, warfare, sanitation levels, immunological resistance and physiological stress. The factors affecting the prevalence of infectious conditions in populations are many and varied: they include the immune system of the host, the virulence of pathogens, ecological considerations, adequacy of nutrition and population density. A well-recognized aspect of the ecology and epidemiology of infectious diseases is the synergy between infection, malnutrition and population density. Close contact in a densely occupied settlement, coupled with the ill effects of poor sanitation, favors the spread of infectious conditions.[50]

48 Stravopodi et al. 2009.

49 Jacobi and Danford 2002; Hapiot 2003.

50 Armelagos 1990; Lambert 1993.

Researchers interested in the history and patterns of infectious diseases are confronted with problems in the analysis of skeletal remains that complicate the interpretation of data. Since bone is a very dynamic and sensitive tissue, relatively few infectious diseases produce recognizable lesions; some infectious diseases provide pathognomonic skeletal changes that could potentially contribute to a specific diagnosis (for example, syphilis), while others do not. In addition, the pattern of bone involvement can be further complicated, since several diseases can affect the skeleton in similar ways. Virtually all infectious diseases recognized in human skeletal remains have resulted from chronic conditions in which the patient survived for many years and skeletal involvement was late in the disease process. Hence, only a small number of individuals who have infectious diseases will exhibit evidence of the condition in the gross anatomy of the skeleton. In a skeletal sample, then, those skeletons showing evidence of infection are not representative of all individuals in the total sample that had infectious disease.[51] Furthermore, individuals presenting skeletal lesions have different immune responses to infection than individuals without skeletal lesions, and the more effective immune response to infection by females further complicates this difference.

Periostitis

Periosteal new bone formation has been commonly interpreted as evidence of non-specific infectious disease, and played a significant part in the 'stress-indicator hypothesis' as a sign of infectious conditions.[52] Perhaps the term 'periostitis' is poor for describing periosteal new bone formation, because it assumes by definition that inflammation has occurred. Although inflammation is not always present when a periosteal reaction arises, it frequently occurs as a general response to intrinsic and extrinsic stimuli such as trauma, neoplastic disease and infectious agents.[53] A study of pathology museum specimens failed to link definite qualitative or quantitative macroscopic and radiological characteristics of the periosteal reactions to specific diseases.[54] This finding – that lesion characteristics are shared among various diseases – is particularly important as it highlights the caution necessary in the interpretation of periosteal lesions. In particular, diagnosis of periosteal reactions from incomplete skeletons may lead to a false impression of the types of lesions occurring throughout the body, and to an overestimation of pathogen load models in past populations.

51 Ortner 1998.

52 Goodman et al. 1988.

53 See discussion in Weston 2006, 48–9.

54 Weston 2006.

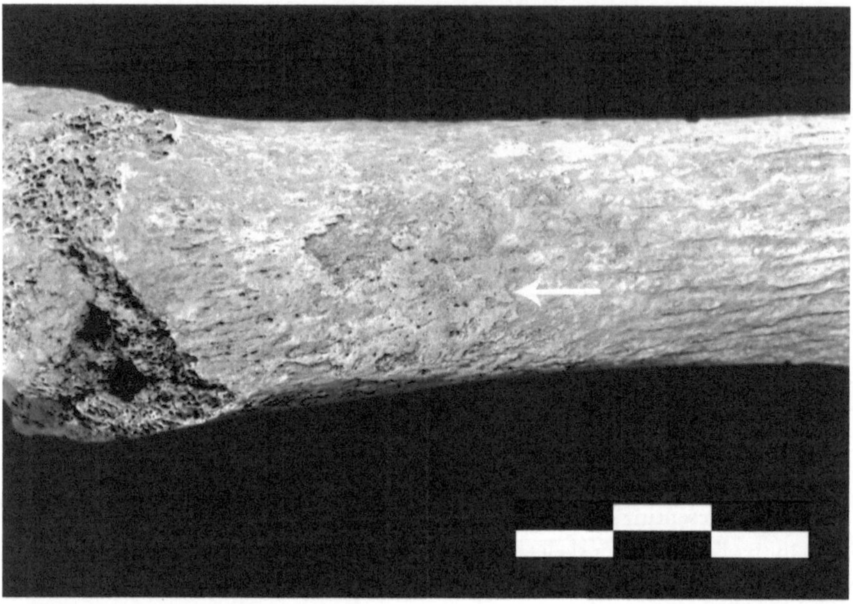

Figure 2.26 Eleutherna: Skeleton 001g, periosteal reaction (arrow) on the distal end of the tibial shaft (photo: K. Painesi. Courtesy of Prof. P. Themelis and the Society of Messenian Archaeological Studies)

Table 2.18 Periostitis in the adult sample (individuals affected)

Site	Total no.	Affected	M	F	I	CPR%
Eleutherna	100	7	5	2	0	7.0
Kastella	35	2	0	2	0	5.7
Kefali	49	5	4	0	1	10.2
Total	*184*	*14*	*9*	*4*	*1*	*7.6*

M=Male, F=Female, I=Indeterminate

Fourteen people (5.1%) exhibited periosteal lesions (Figure 2.26), mainly on the long bones of the lower limbs, nine being males (4.6%) and four females (2.0%) of 195 sexed individuals (Table 2.18) and (Figure 2.27). Absolute frequency rate is 5.0% or 25 affected bones of 498 (Table 2.19). Periosteal lesions are observed on individuals of both sexes and all age categories, with a cluster noted for the age group 31–40 years (Figure 2.28). When comparing between time periods, 12 people (5.7%) and two people (3.1%) are attested for the early and middle Byzantine period, respectively. Absolute frequency rate is 4.7% or 22 affected bones of 461 for the early Byzantine sites, and 8.1% or three affected bones of 37 for the middle Byzantine sites (Figure 2.29).

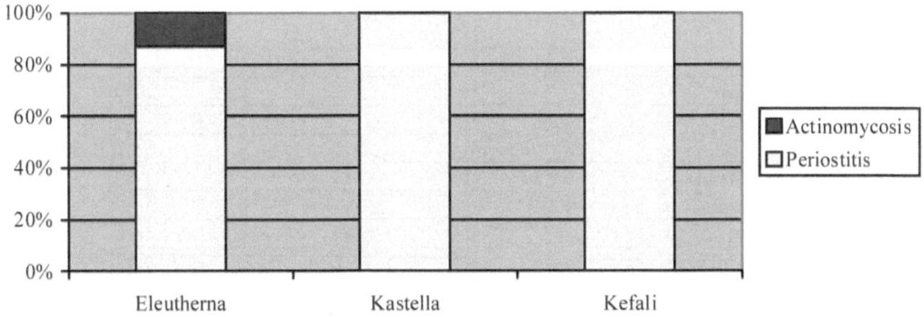

Figure 2.27 Distribution of infectious conditions by site (individuals affected)

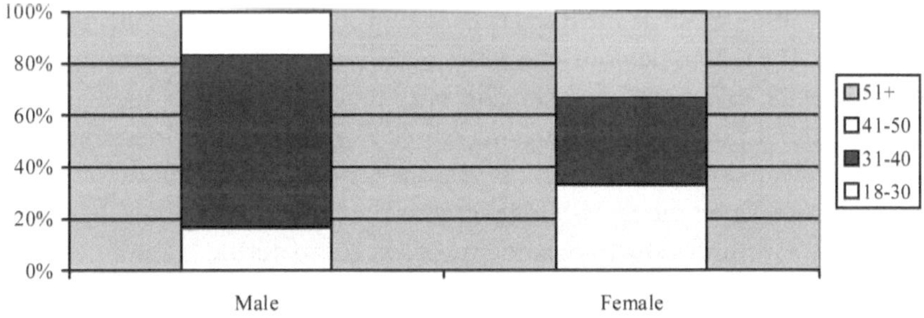

Only individuals of known sex and age are represented

Figure 2.28 Distribution of infectious conditions by sex and age (individuals affected)

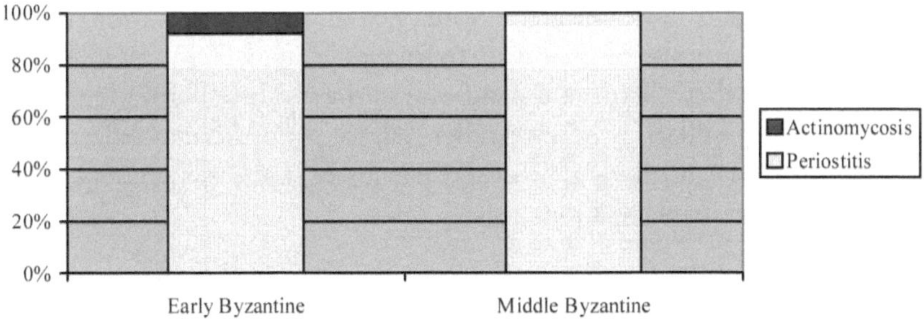

Figure 2.29 Distribution of infectious conditions by time period (individuals affected)

Table 2.19 Periostitis in the adult sample (bones affected)

Site	Total bones	Bones affected	TPR%
Femur			
Kefali	61	5	8.1
Tibia			
Eleutherna	180	5	2.7
Kastella	37	3	8.1
Kefali	55	4	7.2
Total (tibia)	*272*	*12*	*4.4*
Fibula			
Eleutherna	165	8	4.8
Total	*498*	*25*	*5.0*

Skeletal changes in the samples of Eleutherna, Kastella and Stylos studied by the author consist primarily of elevated periosteal lesions with linear striations and pitting along the shaft and distal ends of long bones, most frequently the tibia and fibula. The lesions demonstrate active but chronic inflammations suggestive of non-specific infections of presumably systemic hematogenous origin, or of a bony reaction to overlying skin trauma caused by everyday activities. There has been considerable speculation on the reasons for the localization of periosteal lesions, especially on the tibia.[55] Bones such as the tibia and the fibula, not being completely surrounded by large amounts of soft tissue during life and therefore at slightly cooler temperatures, are more susceptible to infection than bones with greater amounts of soft tissue. It is also true that bones near the skin are at greater risk of direct trauma than bones with overlying muscle. Large chronic ulcers on the skin, especially those due to venous stasis, not uncommonly result in periostitis in local bone lesions on the tibia.[56] Subcutaneous and subperiosteal bruises from trauma in some cases promote bacterial proliferation through release of blood and intracellular fluids from ruptured cells and vessels. Additionally, the anterior and lateral aspects of the tibial diaphysis have the largest and perhaps most vascular and physiologically inactive surfaces of the skeleton, which may also be conducive to bacterial colonization and infection.[57] Perhaps both of these factors are significant in the localization of the observed periostitis. The predilection of male individuals for periostitis may reflect greater exposure to repeated minor trauma to their lower limbs as a consequence of gender influences on occupations.

---

55 See, e.g., Coughlan and Holst 2000; Holst et al. 2001; Lee 2001.

56 Ortner 2003, 207.

57 Steinbock 1976; Martin et al. 1991; Cotran, Kumar and Robbins 1994.

Actinomycosis(?)

Actinomycosis, a chronic granulomatous, suppurative disease of humans and cattle that may be systemic or localized, is caused by the bacterium *Actinomyces israelii*, which is endogenous to the oral cavity.[58] While this pathological condition may occur at any age, cases cluster in individuals between the ages of 15 and 35 years and the male–female ratio is 2:1. The condition presents in three different forms depending on the location of the lesion: cervicofacial, abdominal and pulmonary or thoracic.[59] The thoracic and lumbar regions, the ribs, the cervical vertebrae and the sacrum are the principal sites affected in the post-cranial skeleton, although any bone may be involved.

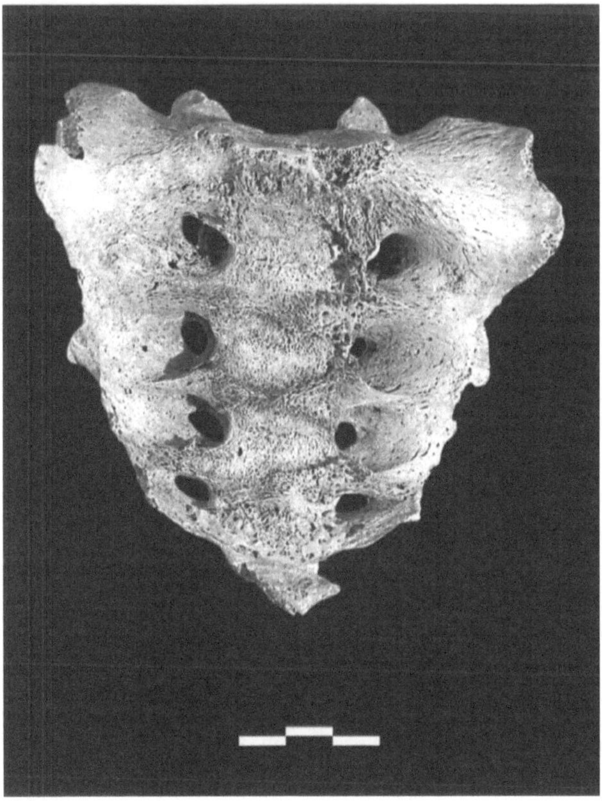

Figure 2.30 Eleutherna: Skeleton 005kg, a possible case of actinomycosis on the sacrum (photo: K. Painesi. Courtesy of Prof. P. Themelis and the Society of Messenian Archaeological Studies)

58 Aufderheide and Rodríguez-Martín 1998, 193.
59 Robbins 1975.

A possible case of actinomycosis was recorded for the sacrum of skeleton 005kg from Eleutherna (0.3%), a young adult male around 25 years old (Figure 2.30). Excessive formation of new bone in an abnormal pattern of sharp extending spicules was noted along the transverse lines of the anterior aspect from the first to the fourth sacral foramina. The differential diagnosis of fungal infection must be excluded, since bone infection amounts to only a very small percentage of these cases, in which the morphology of the skeletal lesions is mainly lytic, with little if any perifocal bone reaction, similar to that of neoplastic disease and tuberculosis.[60] The possible case of actinomycosis reported for the Eleutherna skeleton most likely resulted from interaction between the population and its environment, specifically close contact with cattle resulting in poor sanitation.

Trauma

The record of traumatic incidents imprinted upon a skeleton may contain a wealth of information about a lifetime of encounters with the environment and fellow humans. Trauma affects the skeleton by partial or complete break in a bone, abnormal displacement or dislocation of joints, disruption in nerve and/or blood supply, and artificially induced abnormal shape of bone.[61] Trauma most commonly represents extrinsic influences on the skeleton, such as accidental or intentional violence, cultural (dental mutilation) or therapeutic practices (trepanation) and pathological conditions that might increase the vulnerability of bone to biomechanical stress (cancer and osteoporosis). Clearly, the prevalence and location of traumatic incidents are influenced by cultural factors (lifestyle), while sex and age also play an important role in the distribution of trauma patterns within a population.

Because they are among the most easily diagnosed and common types of skeletal trauma, fractures have traditionally attracted the most interest from paleopathological investigators.[62] The term 'fracture' in its broad sense describes

---

60 Aufderheide and Rodríguez-Martín 1998, 213.

61 See Ortner 2003, 119.

62 Systematic work on fracture prevalence was undertaken as early as the beginning of the 20th century; see Wood-Jones 1910. During the last decades a number of papers stimulated wider interest in population studies of fractures; see, e.g., Lovejoy and Heiple 1981; Merbs 1989; Walker 1989; Roberts 1991; Berger and Trinkaus 1995; Grauer and Roberts 1996; Smith 1996; Stirland 1996; Kilgore, Jurmain and van Gerven 1997; Jurmain and Bellifemine 1997; Lambert 1997; Judd and Roberts 1999; Neves, Barros and Costa 1999; Jurmain 2001; Judd 2004; Domett and Tayles 2006; Djuri et al. 2006; Mitchell, Nagar and Ellenblum 2006;

any traumatic event that results in partial or complete discontinuity of a bone.[63] Fracture healing is a complex process that includes a number of variables, such as the bone involved (skull fractures heal more slowly than long bones), the severity of the fracture, the apposition of the ends, the stability of the fractured ends, the age of the individual (fractures heal more rapidly in children) and their nutritional status. Absence of medical treatment and inadequate immobilization of the fracture during the healing phase can result in a number of complications such as infection, bone deformity, non-union traumatic arthritis and joint fusion.[64]

The distribution of fractures in the adult sample is presented in Tables 2.20, 2.21 and 2.22. Twenty-four people (8.8%) sustained one or multiple fractures, 16 being males (8.2%) and three females (1.5%) of 195 sexed adults (Figure 2.31). Absolute frequency rate is 3.5% or 43 fractured bones of the 1,199 examined bones, with a range of 0.4% (Kefali, spine) to 11.7% (Kastella, parietal bone). As evidenced by the raw fracture data, the majority of cases occurred at the site of Kastella. In general, the majority of traumatic lesions were observed on the upper limbs and in the middle and mature adult age groups; males exhibited more fractures than females, possibly reflecting sex-based differences in activity or risk of fracture (Figure 2.32). When comparing between sites, 10 people (4.8%) and 14 people (21.8%) are attested for the early and middle Byzantine period, respectively. Absolute frequency rate is 2.1% or 13 fractured bones of 618 for the early Byzantine sites, and 5.1% or 30 fractured bones of 581 for the middle Byzantine sites (Figure 2.33).

Table 2.20 Fractures in the adult sample (individuals affected)

Site	Total no.	One fracture				Two fractures				Three or more fractures			
		M	F	I	CPR%	M	F	I	CPR%	M	F	I	CPR%
Eleutherna	100	5	0	0	5.0	0	0	0	0	0	0	0	0
Gortyn	29	0	0	0	0	0	0	0	0	1	0	0	3.4
Kastella	35	6	1	0	20.0	1	0	0	2.8	1	1	0	5.7
Kefali	49	2	1	1	8.1	0	0	0	0	0	0	0	0
Stylos	29	0	0	4	13.7	0	0	0	0	0	0	0	0
Total	*242*	*13*	*2*	*5*	*8.2*	*1*	*0*	*0*	*0.4*	*2*	*1*	*0*	*1.2*

M=Male, F=Female, I=Indeterminate

Brickley 2006; Torres-Rouff and Costa Junqueira 2006; for a thorough bioarchaeological analysis of the history of violence, see Walker 2001; Brickley and Smith 2006.

63 For a thorough review of fractures, see Resnick 1995, 2570–77; Ortner 2003, 120–26.

64 Ortner 2003, 126–36.

Table 2.21 Fractures in the adult sample (bones affected): skull, upper limbs and thorax

Site	Total bones	Bones affected	TPR%
Skull			
Parietal			
Kastella	17	2	11.7
Kefali	40	2	5.0
Total (parietal)	*57*	*4*	*7.0*
Occipital			
Kastella	19	1	5.2
Clavicle			
Kastella	24	2	8.3
Stylos	16	1	6.2
Total (clavicle)	*40*	*3*	*7.5*
Scapula			
Kastella	20	1	5.0
Humerus			
Kastella	37	3	8.1
Ulna			
Eleutherna	104	1	0.9
Stylos	24	1	4.1
Total (ulna)	*128*	*2*	*1.5*
Radius			
Eleutherna	92	2	2.1
Gortyn	19	2	10.5
Kastella	34	2	5.8
Stylos	24	1	4.1
Total (radius)	*169*	*7*	*4.1*
Hand			
2nd mcp			
Kastella	30	1	3.3
5th mcp			
Kastella	35	2	5.7
Total (hand)	*65*	*3*	*4.6*
Ribs			
Kastella	110	8	7.2
Spine			
Gortyn	44	2	4.5
Kastella	104	1	0.9
Kefali	220	1	0.4
Total (spine)	*368*	*4*	*1.0*
Total	*1,013*	*36*	*3.5*

2nd mcp=second metacarpal; 5th mcp=fifth metacarpal

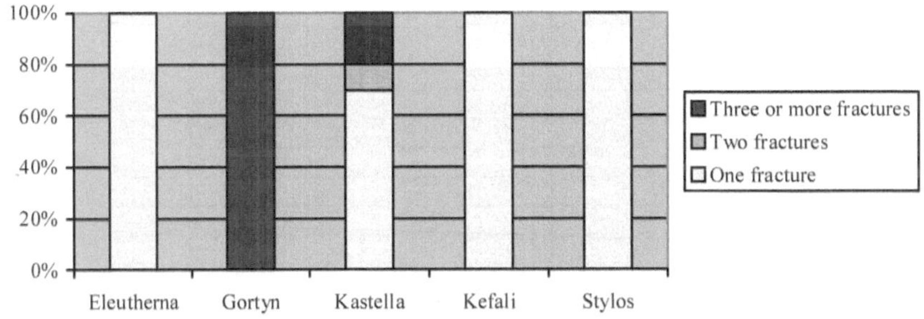

Figure 2.31 Distribution of fractures by site (individuals affected)

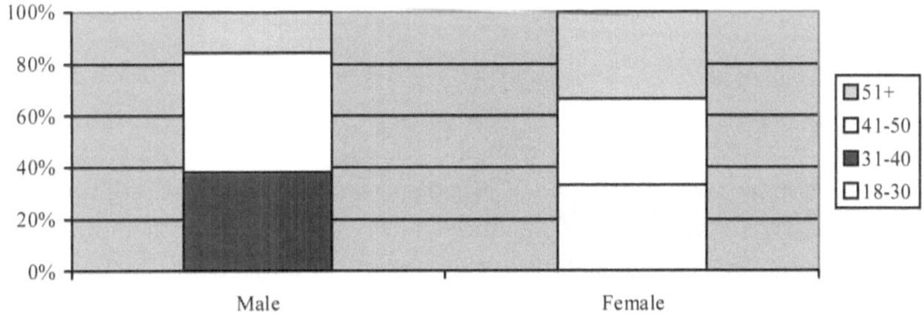

Only individuals of known sex and age are represented

Figure 2.32 Distribution of fractures by sex and age (individuals affected)

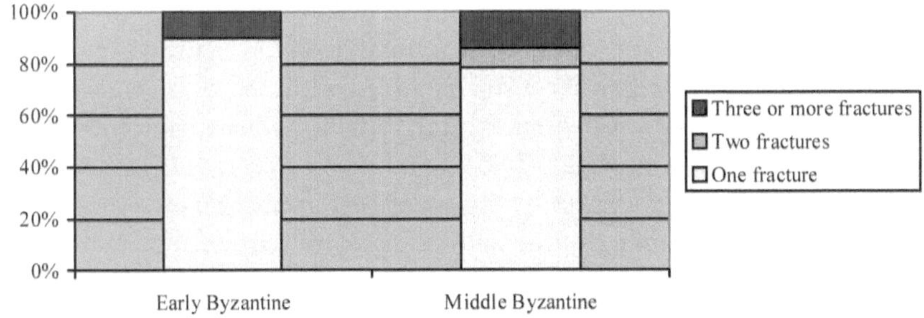

Figure 2.33 Distribution of fractures by time period (individuals affected)

Table 2.22 Fractures in the adult sample (bones affected): lower limbs

Site	Total bones	Bones affected	TPR%
Tibia			
Kastella	37	2	5.4
Stylos	22	1	4.5
(Total tibia)	*59*	*3*	*5.0*
Fibula			
Kastella	28	1	3.5
Foot			
5th mtt			
Eleutherna	99	2	2.0
Kefali	-	1	-
Total (foot)	*99*	*3*	*3.0*
Total	*186*	*7*	*3.7*

5th mtt=fifth metatarsal

Multiple Fractures

Four individuals (1.4%) from Gortyn and Kastella experienced more than one fracture. A male individual aged c. 60 from Gortyn sustained compression fractures in two thoracic vertebrae and Colles' fractures in both radii. Three individuals in the Kastella sample experienced multiple fractures (skeletons 001, 011a and 017).[65] Skeleton 001, a female c. 25 years old, suffered from a compression fracture on the fifth lumbar vertebra (Figure 2.34). Protrusion of the spinal cord and ossified nodules were observed on the superior body, while the inferior body was normal. Slight marginal osteophytosis was also present on the superior body. Five left ribs (the fifth to eighth and the eleventh) presented transverse fractures toward the neck (Figure 2.35). Callus formation is visible in all cases. Involvement of the pleura sheath in the healing process was noted in the fifth to the seventh ribs, and woven bone formation on the eighth. A transverse fracture was also observed on the distal one-third of the left tibia (Figures 2.36 and 2.37). Callus formation is visible, and the affected bone is shorter than the contralateral (Left=34 cm/ Right=36 cm). Secondary osteoarthritis at the ankle joint had developed, as evidenced by the osteophytic formation on several tarsal bones: on the plantar surface of the talus, the posterior articular surface of the calcaneus and the plantar surface of the navicular. Finally, a transverse fracture is also present at the distal end of the left clavicle (Figures 2.38 and 2.39). The affected clavicle was shorter than the contralateral (Left=10.1 cm/ Right=11 cm) and the bone exhibited angular alignment.

65 For the analysis of fractures observed in the Kastella sample, see Bourbou 2009.

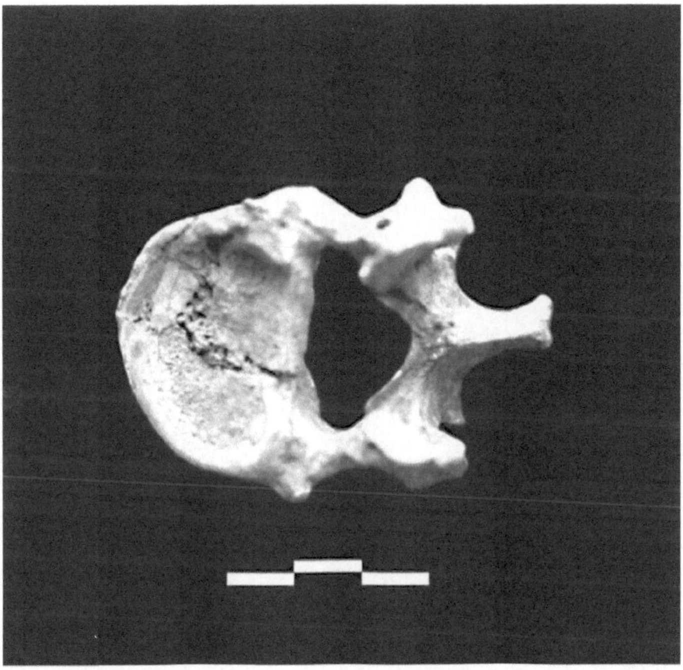

Figure 2.34 Kastella: Skeleton 001, compression fracture on the fifth lumbar vertebra (photo: C. Bourbou)

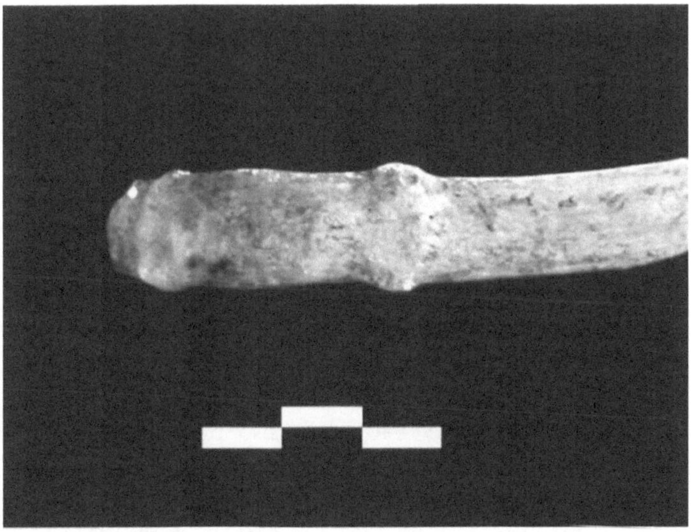

Figure 2.35 Kastella: Skeleton 001, transverse fracture towards the neck of the eighth left rib (photo: C. Bourbou)

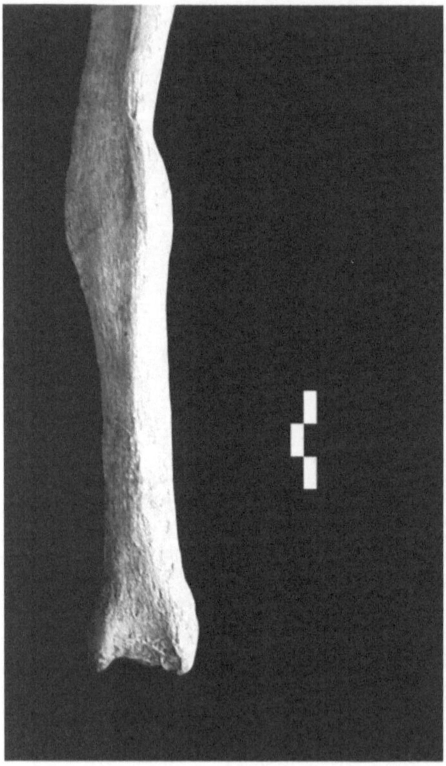

Figure 2.36 Kastella: Skeleton 001, transverse fracture at the distal one-third of the left tibia (photo: C. Bourbou)

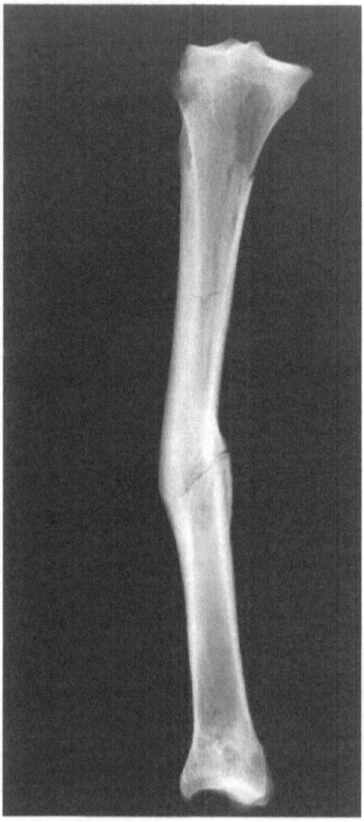

Figure 2.37 Radiograph of the tibial fracture of skeleton 001 from Kastella

Skeleton 011a, a male of 44 years, sustained a transverse fracture on the mid-shaft of the fifth left metacarpal (Figure 2.40). Slight callus formation is visible. In addition, the left scapula presents a sharp cut on the body (Figures 2.41 and 2.42). Complications in the healing process included a displacement of the bone fragments in the lateral border and ossified nodules due to possible involvement of the infraspinatus muscle.

Skeleton 017, a male of 35–40 years, also presents multiple fractures. Transverse fractures were observed at the mid-shaft of the right humerus, the distal one-third of the left radius, the mid-shaft of the left fifth metacarpal, the distal one-third of the left fibula, the distal end of the left tibia (Figure 2.43) and in two right and one left fragmentary ribs. Callus formation is present in all cases and complications were noted in the fractured tibia: ossified nodules are present

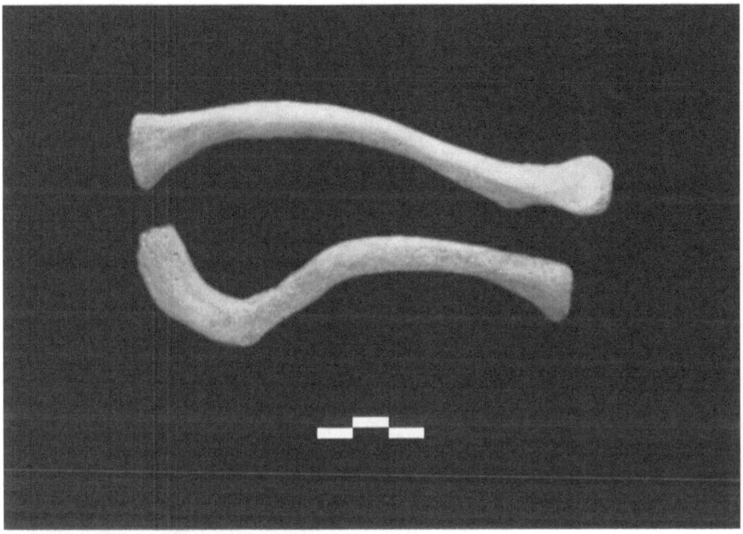

Figure 2.38 Kastella: Skeleton 001, transverse fracture at the distal end of the left clavicle (photo: C. Bourbou)

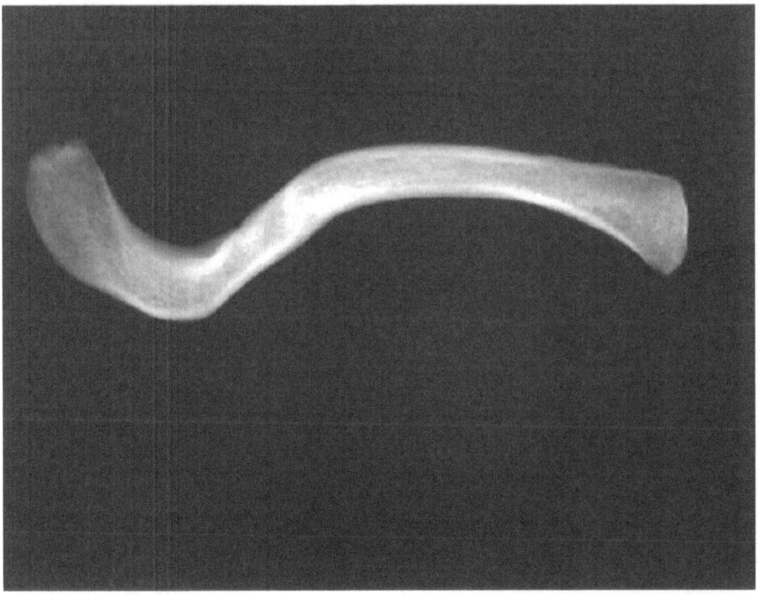

Figure 2.39 Radiograph of the fractured clavicle of skeleton 001 from Kastella

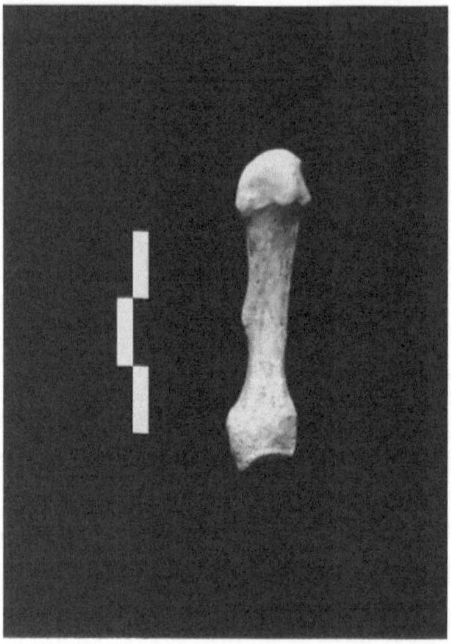

Figure 2.40 Kastella: Skeleton 011a, transverse fracture on the midshaft of the fifth left metacarpal (photo: C. Bourbou)

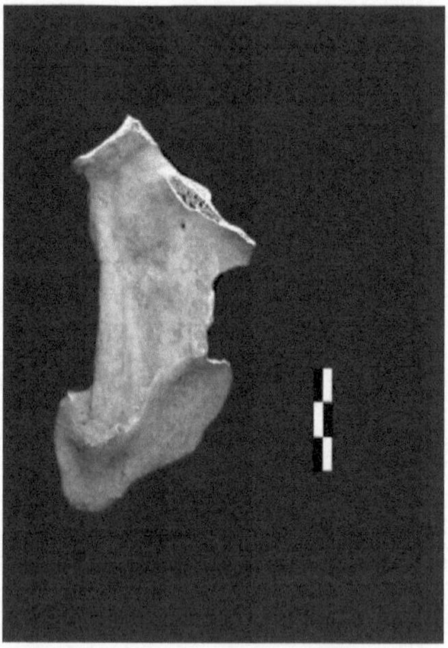

Figure 2.41 Kastella: Skeleton 011a, fracture on the body of the left scapula (photo: C. Bourbou)

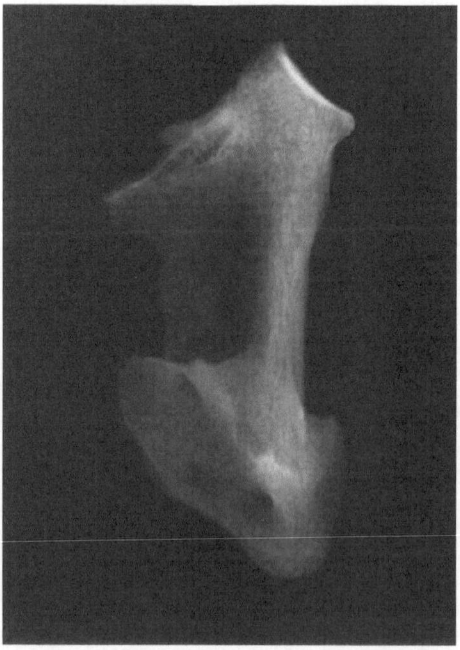

Figure 2.42 Radiograph of the scapular fracture of skeleton 011a from Kastella

on the insertion of the interosseous ligament, and there is osteoarthritis of the ankle joint (marginal osteophytosis at the distal end of the tibia and the talus).

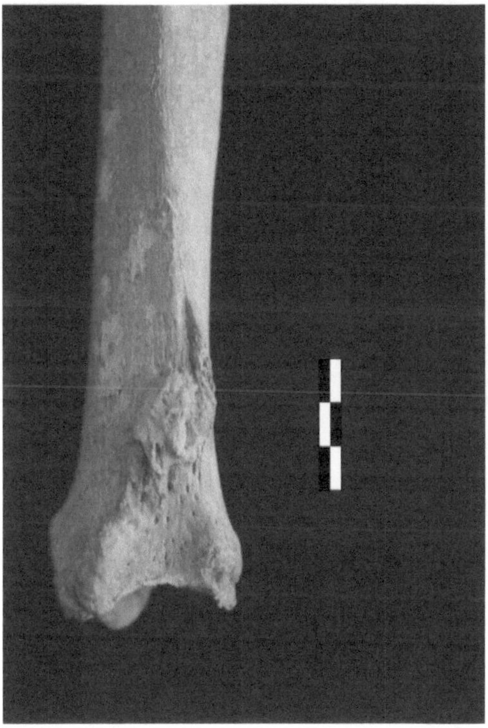

Figure 2.43 Kastella: Skeleton 017, transverse fracture at the distal end of the left tibia (photo: C. Bourbou)

Skull Fractures

Two cranial fractures were recorded for Kastella, both involving male individuals aged 30–35 years (skeleton 002) and 39 years (skeleton 014). Skeleton 002 exhibits a diagonal cut from the left parietal to the central part of the occipital bone (Figures 2.44 and 2.45). The sharp-edged defect is 10.1 cm long with a maximum width of 1.5 cm. The internal edges are sharp with no evidence of healing. Skeleton 014 presents an oval depressed skull fracture (1.1 × 0.5 cm) on the right parietal, just above the lambdoidal suture (Figures 2.46 and 2.47). Two possible depressed fractures are also observed in the right parietals of two male individuals (both aged 41–50 years) from Kefali.

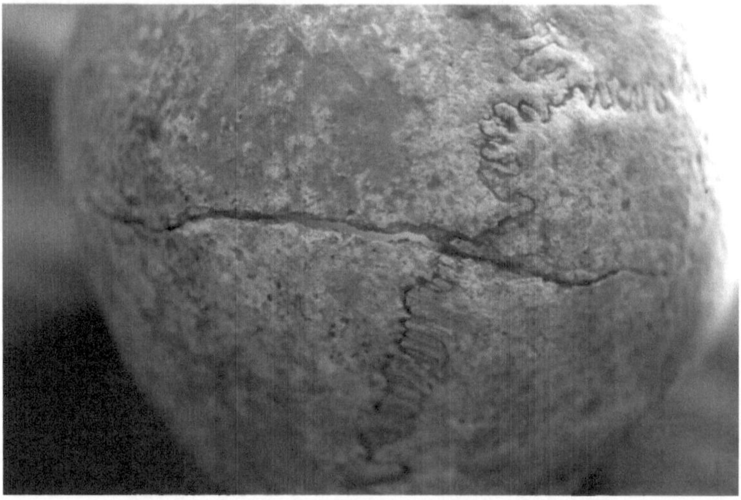

Figure 2.44 Kastella: Skeleton 002, fracture extending from the left parietal to the central part of the occipital bone (photo: C. Bourbou)

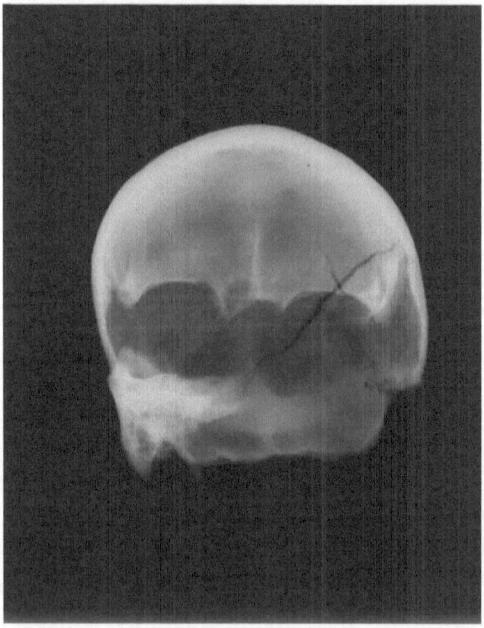

Figure 2.45 Radiograph of the fracture on the skull of skeleton 002 from Kastella

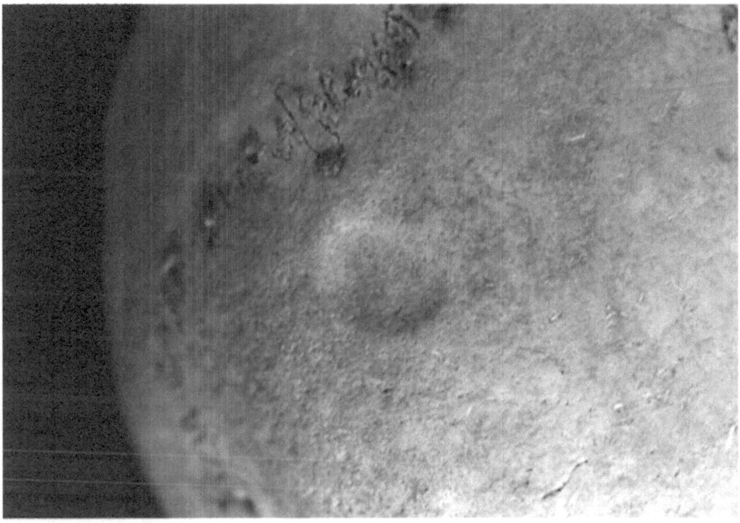

Figure 2.46 Kastella: Skeleton 014, depressed fracture on the right parietal (photo: C. Bourbou)

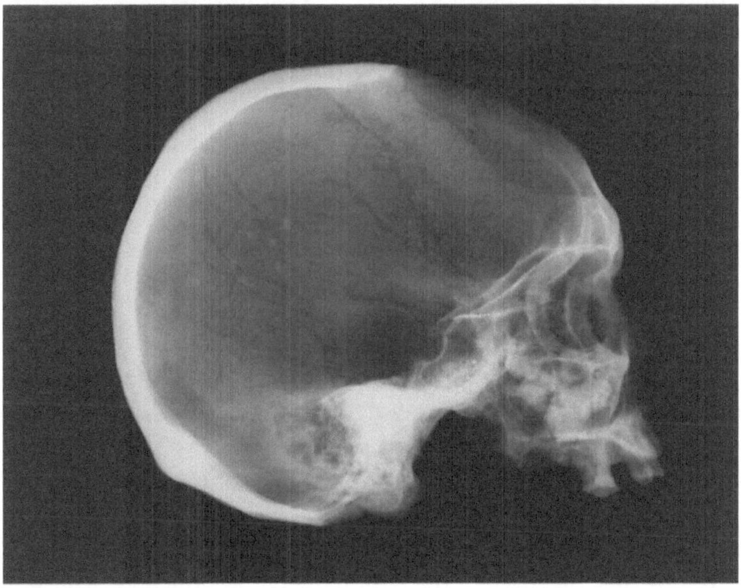

Figure 2.47 Radiograph of the depressed fracture on the skull of skeleton 014 from Kastella

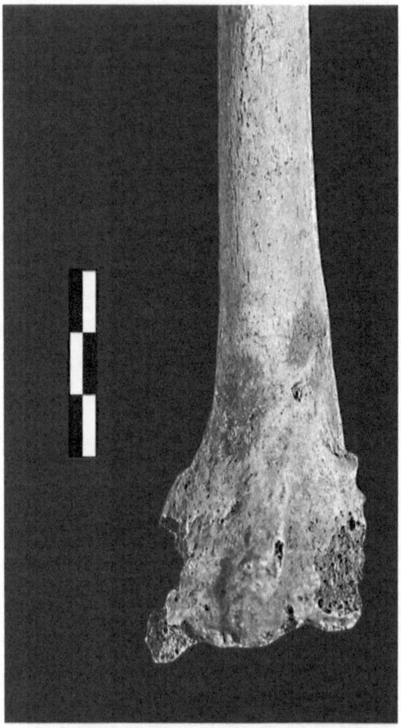

Figure 2.48 Eleutherna: Skeleton 005ke, Colles' fracture on the distal end of the left radius (photo: K. Painesi. Courtesy of Prof. P. Themelis and the Society of Messenian Archaeological Studies)

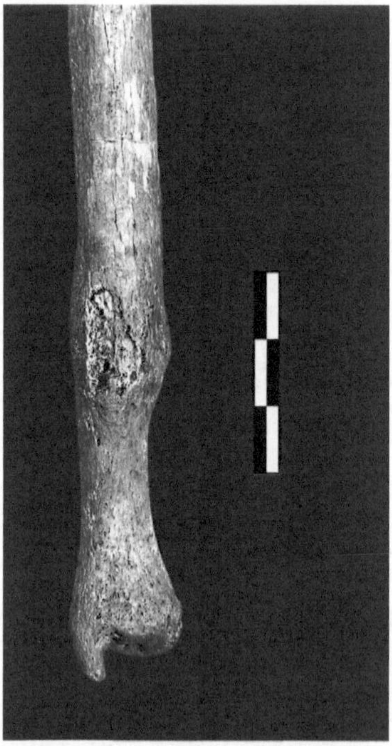

Figure 2.49 Eleutherna: Skeleton 001d, parry fracture at the distal end of the right ulna (photo: K. Painesi. Courtesy of Prof. P. Themelis and the Society of Messenian Archaeological Studies)

Upper Limb and Thorax Fractures

Skeleton 022, a male of 35 years from Kastella, presents a transverse fracture at the distal end of the left clavicle. Angular alignment and shortening of the bone were noted (Left=14 cm/ Right=14.5 cm). Transverse fracture on the mid-shaft of the left clavicle is also recorded for an adult individual from Stylos (burial 28/1997). Skeleton 008b, a mature adult male, and skeleton 025, an adult male from Kastella, present a well-remodeled transverse fracture at the one-third proximal diaphysis of the right humerus and the mid-shaft of the left humerus, respectively. In the latter case callus formation is visible, as is additional shortening of the bone (Left=30 cm/ Right=32 cm). Skeleton 013, a male of 44 years from Kastella, suffered from a Galleazi's fracture at the distal end of the left radius. Angular alignment was observed, as well as osteoarthritis on the wrist joint in the presence of marginal osteophytosis and slight eburnation on the radius. Another adult individual from Stylos (burial 28/1997) exhibits a Galleazi's fracture at the distal end of the left radius. Colles' fractures at the distal end of their left radii are reported for two individuals from Eleutherna – skeleton 005ke, a male of 45 years, and skeleton 018, another adult male (Figure 2.48). Parry fractures are reported for Stylos: an adult individual (burial 1/1990) presents a well-remodeled parry fracture at the distal end of the right ulna, and a male individual of 54 years (skeleton 001d) from Eleutherna at the distal end of the left ulna (Figure 2.49). Regarding the bones of the hand, skeleton 023, a female of 50–60 years from Kastella, sustained a transverse fracture on the mid-shaft of the left second metacarpal. Callus formation is present, and the affected bone appears shorter than the contralateral (Left=5 cm/ Right=6 cm). Finally, a thoracic vertebra of a mature female from Kefali exhibits a compressed fracture.

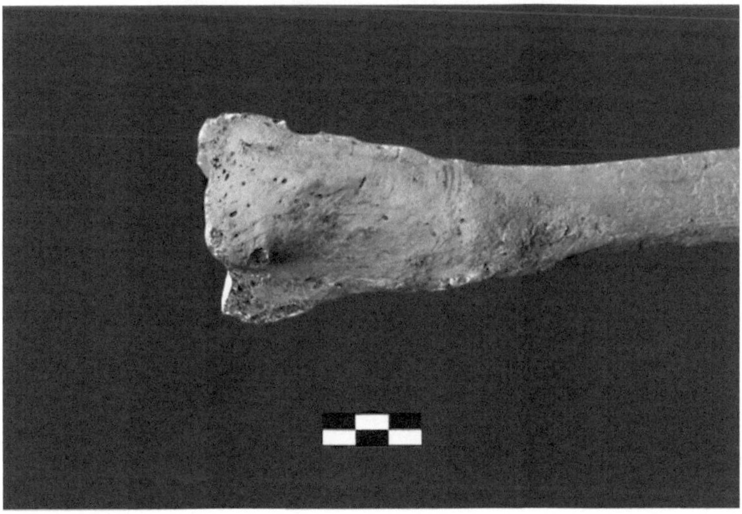

Figure 2.50 Stylos: Burial 26a/1989, transverse fracture on a distal left tibia (photo: C. Bourbou)

Lower Limb Fractures

One distal left tibia of an adult individual from Stylos (burial 26a/1989) exhibits a transverse fracture (Figure 2.50). Gross callus formation is present, and is characterized by thick layers of lamellar bone covering the entire surface of the distal end. The fracture does not seem to have healed well due to the slight deformation of the bone, which has an inclination toward the medial aspect. The absence of a cloaca excludes the differential diagnosis of osteomyelitis. Three cases of fractures at the fifth metatarsal are reported: for Eleutherna a male individual, 35 years old (skeleton 001st), and another adult male (skeleton 009a) sustained transverse fractures on the left and right bones, respectively (Figure 2.51). The case from Kefali is a diagonal fracture sustained by an adult individual of unknown sex.

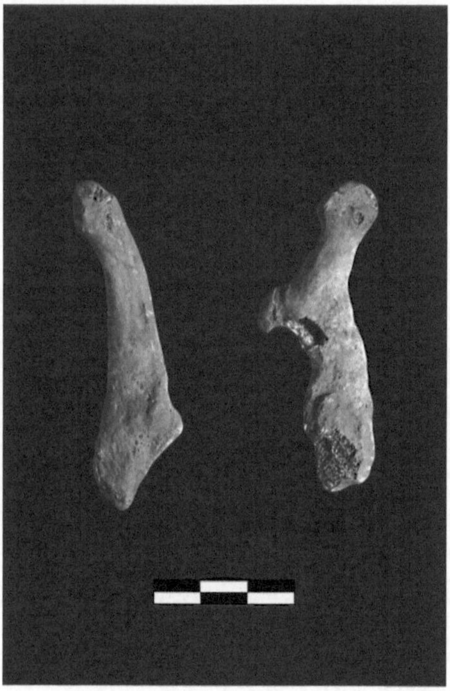

Figure 2.51 Eleutherna: Skeleton 009a, transverse fracture on the left fifth metatarsal (photo: K. Painesi. Courtesy of Prof. P. Themelis and the Society of Messenian Archaeological Studies)

The ancient world was a difficult place to live and the Byzantine period was no exception; people must have been prone to accidents in daily life and have been victims of violent attacks. It is not surprising that Byzantine medical writers devoted entire chapters to the diagnosis and treatment of fractured bones, exhibiting great expertise in surgical operations (for example, amputations) when needed.[66]

The ability to detect which injuries occurred simultaneously is restricted in the case of multiple trauma observed in ancient populations, and these

66 See, e.g., *Paul of Aegina* (ed. Heiberg 1921 and 1924; tr. Adams 1834).

injuries may represent injury recidivism rather than a single traumatic episode. In modern clinical literature, injury recidivism refers to individuals who accumulate a number of traumatic lesions over their lifetime. Bioarchaeologists are currently applying the criteria developed by modern clinical researchers to determine whether characteristics of injury recidivism existed in past societies.[67] Although our cases of multiple fractures in the same individual may suggest an exceptionally dangerous life with repeated traumatic events, it seems unlikely that these individuals sustained constant physical abuse, since the observed fractures do not present different stages of healing. The advanced healing and, in some cases, secondary changes (for example, arthritic changes) indicate that the injuries occurred some years before the individuals' deaths, and were most likely associated with an accidental event. Such an interpretation appears even more plausible as the observed fractures provide no evidence that they resulted from an underlying disease. For example, the fractures of the lower radial shaft (Galleazi's fracture) and associated subluxation/dislocation of the distal radio-ulnar joint are typically produced by a fall on the hand with rotation force. Similarly, Colles' fracture is almost always due to a fall onto an outstretched hand.[68] Fractures of the clavicle – most commonly the middle segment – also usually result from a fall onto an outstretched hand or a fall on the shoulder. The high frequency of these fractures can be at least partially associated with the subcutaneous location of the bone.[69]

The possibility of injuries due to conflict must also be considered in some cases. Injuries most frequently associated with interpersonal violence and observable in archaeological remains include cranial injuries that can be attributed to direct blows,[70] multiple lesions from habitual or severe assault and distal ulna shaft fractures (parry fracture) resulting from defending a blow to the head.[71] The ulna parry fracture is perhaps the most controversial injury, owing to its implications for social behavior in past societies (interpersonal

67 See, e.g., Judd 2002.

68 For a detailed paleopathological analysis and interpretation of Colles' fracture, see Mays 2006.

69 Resnick 1995, 2715–18.

70 See, e.g., Walker 1989; Powers 2005; Mays 2006; Torres-Rouff and Costa Junqueira 2006; Paine et al. 2007.

71 See, e.g., Walker 1989, 2001; Smith 1996; Bridges 1996; Anderson 1996; Hutchinson 1996; Jurmain and Bellifemine 1997; Jurmain 2001; Judd 2004; Powers 2005; Mays 2006; Torres-Rouff and Costa Junqueira 2006; Paine et al. 2007. According to Lovell 1997, 166, fractures of the skull (especially the nasal and zygomatic bones and the mandible), posterior rib fractures, vertebral spinous process fractures and fractures of the hand and foot bones, which can result from the direct trauma of punches and kicks, are considered to have a high specificity for a clinical diagnosis of assault.

violence, female abuse).[72] Judd, in her study on parry fractures, set a number of quantitative and qualitative criteria that could enhance the identification of the proximate mechanism of the fracture (direct or indirect force).[73] Nevertheless, any attempt to interpret such fractures as indications of interpersonal violence should be made with caution, as the interpretation affects how we perceive the familial, social and other relationships of a specific society. Limitations still remain in identifying the ultimate mechanism and the sequence of the healed injuries. It is, for example, impossible to know whether the individual acquired the injury during a fall caused by the individual's own clumsiness, an activity or a push during an altercation.

In the case of the cranial fracture of skeleton 002 from Kastella, the sharp, clearly defined edges could not have been produced postmortem in a dry skull. There is no evidence of remodeling or secondary infection. The individual does not seem to have survived long enough for the healing process to begin, thus the injury appears to have been perimortem. The sharp edge, as well as the lack of microfracture, is suggestive of a long, straight, sharp-edged weapon, such as a blade or sword.[74] The depressed fracture observed on the skull of skeleton 014 from Kastella is not typical of those from falls from high places, or those involving striking the head against a large mass, such as a rock or a hard surface, which would result in a large comminuted or linear fracture.[75] Most probably, this fracture pattern indicates a blow with a small weapon such as a sling-shot, small club or tool. Finally, in the paleopathological record fractures to the scapular body are relatively rare, most probably because this bone does not usually survive intact. Clinical cases of scapular fractures, also infrequent, demonstrate that the scapular body is mainly involved.[76] The type of fracture recorded for the scapula of skeleton 011a from Kastella can most probably also be attributed to a case of interpersonal violence – a direct force of considerable magnitude – where again a long, straight, sharp-edged weapon such as a blade or sword was used.

With the exception of the cranial trauma mentioned above, which was probably fatal, all the other fractures – albeit exhibiting complications (periosteal reaction, osteoarthritis, loss of normal shape of bone) and no evidence of medical treatment – demonstrate healing process, indicating that the individual survived the incident. It should be noted, though, that besides complications that should have affected the health status of the individual, the impact of each fracture and its sequelae upon lifestyle in general would have depended upon the range of

72 Grauer and Roberts 1996; Lovell 1997, 165; Jurmain 1999.

73 Judd 2008.

74 See the publication by Lewis 2008 on the identification of sword marks on bone.

75 Galloway 1999, 67–8.

76 Resnick 1995, 2718–20.

activities to which the individual was previously accustomed. Individuals whose lifestyles involved manual labor (for example, farming) would have found their activities significantly restrained by the type of injuries sustained, due to pain, weakness and reduced range of motion.

Humerus varus

Primary humerus varus is a rare condition.[77] It can occur due to trauma during birth, perhaps as a result of injury to the medial aspect of the growth plate.[78] The humeral shaft is where birth injury most often occurs. Displacement of either the humeral or femoral head is seldom found and is normally unilateral; bilateral involvement, if not due to intrauterine trauma, can occur if a child falls backward with arms extended and hands caught behind the buttocks.[79]

A young adult male from Eleutherna, approximately 19 years old (skeleton 001b), presents a distinctive pathological condition (0.3%). The head of the left humerus was displaced disto-medially, with resultant shortening of the anatomical neck that can be seen more clearly from the anterior aspect (Figure 2.52). There is no evidence of fracture and the metaphysis was not involved. The glenoid surface of the scapula is normal, but the acromion shows evidence of marginal osteophytosis and slight porosity. Because of the fragmentation of both humeri, measurements could not be taken. The preserved epiphyses of the other long bones were unaffected and no other pathological conditions are recorded. The appearance of this displacement is suggestive of unilateral slipped epiphysis, a well-known finding in the proximal femur.[80] The anomalous position of the humeral head, however, has led to a reduction in the angle of the neck, producing a so-called varus deformity, so that the term 'humerus varus' has been preferred.[81]

A variety of pathological conditions can produce humerus varus, among them osteomalacia and rickets, neonatal infection, tumor formation, thalassemia, cretinism and generalized spondyloepiphyseal dysplasia.[82] Skeleton 001b from Eleutherna shows no evidence of underlying disease or recent trauma; all other epiphyses present have developed and/or fused normally, and this isolated deformity does not correspond to any established syndrome. The condition appears to have been caused by untreated intrauterine or early childhood trauma, resulting in a deformity moderate to severe in degree, with impingement upon

77 Anderson 1997; Merbs and Vestergaard 1985; Capasso 1989.

78 Lucas and Gill 1947; Langenskiold 1953.

79 Tachdjian 1972.

80 Ortner and Putschar 1985.

81 Ogden, Weil and Hempton 1976.

82 Davies 1956; Ogden, Weil and Hempton 1976; Ellefsen et al. 1994.

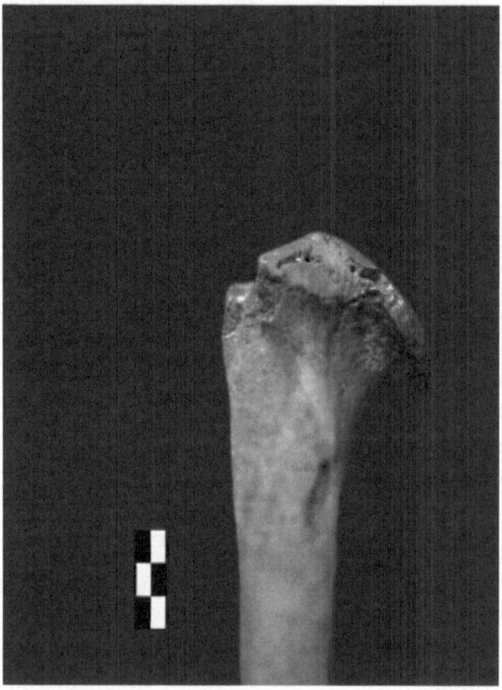

Figure 2.52 Eleutherna: Skeleton 001b, displaced head of the left humerus (humerus varus) (photo: C. Bourbou)

the acromion.[83] Marked humerus varus frequently presents with symptoms during adolescence, and this 19-year-old individual from Eleutherna is likely to have lived with a slightly disabled shoulder and arm.[84]

Circulatory Disorders

A broad number of lesions can affect arteries and veins, and their etiologies range from infectious to autoimmune conditions. Most of the circulatory disturbances that affect the human skeleton occur in the long bones and can be associated with necrosis (cellular death), for example of the femoral neck, or with trauma and vascular deficiency.[85]

---

83 Bourbou 2001b.

84 Burman 1938; Davies 1956.

85 For a review of circulatory disorders, see Ortner 2003, 343–57.

Osteochondritis dissecans

Osteochondritis dissecans is a benign, non-inflammatory condition affecting young adults in which small, focal epiphyseal areas of necrosis appear on the convex surfaces of diarthrodial joints and result in the partial or complete detachment of a section of the subchondral bone and articular cartilage.[86] For the most part osteochondritis dissecans affects individuals between the ages of 10 and 25 years, with males affected two to three times more often than females. Any diarthrodial joint may be involved, but 85–90% of cases present in the medial femoral condyle; the remaining 10–15% have been found in the elbow (humeral condyle, radial head or coronoid fossa), tibial plateau, talus, hip joint (femoral head and/or acetabulum) and shoulder (glenoid cavity or humeral head).

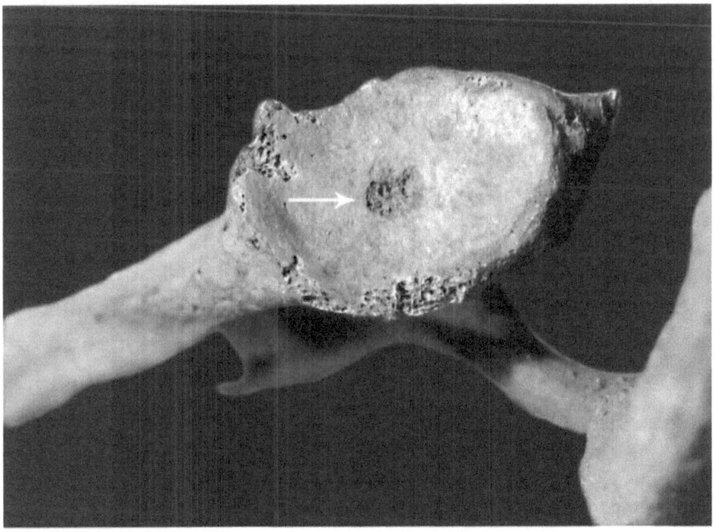

Figure 2.53 Eleutherna: Skeleton 008b, osteochondritis dissecans (arrow) on the glenoid surface of the left scapula (photo: K. Painesi. Courtesy of Prof. P. Themelis and the Society of Messenian Archaeological Studies)

Only one case of osteochondritis dissecans (0.3%) is observed in the skeletal samples studied here, on a 35-year-old male individual (skeleton 008b) from Eleutherna.[87] A porous, almost circular lesion is noted on the glenoid surface of

86 Aufderheide and Rodríguez-Martín 1998, 81–3; Ortner 2003, 351–2.

87 The diagnosis of this lesion is problematic and the data provided is usually ambiguous; therefore the single reported case probably significantly under-represents the actual frequency of the condition in Byzantine Crete. The sample from Stylos included four

the left scapula (Figure 2.53). The condition is regarded as idiopathic, since none of the suggested etiologies is sufficiently convincing: trauma or microtrauma, circulatory disturbances of the bone, inflammation, endocrine disturbances and genetic factors.[88] Familial incidence has recently been observed, which may be the consequence of a genetic predisposition.[89]

Congenital Abnormalities

A large number of congenital abnormalities can occur in the skeleton. Typically, these abnormalities are the result of a problem in embryological development; while some are incompatible with prolonged life, many are compatible with life and maturity.[90] The etiology of many of these abnormalities is poorly understood, but there is at least a strong probability that their pathogenesis involves a genetic predisposition (single gene disorders, chromosomal disorders or an interaction between genetic and environmental factors).

Spina bifida occulta

The condition is characterized by a failure of the vertebral neural arches, usually of the lower lumbar vertebrae, to fuse because of a neural tube defect. In spina bifida occulta the posterior parts of the vertebrae enclosing the spinal cord are absent; thus, in skeletal samples, the spinal canal is exposed, while in life it would have been bridged by cartilage or membrane.[91] The condition commonly involves one or more segments of the sacrum, but may occur in other parts of the spine.

The cases of spina bifida occulta in the adult sample are presented in Table 2.23. Five individuals (1.8%) presented spina bifida occulta; absolute frequency rate for the condition is 9.8% or five affected sacra of 51. For the skeleton 001h from Eleutherna, incomplete fusion of the posterior neural arch involved all sacral segments; two cases

cases of pseudo-osteochondritis dissecans observed on the glenoid and tibial plateau of a female, 30–35 years old (skeleton 001), the glenoids of a 35-year-old male (skeleton 019), the glenoids and distal femoral ends of a mature male (skeleton 021) and the patella of a 51-year-old male (skeleton 022). Although the lesions resemble the circular porous lesions encountered in cases of osteochondritis dissecans, they actually represent taphonomic alterations on the bones' surface.

88 Helms 1989; Forrester and Brown 1990; Brower 1990; Kulund 1990; Bullough 1992; Martín-Oval and Rodríguez-Martín 1994.

89 Jaffe 1972.

90 See Barnes 1994, 1–31; Aufderheide and Rodríguez-Martín 1998, 51; Ortner 2003, 453; Roberts and Manchester 2005, 55.

91 Roberts and Manchester 2005, 55.

from Kefali involved all sacral segments as well; while, in the third case from Kefali, the neural arch is not completed at the fourth and fifth sacral vertebrae.

Table 2.23 Spina bifida occulta in the adult sample (individuals and/or sacra affected)

Site	Total no.	Affected	M	F	CPR%	Total no. of sacra	Sacra affected	TPR%
Eleutherna	100	1	1	0	1.0	35	1	2.8
Gortyn	29	1	1	0	3.4	4	1	25.0
Kefali	49	3	2	1	6.1	12	3	25.0
Total	*178*	*5*	*4*	*1*	*2.8*	*51*	*5*	*9.8*

M=Male, F=Female

Spina bifida occulta has often been diagnosed in archaeological populations and is known to have a genetic base.[92] Since it is found in adult skeletons from antiquity, the condition clearly did not cause its possessors difficulty in functioning satisfactorily. Today, spina bifida occulta is discovered only in the course of routine radiological examination.[93] It has been affirmed that when this defect is found in an adult individual from an archaeological context it can be assumed that the condition is spina bifida occulta, since the more severe form of the condition, spina bifida cystica, features a meningocele or a myelomeningocele that is accompanied by severe neurological problems that make long life unlikely.[94]

Sacralization

Shifting in the vertebral column is not rare, primarily at the less stable lumbosacral and occipitocervical borders. The affected vertebra (or transitional vertebra) takes on the characteristics of an adjacent vertebra. Such a shifting is possibly triggered by a delay in the formation of the intervertebral disc space and adjacent vertebral segments that border two regions of the vertebral column.[95] Sacralization refers to the complete or incomplete incorporation of the last lumbar vertebra into the sacrum, when shifting occurs on the superior part of the lumbosacral border.[96] It is more likely to occur unilaterally and more commonly on the right side, or

[92] For cases in the paleopathological record, see Aufderheide and Rodríguez-Martín 1998, 62; Ortner 2003, 469.

[93] Aufderheide and Rodríguez-Martín 1998, 61. The disorder is usually asymptomatic in the living individual.

[94] Morse 1978.

[95] Barnes 1994, 79–80.

[96] Barnes 1994, 108–10.

asymmetrically. Symptoms include low back pain, severe pain radiating from the sacral area and down the leg and, since the condition causes curvature and rotation of the lumbar spine, it can lead to a progressive scoliosis.

Table 2.24 Sacralization in the adult sample (individuals and/or sacra affected)

Site	Total no.	Affected	M	F	CPR%	Total no. of sacra	Sacra affected	TPR%
Eleutherna	100	1	1	0	1.0	35	1	2.8
Kefali	49	1	1	0	2.0	12	1	8.3
Total	*149*	*2*	*2*	*0*	*1.3*	*47*	*2*	*4.2*

M=Male, F=Female

Table 2.24 presents the cases of sacralization in the adult sample. One individual from Eleutherna and one from Kefali (0.7%) present sacralization; absolute frequency rate for the condition is 4.2% or two affected sacra of 47. The fifth lumbar vertebra of skeleton 001st from Eleutherna (Figure 2.54) is fused with

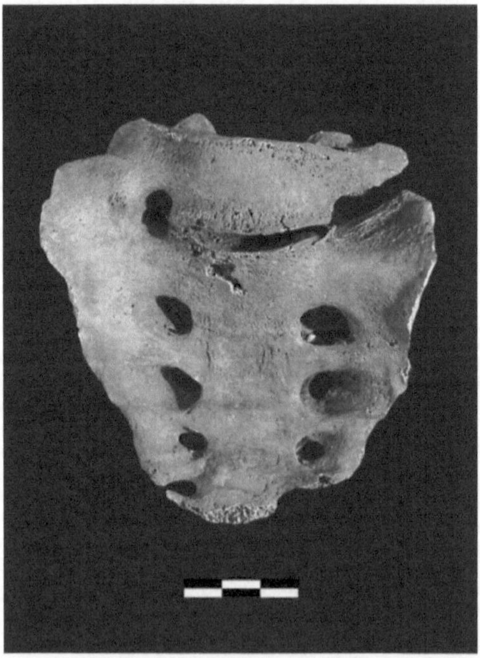

Figure 2.54 Eleutherna: Skeleton 001st, fusion of the fifth lumbar vertebra with the first sacral vertebra (sacralization) (photo: K. Painesi. Courtesy of Prof. P. Themelis and the Society of Messenian Archaeological Studies)

the first sacral vertebra. The sacralization is partial, involving only the right side of the sacrum. No detailed description of the defect is given for the Kefali case.

Tumors of Bone

Uncontrolled proliferation of bone, cartilage, fibrous tissue or blood vessels can generate tumors in bone. Benign tumors consist of well-differentiated, localized tissue, while malignant tumors consist of poorly differentiated tissue that continues to grow uncontrolled and potentially metastasizes to other parts of the body via the blood or lymphatic stream.[97] Malignant tumors affecting bone include carcinomas and sarcomas, either of which can spread from the primary site to other parts of the body (metastatic tumors). Bone sarcomas are rare but onset tends to be during young age, with the result that the prevalence between archaeological and modern skeletal samples is likely to be similar. Metastatic carcinoma to bone is much more common in archaeological human skeletal remains and, although the paleopathologist cannot perform the clinical test available to the modern pathologist, careful analysis of the type and distribution of lesions, age at death and sex of the skeleton facilitates the diagnosis.[98] In contrast, metastatic tumors of bone tend to be associated with old age, and their prevalence in ancient human populations is likely to be less than in modern western populations, as individuals in the past usually died of other causes before cancer could cause their death.[99] In our sample, only two cases of a benign primary osteoblastic tumor are observed.

Button osteoma

Button osteoma is a small, smooth lump of compact bone on the skull, and is one of the most common bone abnormalities encountered in both archaeological and modern populations. It consists of mostly dense lamellar bone and is usually located on the outer table of the cranial vault (mainly on the frontal and parietal bones). Usually the lesion is single, not more than 2 cm in maximal diameter, although multiple lesions can occur.[100] Eshed et al. proposed that what has been commonly described as 'button osteoma' in the anthropological literature is in

97 Ortner 2003, 503.

98 For a review of bone tumors, see, e.g., Dorfman and Czerniak 1998; Greenspan and Remagen 1998; Ortner 2003, 504–44. For cases in the paleopathological record of Greece, see Bourbou 2003b, 182–4.

99 Ortner 2003, 504.

100 Ortner 2003, 506.

fact not an osteoma, but rather a unique aberration, classified as hamartoma, so that the term 'button hamartoma' is suggested.[101]

Two button osteomas were recorded for the skull of a male individual (skeleton 015a) from Eleutherna (0.3%). One osteoma (1 × 1 cm) is located on the right frontal bone, while the other (0.5 × 1 cm) is located on the left parietal bone (Figure 2.55). Osteomas are predominantly asymptomatic, independent of sex and race, but age dependent.[102] Some researchers have suggested that these osteomas have neoplastic qualities.[103] Their etiology is unknown; theories invoke genetic, developmental, traumatic and infectious factors, although none of these have been verified.

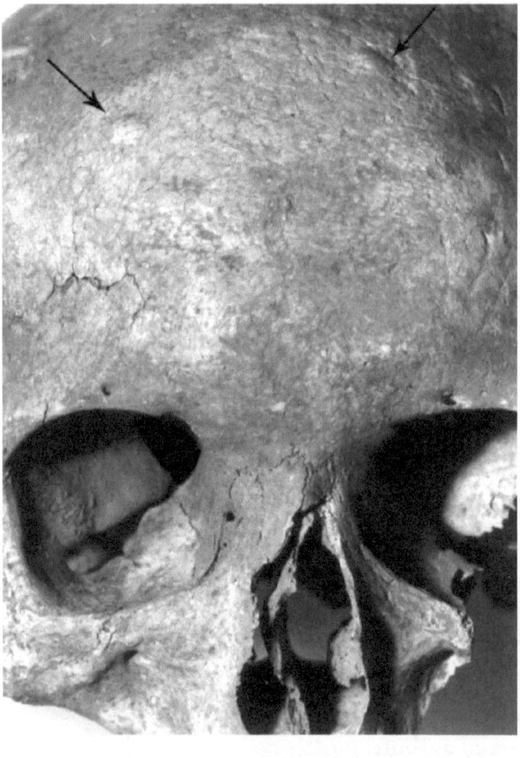

Figure 2.55 Eleutherna: Skeleton 015a, button osteomas (arrows) on the frontal and parietal bones of the skull (photo: K. Painesi. Courtesy of Prof. P. Themelis and the Society of Messenian Archaeological Studies)

101 Eshed et al. 2002.

102 Aufderheide and Rodríguez-Martín 1998, 375.

103 Perou 1964; Aufderheide and Rodríguez-Martín 1998.

Chapter 3

Tiny Occupants in Shallow Graves: The Bioarchaeology of Non-Adult Individuals

Childhood, whilst a biological stage of human development, is also a social construct. Many cultures have different attitudes towards the younger members of the population, and treat them differently in both life and death.[1] Children were once invisible in the archaeological record, but have come into view through an increase in relevant published material in recent years.[2] Researchers engaged in the study of children in the archaeological context often criticize archaeologists for tending to ignore children completely, or, when they are included in archaeological interpretations, for often depicting them in stereotypical ways that cast them in peripheral roles within the society. This point of view, that children are 'variables' rather than 'cultural actors,' appears to have stemmed from the notion that children were not really important because their activities did not make a significant contribution to the society and because, with the exception of mortuary evidence, their behavior left few material traces.[3] However, the application of gender-based approaches to archaeology has greatly enhanced our understanding of how families and societies were organized in the past, and children have emerged as making significant cultural contributions in areas considered important to archaeological research.[4] Whether researchers have diverse approaches for the inclusion of children and childhood in archaeological interpretations, or still struggle with how to identify their activities, the need to consider the biological and the cultural aspects of childhood is fundamental.

Survival of non-adult individuals is the most critical barometer of population fitness and biocultural changes within a society. However, it is only in the last decade that studies on growth and development, as well as on disease and

---

1 For theoretical perspectives of childhood, see e.g., Scott 1999, 1–51; Sofaer Derevenski 2000, 3–16; Lewis 2007, 4–8.

2 Lillehammer 1989; Moore and Scott 1997; Kamp 2001; Dasen 2004; Bakke 2005; Baxter 2005a, 2005b; Wileman 2005.

3 Baxter 2005b.

4 Nelson 1997.

mortality patterns, have increased in number.[5] Earlier lack of studies has been merely explained by the repetitively cited argument that non-adult remains do not survive the burial environment. This argument is now proved to be ill-founded, as indicated by the large number of non-adult remains retrieved from archaeological excavations sometimes even better preserved than those of adults.[6] It is widely accepted, though, that non-adult remains are subject to factors inherent to the nature of their bones, burial conditions, excavation and recovery techniques, as well as social attitudes towards their disposal and associated funerary practices. Their porous bones are more susceptible to disarticulation, scavenging and color change; highly alkaline or acidic soils result in poor preservation; and lack of expertise on the part of the excavator to identify their tiny skeletal elements further hinders the optimal recovery of non-adult remains.[7] Another concern of bioarchaeologists stems from bias in the representativeness of the skeletal sample, as mortuary, cultural, economic and other variables influence the final resting place of the non-adults. In classical Greece, for example, the rites of passages in childhood were clearly defined, peaking with the formal recognition of the child as a full member of the society at the age of 3 years. Thus, children dying before that age may not have received a formal burial ritual, and may have been buried in different areas from the rest of the community.[8]

Besides these potential biases and although the debate on the 'gold standard' that 30% of the mortuary sample should contain non-adult individuals is still open to discussion, it is well understood that bioarchaeology can provide an important element to research on non-adult individuals in the past.[9] It is particularly the age at death of non-adults that potentially provides useful information on the population's ability to adapt to its environment, socio-economic transitions, cultural practices for feeding and weaning the infant, maternal health and obstetrics, as well as disease patterns. In the protected uterine environment the fetus receives essential nutrients from the mother and is protected from external

---

5 For a thorough review on advances in children's bioarchaeology, see Lewis 2007, 10–13.

6 See, e.g., Saunders 2000, 135–8.

7 See, e.g., Gordon and Buikstra 1981; Herring, Saunders and Boyce 1994; Guy, Masset and Baud 1997; Jones and Ubelaker 2001; Robinson et al. 2003; Ingvarsson-Sundström 2003. The publication of specialized texts on fetal and juvenile anatomy see, e.g., Fazekas and Kósa 1978; Scheuer and Black 2000, 2004; Baker, Dupras and Tocheris 2005 facilitate the challenging task of identifying the morphologically complex non-adult skeletal parts.

8 This topic currently stimulates new investigations; see, e.g., Lagia 2007; Bourbou and Themelis in press.

9 Saunders and Barrans 1999; Saunders 2000; Perry 2005; Lewis 2007.

pathogens and other stimuli by her immune system. The response of the mother to a variety of environmentally and culturally induced stimuli indirectly affects the fetus. Neonatal deaths are attributed to the endogenous state of the infant, mainly genetic influences such as congenital abnormalities and the health status of the mother. Once born, it is the environment that has a direct effect on the child who is still protected, though for a short period, by breastfeeding. Postnatal deaths are considered to reflect the influence of the physical and cultural environment, such as poor sanitation and nutrition.[10] Any possible failure to adapt to this new environment has fatal effects. The ability of a population to provide the necessary biocultural means for a child's survival after birth is the most sensitive indicator of that population's overall fitness.

Children in Byzantine Society

The practical division of life in Byzantium into stages (educational periods and cultural transitions, such as marriage, entering civil or military service) is an inheritance from antiquity.[11] The classical Greek term *pais* was also broadly used by the Byzantines, along with *neogonon paidion* and *brephos* for the newborn, *nēpion* and *paidion* for the little child, *pais* and *teknon* for any child, boy or girl, *meirakion* for boy and *neaniskos* for young man.[12] In many cases, physiological age integrates with social age, and these two elements – the biological 'child data' and the sociocultural 'data child' – may be linked through careful consideration of how body changes in children correspond to alterations in their social and cultural identity.[13] Hence, children in every society can be manipulated to make statements, reflect cultural and religious beliefs, and affect existing ideological schemes, social concerns and political tensions; they can be given special associations with the rituals of life and death, embodying a number of contradictory forces which make them a powerful symbol within the human culture.

The role of beliefs, especially those connected with Christianity, is traceable on burial rituals, as non-adults are more likely to be found in communal

---

10 The implications of endogenous and exogenous causes of death in infants have been investigated in a study by Lewis and Gowland 2007, who compared infant mortality profiles from medieval and post-medieval rural and urban sites in England (AD 850–1859).

11 For the practical divisions of life in antiquity, see, e.g., Néraudau 1984, 47–9; Eyben 1993, 6–9.

12 Kiousopoulou 1997, 48, 53–4, 61–6; Hennessy 2008, 10–11; Prinzing 2009, 16–23.

13 Sofaer Derevenski 2000, 9–11.

cemeteries and burial grounds. Although, at least during the early Christian era, making clear-cut distinctions between pagan and Christian rituals is sometimes difficult, Lucy comments that:[14]

> It seems to be the general pattern that Christian cemeteries contain high proportions of younger burials, while pre-Christian sites can be typified by their general absence.

Detailed descriptions of the preparation of a child's body for burial and the relevant funerary ceremonies can be found in literary texts (cf. *Psellos'* oration on the death of his daughter Styliane), but when it comes to the actual procedure for the digging of graves for children, written texts remain silent and one can only turn to the archaeological evidence.[15] Segregation of non-adult burials within a Christian cemetery was not uncommon; however, child burials are usually found scattered among those of adult individuals. Burials in simple pits, cists or tile graves and in pottery vessels are usually encountered; non-adults are also recovered from ossuaries.[16] Commonly, non-adults were buried together with adult individuals: the pairing of mother and child, and two or more adult individuals and child are the most characteristic occurrences. Accompanying goods are also found within non-adult burials, such as jewelry (glass and bronze bracelets, necklaces, earrings) and toys.[17]

Christianity changed attitudes towards other practices such as contraception, abortion and infanticide, and already in the fourth century Christian writers condemned abortion and infanticide.[18] The Church not only condemned infanticide as a mortal sin but also developed a rite of exorcism to deal with human spirits which might be haunting the living. Valentinian I (AD 364–375) first made infanticide illegal in the western Roman Empire in AD 370 and later

---

14 Lucy 1994, 24–7. A good example is the late Roman infant cemetery at Lugnano, Italy, which is suggested to have resulted from a single outbreak of malaria: see Soren, Fenton and Birkby 1995; Soren 2008. The unusual pagan objects found scattered among the graves (e.g., headless puppies, a raven's claw) may reflect the desperation of people who were nominally Christians but who resorted to magical practices, including superstitious offerings, in moments of stress.

15 *Psellos* (ed. Sathas 1876); Talbot 2009.

16 Laskaris 2000, 288–290; Lewis 2007, 32–3; Tritsaroli and Valentin 2008.

17 Koukoules 1948, 161–224; Rahmani 1981, Laskaris, 2000, 290; Lazos 2002, 57–84, 119–127; Pitarakis 2009; Anagnostakis and Lambropoulou 2009; examples of accompanying goods are illustrated in Papanikola-Bakirtzi 2002, 208, 419, 493–5.

18 For a general discussion on abortion and contraception, see e.g., McLaren 1990; Riddle 1994; Talbot 1997, 125–6; McClanan 2002; Fulghum-Heintz 2003, 277; for a thorough overview on the bioarchaeology of infanticide, see Lewis 2007, 87–94.

Justinian (AD 527–565) recognized the fetus in the womb as a fully human being.[19] One of the best-known archaeological finds associated with infanticide is reported for the late Roman/early Byzantine site of Ashkelon in Israel.[20] The skeletal remains of nearly one hundred infants were found in the sewer beneath a bathhouse, suggesting a very abnormal attitude towards them, since all previous reports of the discovery of infant remains in Israel have described their careful burial. DNA analysis conducted at the Hebrew University resulted in the identification of a large number of males.[21] Textual evidence indicates that, although female infanticide was commonly practiced in ancient Roman society, female children were occasionally saved and raised to become prostitutes. The high number of dead male babies suggests that female infants were selectively preserved because they were of greater economic value. All these infants in the site of Ashkelon may have been offspring of prostitutes working in the bathhouse, which functioned as a brothel.

Research on Byzantine children is not entirely out of the realm of gender studies, but it has recently reached a greater level of sophistication, covering aspects such as social identity and legal status, education, material culture and influences of the cultural and religious environment.[22] However, it has been recently understood that the integration of biological data and documentary sources is the most holistic approach so to better perceive the life-course and the way in which Byzantine society treated its younger members.[23]

---

19 *Codex Justinianus* (ed. Krueger and Mommsen 1928), IV.XLIII.1; see also Patlagean 1973, 85; Moffat 1986, 714–15; for the genesis of early Christian thought on the embryo, see Congourdeau 2004; Brisson, Congourdeau and Solère 2008.

20 Smith and Kahila 1992.

21 Faerman 1997. Infants thought to be the victims of infanticide have been occasionally tested using DNA sex typing; see, for example, Waldron, Taylor and Rudling 1999; Mays and Faerman 2001.

22 It is beyond the scope of this chapter to thoroughly explore the Byzantine literature referring to the life and role of children in Byzantine society. A number of publications cover some of these aspects; see, e.g., a broad overview of Byzantine childhood in Moffatt 1986; Papaconstantinou and Talbot 2009; on the legal status of children, Antoniadis-Bibicou 1973; Patlagean 1973; Beaucamp 1977; on children's education, Buckler 1948; Guilland 1953; Moffatt 1977; Kalogeras 2000, 2001; on the legal, ecclesiastical and monastic status of orphans, Miller 1996, 2003; on children and the Church, Leloir 1980; on the representation of children in Byzantine art, Antonopoulos 1986; Hennessy 2008.

23 Bourbou 2001a. In 2006 the Dumbarton Oaks Spring Symposium *Becoming Byzantine: Children and Childhood in Byzantium* tackled for the first time the subject in much more detail, also including papers on bioarchaeological evidence for the reconstruction of mortality profiles, Bourbou 2006c, and isotopic data for the detection of breastfeeding and weaning patterns, Bourbou and Garvie-Lok 2006. Byzantine children have recently drawn the attention of other researchers, see, e.g., Tritsaroli and Valentin 2008.

Byzantine children were expected to continue the family line, transmit family property from one generation to the other and care for their parents, assuring as well their burial and postmortem commemoration. As in every past or modern society worldwide, children must have been noisy, enjoyed playing and were prone to accidents, sometimes while performing household tasks.[24] Psellos' funeral oration, written in a quite different style from his other works, is a poignant example of emotions toward children, indicating that Byzantine parents expressed their love and grief in ways similar to our modern conceptions.[25]

Making It To Adulthood? Reconstructing Non-Adult Mortality Patterns

Pregnancy and delivery were thought by the Byzantines to be critical periods for both mother and child, since complications during pregnancy (for example, maternal illness, congenital abnormalities) or childbirth (for example, baby in breech position with its feet first) are frequently attested. Physiological problems or diseases that could interfere with a healthy pregnancy and birth were often thought to be the work of evil spirits, particularly the female demon Gylou. The demon was thought to appear to pregnant women and cause miscarriages, kill newborns because she was envious for not being able to have any children of her own, or was responsible for post-partum fever.[26] From the early Byzantine period, bronze or lead amulets depict a half-woman, half-serpent figure with disheveled hair being speared by a rider saint, the so-called Holy Rider.[27] Similarly, on the reverse of some of the Holy Rider amulets appears the depiction of various animals attacking the so-called 'Evil Eye' or the 'Evil Eye of Envy', which is connected to the notion that envy could inflict harm. Parents may have put the Holy Rider/Evil Eye amulet on a newborn or hung it near the baby's cradle.[28]

---

24 Byzantine literature includes numerous accounts of accidents; Moffatt 1986, 707 refers to children falling down wells, falling off buildings, cracking their heads on rocks; Abrahamse 1979, 506–7 notes falls into boiling cauldrons, pits and cisterns, eating eggs of serpents, crawling to the edge of windows; see also examples in, e.g., the *Vita of Symeon Stylites the Younger* (ed. van de Ven 1962), chs 149, 196, 238.

25 See Patlagean 1996, 487–8.

26 Gylou was based on a prototype of Lilith, the barren first wife of Adam in the Jewish tradition, and on baby-snatching nymphs from ancient Greek lore; see Greenfield 1988, 182–90; Hurwitz 1992, 90, 96; Fulghum-Heintz 2003, 278–80.

27 See Vikan 1984; Russell 1995.

28 On the attitude of the Church towards such popular notions, see Dickie 1995. Besides taking these anti-demonic measures, women also appealed to the Virgin Mary and

Byzantine illustrations of childbirth depict the young mother against an architectural background, dressed in a short, lightweight tunic, drawn above the knees, free of the usual constraining band for the breasts and with disheveled hair, giving birth in seated and standing positions, lying on a bed or using a birthing chair.[29] Koukoules indicates another method with the woman on her knees, as recommended by the second-century AD physician Soranus, especially when the woman suffered from degeneration in the lumbar region.[30] Although these images usually represent the birth of holy figures, they can be seen as depicting the everyday reality of such an event, since the artists must have drawn upon the world around them for inspiration. No evidence exists that Byzantine surgeons performed Caesarean sections, but their excellent surgical skills are evidenced in operations such as embryotomy (physical dismemberment and removal of the fetus from the uterus) or the separation of Siamese twins as early as the tenth century AD.[31] Gynecology does not seem to have made great advances in the Byzantine era, and, in many medical texts from the period, specifically female concerns are beclouded or even omitted.[32] The relationship between menstruation, conception and the uterus was not fully understood by the Byzantines. The womb was considered as an enigmatic organ or as the cause of pathological conditions (for example, migraines and erratic behavior) and was assigned almost magical powers.[33] Several surviving amulets depict the 'wandering womb' as an octopus-like creature with a female face and include specific inscriptions, or the Holy Rider motif, emphasizing the connection between the womb and the risks of childbirth.[34] Male doctors

---

saints such as Hagia Marina for help during childbirth, see Fulghum-Heintz, 2003, 276, 279–80.

29 Koukoules 1951, 22–3; Talbot 1997, 124–5; Meyer 2005, 312–13; cf. the manuscript illustrations of Rachel giving birth to Benjamin (Vatican City, Vatican Library, *gr*. 747, fol. 56v); Lot's daughter bearing Ben-Ammi (Vatican City, Vatican Library, *gr*. 746, fol. 77v); Rebecca giving birth to Esau and Jacob (Vatican City, Vatican Library, *gr*. 747, fol. 46v).

30 Koukoules 1951, 23.

31 Examples of tools used for embryotomy (e.g., pierlike carnioclasts and embryo hooks) were excavated at Ephesus and probably date to the fifth century; see Bliquez 1984; McClanan 2002. Pentogalos and Lascaratos 1984, and Matsaggas and Marketos 1985 brought to attention the case of the Siamese twins.

32 Certainly, a number of Byzantine physicians refer in their works to specific diseases suffered by women (tumors, menstruation problems, inflammations etc); see discussion in, e.g., Ricci 1950; Harstad 1986.

33 Aubert 1989.

34 Metal amulets, the cheapest being of bronze, as well as semi-precious stones such as hematite, commonly known as 'bloodstone' for its red color and thought to aid in stopping

who had the formal education to deal with gynaecological issues often did not examine women patients, leaving their examination to midwives or the patients themselves.[35]

Evidence of high infant and childhood mortality is often attested in the Byzantine sources. The following examples – to give but a few – are derived from hagiography of the ninth century. In the Vita of St Evaristos mention is made of an unfortunate father who has lost four children in a row at birth; the Vita of St Peter of Atroa speaks of a couple whose 13 children all died prematurely; the Vita of Theodora of Thessalonike refers to Theodotos, a benefactor of Theodora's monastery, who saw four of his children die young.[36] Besides these anecdotal indications of high non-adult mortality in hagiography, the studies based on documentary evidence by Patlagean and Laiou, although looking at a specific area and time period, give an indication of what we might generally expect on non-adult mortality patterns.[37] Patlagean surveyed grave stelae of children from fourth-century Asia Minor and the area between Egypt and Syro-Palastine and found that only 50% of the children survived to the age of 15 years. Laiou examined census records concerning fourteenth-century Macedonian peasants living on monastic lands and found that half of the children died before the age of 5 years.[38] If we turn to the bioarchaeological record for early and middle Byzantine Crete, the non-adult sample under study includes 174 individuals, representing 39.1% of the total number of individuals under study. The distribution of non-adult deaths by age group is presented in Figure 3.1. Non-adults up to 1 year of age include 37 individuals (21.2%), while a clustering of deaths is observed for children aged 1 to 14.6 years, with 99 individuals (56.8%); the number of deaths for adolescents aged 14.6 to 17 years decreases to 24 individuals (13.7%). Comparing time periods, non-adults up to 1 year of age include 24 individuals

---

hemorrhage, are known; see Hanson 1995; Fulghum-Heintz 2003.

35 For a presentation of the manual of gynecology transmitted under the name of Metrodora (who has been traditionally considered as living in the seventh century AD), see Congourdeau, 1993b; for its analysis as an *iatrosophion*, see Touwaide 2006; for female physicians and midwives see, e.g., Kislinger 1989; Bourdara 1989; Margarou 2000, 223–6, 235–6; Nikolaou 2005, 286–329; Fulghum-Heintz 2003, 139–40.

36 *Vita of Saint Evaristos* (van de Vorst 1923), p. 317, ch. 34; *Vita of Saint Peter of Atroa* (ed. Laurent 1956), ch. 59; *Vita of Theodora of Thessalonike* (ed. Paschalides 1991), ch. 8–9, 78–84, and the English translation by Talbot 1996, 228–30. It is noteworthy that a common *topos* of hagiography is for parents to dedicate to monastic life a child who manages to survive after siblings born earlier have all died. In the case of the couple who have lost all of their 13 children, their fourteenth child who survived became a monk; similarly, the fifth child of Theodotos, a girl who miraculously recovered, was raised in Theodora's nunnery.

37 Laiou 1977; Patlagean 1977.

38 On life expectancy estimations, see Laiou 1977, 293–4; Patlagean 1977, 95–100.

(17.9%) and 13 individuals (32.5%) for the early and middle Byzantine period respectively. The next age category includes 79 children (58.9%) for the early Byzantine period and 20 (50.0%) for the middle Byzantine period. Deaths of adolescents count for 17 individuals (12.6%) for the early Byzantine period and seven (17.5%) for the middle Byzantine period (Figure 3.2).

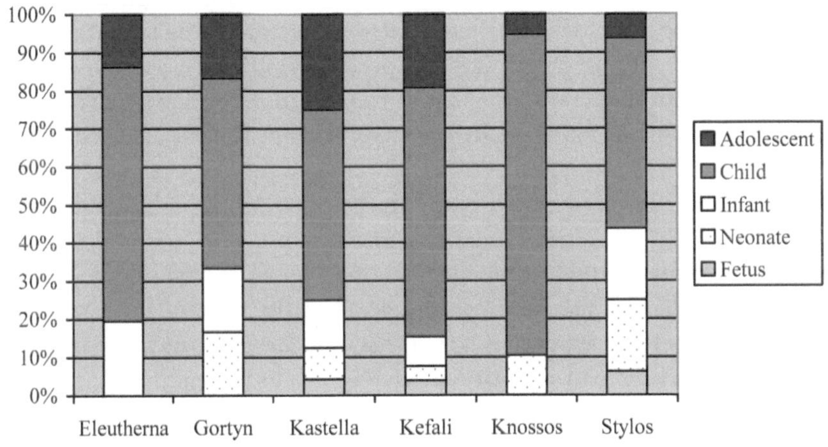

Figure 3.1 Non-adult mortality in the sample

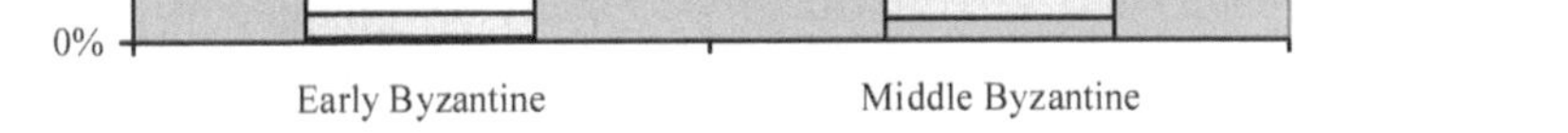

Figure 3.2 Non-adult mortality by time period

It is commonly expected that in any mortality sample the highest proportion of deaths will be among infants. Infant mortality is calculated as the number of infant deaths in one calendar year per 1,000 live births.[39] Modern data derived from the World Health Organization (WHO) suggest that infant mortality, especially during the first four weeks after birth, is still a major problem for

[39] Stockwell 1993.

developing countries, as in Africa, for example, where there are 41 deaths per 1,000 live births. Overall, in developing regions the risk of death is more than six times that of developed countries, while in the least developed regions it is more than eight times higher.[40]

As argued above, early deaths are generally attributed to the endogenous state of the infant and the health status of the mother. A number of factors could have affected both the mother and the fetus during pregnancy and at the time of and after delivery. Poor maternal health and nutritional status, inadequate care during pregnancy and possibly restricted access to medical treatment, inappropriate management of complications during pregnancy and delivery (for example, infection, hemorrhage, eclampsia, obstructed labor, fetal malpresentation), poor hygiene during delivery and the first critical hours after birth all could have played their part. On the other hand, problems such as a premature birth, difficulties in adapting to extrauterine life, harmful practices after birth that lead to infections (for example, neonatal tetanus) and general lack of newborn care may result in the death of the fetus or the newborn.[41] Sudden Infant Death Syndrome (SIDS) may also have played a role in infant mortality patterns in past populations, as most deaths peak at the age of 2 to 3 months.[42] SIDS cannot be excluded as a possible explanation of infant deaths in archaeological populations, as people in the past described sudden unexplained infant deaths similar to the typical SIDS death today.[43]

Once past the crucial period of infancy, children were generally at risk of death due to weaning, exposure to infectious disease and susceptibility to accidental trauma. In the majority of the sites, and independent of the time period, child mortality exceeded infant mortality (see Figure 3.2). This clustering of child deaths could be rooted largely in environmental factors, such as poor sanitation, and cultural factors influencing weaning practices.[44] If living conditions were harsh and unhygienic, any child could have been at risk, especially one who had already caught their share of early childhood illnesses. Weaning practices and the transition from breastmilk to solid foods exposed the child to an increased number of bacterial and parasitic infections, giving rise to the weanling diarrhea

---

40 WHO 2006, 19.

41 See relevant discussion in Barker and Osmond 1986; Barker 1992a, 1992b; Barker and Martyn 1992; Lewis 2007, 84–6. Neonatal tetanus has been, and remains, a common cause of infant death, particularly in environments where lack of hygiene at birth is prevalent, see WHO 2006, 3.

42 Bourbou 2004, 68.

43 Savitt 1993. For the contribution of anthropological studies to SIDS, see the study by McKenna, Ball and Gettler 2007.

44 Bourbou 2004, 66–7; Lewis 2007, 99–100; see also Chapter 4.

complex.[45] The nutritional value of supplementary foods, sanitary conditions in which feeding took place and the overall state of the child's environment were of vital importance. Malnourished children are more susceptible to infections and, as nutritional stress results in children being less resilient to future infections, successive cycles of infection and malnutrition take place.

Non-Adult Health and Disease Patterns

Although pediatrics in the modern sense did not develop as a separate specialty in Byzantine medicine, Byzantine physicians included in their medical texts sections devoted to perinatal care and nutrition, as well as descriptions and treatments of specific pathological conditions.[46] For example, Oribasius, Aetius of Amida and Paul of Aegina devoted specific sections in their books to the care and feeding of the newborn and the selection of a wet nurse, as well as to the treatment of various common diseases suffered by children, such as aphthae, inflammations of the ear and eyes, cough and congenital abnormalities (for example, hydrocephalus) or health problems during dental eruption.[47] *Vitae* of saints also provide useful information on pathological conditions, as, for example, the case of a crippled boy who could only crawl on all fours, supporting his hands on wooden blocks.[48] A number of specific childhood diseases such as smallpox, measles and scarlet fever would often kill the individual before any skeletal changes could develop. Our knowledge of this type of fatal disease is enriched when studying the literary sources. For example, Michael Psellos describes the fatal disease that afflicted his beloved daughter Styliane, possibly referring to a case of smallpox.[49]

---

45 Lewis 2007, 99–100.

46 For an overview of pediatrics in Byzantium, see Poulakou-Rebelakou 1992. Documentary evidence on perinatal nutrition and the introduction of supplementary foods following cessation of breastfeeding are discussed in Chapter 4.

47 See, e.g., *Oribasius* (Raeder 1928–33), V; *Aetius of Amida* (Olivieri 1935), IV; *Paul of Aegina* (ed. Heiberg 1921 and 1924; tr. Adams 1834), I. The most detailed study on childhood illness found in the Byzantine medical texts is the book by Hummel 1999.

48 *Vita of Makarios of Pelekete* (ed. van den Gheyn 1897), 149–50.

49 This case, as well another possible one attested by Theodorus Prodromus (AD 1100–1170), was brought to scholarly attention by Lascaratos and Tsiamis 2002; see also Leven 1993, 1997. When bone lesions have not developed due to the acute death of the individual, preserved soft tissues of mummified children provide an excellent source for studying the presence and development of childhood diseases, such as smallpox. One case of a 2-year-old child from mid-sixteenth century Italy presenting the exanthema typical of smallpox is reported by Fornaciari and Marchetti 1986. For a brief overview on the

The types of paleopathological data that can be obtained from non-adult remains are both indirect and direct. For example, indirect evidence on obstetric hazards can be retrieved from the presence of fetuses within or expelled from the abdominal cavity of a female.[50] Similarly, a number of lesions present in the teeth and bones of non-adults have been used as indirect evidence for malnutrition (non-specific metabolic stress), such as enamel hypoplasia, cribra orbitalia and porotic hyperostosis. Direct evidence on specific deficiency diseases is provided in cases of scurvy and rickets, while fracture patterns may help identify child abuse, accidental injuries or suggest the type and onset of labor in which non-adults were engaged. The vast majority of pathological conditions that can be detected in the adult skeleton can be also observed on non-adult remains, such as dental diseases, specific infections, neoplasms and metabolic and congenital conditions – to name but a few.[51]

However, the fact that not all diseases leave traces on skeletal remains, coupled with factors associated with the nature, development and preservation of immature bones, limits the diagnosis of pathological conditions in non-adults. Problems also exist regarding the diagnosis and etiology of diseases, leading researchers in some cases to exclude specific age categories from their investigation.[52] Current improved methods and application of innovative techniques facilitate the diagnosis of specific pathological conditions such as scurvy and rickets.[53] The detailed study by Lewis on the nature, distribution

---

pathological conditions observed in child mummies, see Bourbou 2005, 210; Atoche-Peña, Rodríguez-Martin and Ramírez-Rodríguez 2008, 555–83.

[50] See Malgosa et al. 2004.

[51] See, e.g., on rickets: Ortner and Mays 1998; Mays, Brickley and Ives 2006; Blondiaux et al. 2002; on enamel hypoplasia, Boldsen 2007; on leprosy, Bennike et al. 2005; on yaws, Buckley and Tayles 2003; on osteomyelitis, Canci, Tarli and Repetto 1991; on congenital syphilis, Palfi et al. 1992; Ferencz and Józsa 1992; Gladykowska-Rzeczycka and Krenz 1995; Rothschild and Rothschild 1997; Erdal 2006; on neoplastic conditions, Barnes and Ortner 1997; Alt et al. 2002; Anderson 2002; on Binder syndrome, Mulhern 2002; on dwarfism, Tillier et al. 2001; on tuberculosis, Ortner and Bush 1993; Schultz 1999; Santos and Roberts 2001; on trauma, Jiménez-Brobeil, Al Oumaoui and du Souich 2007. For comparative studies on non-adult health patterns, see, e.g., Buckley 2000; Lewis 2002; Blom et al. 2005; Bennike et al. 2005; Boldsen 2007; Schultz, Timme and Schmidt-Schultz 2007.

[52] Ribot and Roberts 1996, excluded non-adults under the age of two when recording the presence of periostitis in their samples, arguing that it is almost impossible to distinguish between normal and abnormal bone porosity in infants and children, as skeletal growth is very intensive during uterine life and the first two years of life.

[53] See, for example, the study by Mays, Brickley and Ives 2006, and Brickley and Ives 2008 on dry-bone criteria for recognition of rickets in non-adults remains, and the studies by Ortner et al. 2001, Brickley and Ives 2006, 2008 on the diagnosis of skeletal lesions attributed

pattern and possible etiology of endocranial lesions provides a solid background for the recording and interpretation of these lesions.[54] Solving the problems of preservation and diagnosis inherent to the study of non-adult remains is fundamental for answering broader questions about health and disease patterns at a wider regional and temporal level.

The pathological conditions observed in our non-adult sample have been carefully evaluated. Pathological conditions for which only vague or inadequate reference exists were excluded. For example, Zygouri refers to a fracture at the distal end of the left fibula of a juvenile (ΚΠα 18-08), 16 to 18 years of age from Kefali, simply arguing that the fracture is well healed; however, no further evidence on the type of fracture is provided, nor was the bone radiographed.[55] Similarly, Musgrave refers to a case of a 10-year-old child suffering from dysplasia on the left femur, with no further description of the case or possible complications. He also argues the presence of 'a great number of Harris lines', as revealed by the radiographic analysis of non-adult long bones, suggesting that their presence can be attributed to metabolic disturbances during growth caused by diseases or malnutrition.[56]

A small number of dental diseases, including a few cases of dental enamel hypoplasias, are recorded for the samples of Gortyn, Kastella and Kefali. Mallegni reports one case of an adolescent exhibiting abscess and ante-mortem tooth loss;[57] Zygouri has observed a carious lesion and periodontal disease in a 5-year-old child, as well as a carious lesion and calculus in an adolescent; calculus is also present in a child and an adolescent from Kefali and in a child from Kastella.[58] Such a small number of cases contribute little to the reconstruction of dental disease patterns in our non-adult sample. However, the appearance of dental pathologies in childhood probably indicates that diet and lack of systematic oral hygiene could have stimulated an early onset. Dental enamel hypoplasias are recorded in the form of striae, mainly on the canines and incisors, in three children from Kastella, and in one adolescent from Kefali. Although dental enamel hypoplasias have long been used as a non-specific indicator of systematic physiological stress during early life, the number of cases is too small to infer possible patterns linking these defects to bouts of malnutrition, weaning, disease,

---

to scurvy. The application of innovative techniques such as paleohistology enhances a more positive diagnosis; see Schultz 2001.

54 Lewis 2004.

55 Zygouri 2005.

56 Musgrave 1976; for a review on Harris lines, see Aufderheide and Rodríguez-Martin 1998, 422; Lewis 2007, 107–11.

57 Mallegni 1988, tables 1 and 2.

58 Zygouri 2005 refers to another two 'subadults' exhibiting dental pathologies.

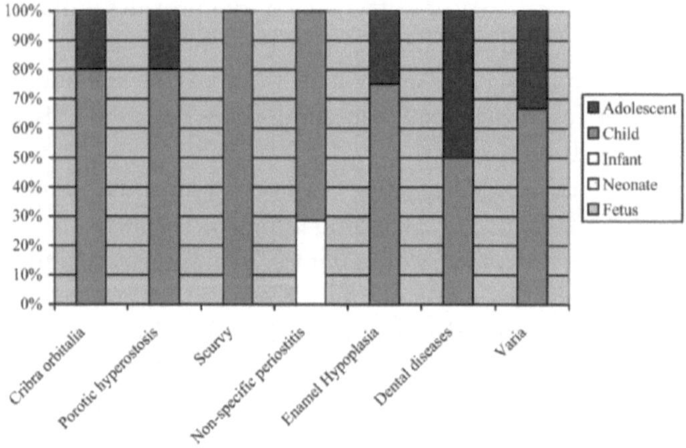

Figure 3.3 Distribution of pathological conditions in the non-adult sample (individuals affected)

Under "Varia" are included: a case of fracture, infantile cortical hyperostosis and a congenital abnormality (femur dysplasia)

fever or intrauterine under-nutrition due to a deficient maternal diet.[59] It is worth noting, however, that recent studies have discredited much of the earlier work that correlates peaks in enamel hypoplasias with weaning stress, arguing that, during the two- to four-year developmental period (frequent peak in the formation of these defects), the enamel is more susceptible to environmental disturbance and that the position of the defects on the tooth crowns may be related to the structure of the enamel layers.[60]

Based on this survey of the pathological conditions in the non-adult sample, our discussion will be limited to the presence of cribra orbitalia and porotic hyperostosis, scurvy, non-specific periostitis and infantile cortical hyperostosis. Figure 3.3 presents the distribution of pathological conditions by age group. From birth to 1 year of age, two individuals (1.1%) demonstrate pathological conditions, while the majority of cases are children, including 26 individuals (14.9%); adolescents number seven individuals (4.0%). Comparing time periods, the breakdown by age categories includes from birth to 1 year of age one individual (2.2%), 20 children (12.6%) and seven adolescents (3.7%) for the early Byzantine period; for the middle Byzantine period only one infant and one adolescent (2.5%) respectively, and seven children (12.5%) are included (Figure 3.4).

59 See, e.g., Goodman and Rose 1990; Guatelli-Steinberg and Lukacs 1999; King, Humphrey and Hillson 2005; Ogden, Pinhasi and White 2007; Triantaphyllou et al. 2008; see relevant discussion in Lewis 2007, 104–7, and Chapter 2 in this book.

60 See, e.g., Reid and Dean 2000.

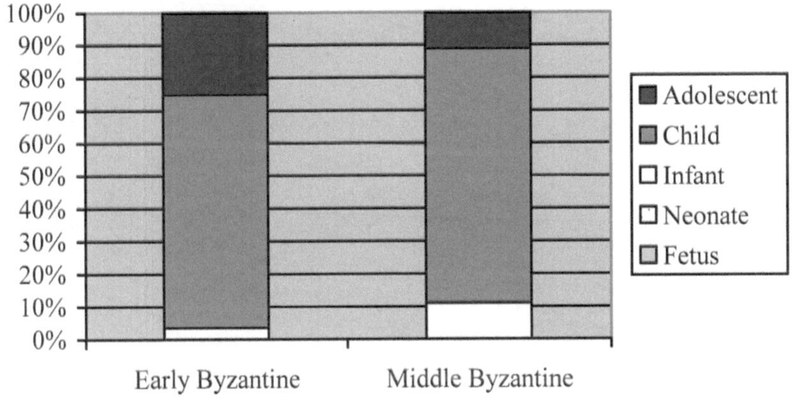

Figure 3.4 Distribution of non-adult pathological conditions by time period (individuals affected)

Hematopoietic and Metabolic Disorders

Cribra orbitalia and porotic hyperostosis

Cribra orbitalia and porotic hyperostosis are the most frequently observed hematopoietic disorders in the non-adult sample (Figure 3.5).[61] The observed cases of cribra orbitalia and porotic hyperostosis are presented in Tables 3.1 and 3.2. Ten non-adult individuals (5.7%) exhibited cribra orbitalia and five (2.8%) exhibited porotic hyperostosis. Absolute frequency rate for cribra orbitalia is 85.0% or 17 affected orbital roofs of 20, and for porotic hyperostosis 15.5% or 12 affected cranial bones of 77. When comparing time periods, cribra orbitalia is observed in ten individuals or 5.7% for the early Byzantine period, while no cases are reported for the middle Byzantine period. Porotic hyperostosis is observed in three individuals (2.2%) for the early Byzantine period, while one individual (2.5%) from the middle Byzantine period exhibits porotic lesions on the cranial vault. Absolute frequency rate can be provided only for the early Byzantine period, where for cribra orbitalia it is 85.0% or 17 affected orbital roofs of 20. Absolute frequency rate for porotic hyperostosis is 15.3% or ten cranial bones of 65 for the early Byzantine sites, and 16.6% or two bones of 12 for the middle Byzantine sites.

61 For a thorough discussion on cribra orbitalia and porotic hyperostosis, see Chapter 2.

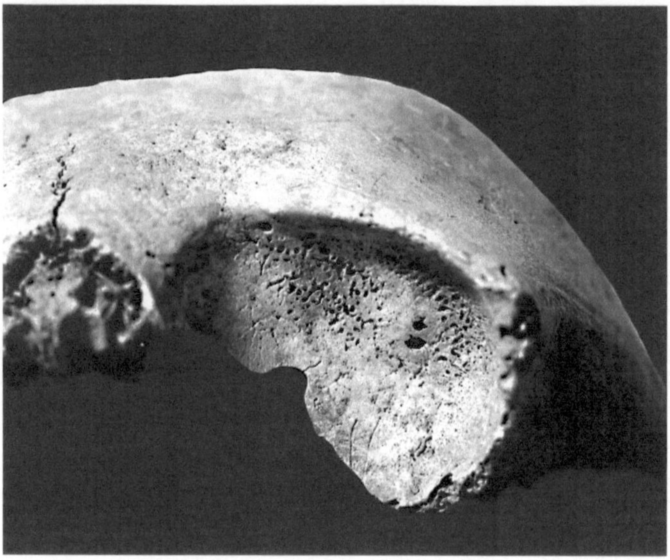

Figure 3.5 Eleutherna: Skeleton 005ie, cribra orbitalia (photo: K. Painesi. Courtesy of Prof. P. Themelis and the Society of Messenian Archaeological Studies)

We noted in Chapter 2 that differential diagnosis of porous lesions is a challenging task, as a variety of conditions may result in similar lesions. However, the anatomical details of the lesions observed in the sample cannot be attributed to infectious conditions or metabolic disorders such as scurvy or rickets.[62] Similarly, the lack of skeletal evidence for genetic anemias excludes this diagnostic option. It seems better to suggest a multifactorial etiology involving the synergistic effects of dietary deficiencies, infections and parasite load, which potentially resulted in marrow hyperplasia in response to anemia. However, if these lesions can be attributed to an anemic reaction, this does not necessarily have to be exclusively attributed to an iron deficiency. In the paper by Fairgrieve and Molto, feeding practices and the quality of supplementary foods introduced after cessation of breastfeeding are considered for the interpretation of cribra orbitalia recorded in the non-adult sample.[63] The authors argue that the introduction of both goat's milk and honey in the infant diet may have had dire consequences, as infants fed on goat's milk develop megaloblastic anemia at about 3–5 months due to folic acid deficiency. Honey, on the other hand, is

62 See Ortner 2003, 375.

63 Fairgrieve and Molto 2000.

a confirmed source of *Clostridium botulinum* spores, resulting in a severe and often fatal form of food poisoning – botulism.[64] As porotic lesions are observed primarily in children (see Figure 3.5), weaning stress must be considered as a plausible explanation for their development.

Table 3.1 Cribra orbitalia and porotic hyperostosis in the non-adult sample (individuals affected)

Site	Total no.	Affected with cribra orbitalia	CPR%	Affected with porotic hyperostosis	CPR%
Eleutherna	51	3	5.8	0	0
Gortyn	24	3	12.5	0	0
Kefali	40	4	10.0	4	10.0
Stylos	16	0	0	1	6.2
Total	*131*	*10*	*7.6*	*5*	*3.8*

Table 3.2 Cribra orbitalia and porotic hyperostosis in the non-adult sample (bones affected)

Site	Total cranial bones	Cranial bones affected	TPR%
Orbits			
Eleutherna	14	5	35.7
Gortyn	-	6	-
Kefali	6	6	100
Total (orbits)	*20*	*17*	*85.0*
Frontal			
Kefali	22	2	9.0
Parietal			
Kefali	25	4	16.0
Stylos	12	2	16.6
Total (parietal)	*37*	*6*	*16.2*
Temporal			
Kefali	18	4	22.2
Total	*97*	*29*	*15.5*

Vitamin C Deficiency (Scurvy)

Scurvy is a dietary deficiency of ascorbic acid (vitamin C). The vitamin is found in a wide range of foods, including numerous vegetables (dark-green leafy vegetables contain 100–150 mg/100 g) and fresh fruits (oranges and lemons contain 50 mg/100 g); small amounts of vitamin C are also available from milk (goat/sheep milk contains 2–3 mg/100 g), organ meat (liver and kidney

64 See also Chapter 4.

contains 10–40 mg/100 g) and fish (cod flesh contains 0.5–2 mg/100 g).[65] It is not required in the diet of most animal species; only humans and a few other species, such as guinea pigs, lack the enzyme necessary to synthesize the vitamin.[66] Vitamin C has a number of roles in the body, including the formation of collagen and cartine synthesis, which is required to produce energy in muscles, blood formation and the metabolism of iron and folate.[67]

Rapidly growing bones – such as the costochondral junctions of ribs, the distal metaphysis of the femur, radius and ulna and the proximal epiphysis of the humerus – demonstrate the most marked skeletal changes. The onset of scurvy results in defective connective tissue and blood vessels, making scorbutic infants and children particularly vulnerable to hemorrhage. Skeletal changes are caused either directly by the vitamin C deficiency or by traumatic effects on the scorbutic bone and associated blood vessels. The condition is rarely observed before 4 months of age, with a peak between 8 and 10 months.[68]

Infantile scurvy has until recently received little attention in the paleopathological record.[69] There may have been problems in recognizing the condition as a distinct clinical entity, and perhaps many cases of scurvy may have been misdiagnosed.[70] Recent advances in the identification of scorbutic skeletal lesions as discussed by a number of researchers enhance the ability to positively recognize the changes attributed to the condition.[71] Table 3.3 presents the macroscopic and radiological features required for the diagnosis of scurvy. Furthermore, the application of innovative techniques such as paleohistological analysis enables researchers to differentiate scorbutic cases from other hemorrhage-inducing pathologies like inflammation and anemia.[72]

---

65 Vitamin C contents following data given in Brickley and Ives 2008, table 4.1; WHO 1999, table G.

66 Hodges 1980.

67 Brickley and Ives 2006, 2008, 47.

68 Ortner 2003, 384.

69 For an early description of scurvy, see Barlow 1883; Fraenkel 1929. Up-to-date paleopathological cases are reported by Ortner 1984; Roberts 1987; Molleson and Cox 1993; Lilley et al. 1994; Mogle and Zias 1995; Ortner and Ericksen 1997; Ortner, Kimmerle and Diez 1999; Ortner et al. 2001; Bourbou 2003c; Melikian and Waldron 2003; Maat 2004; Brickley and Ives 2006; Garvie-Lok 2008; Mays 2008; see also a thorough overview of cases in the paleopathological record by Ortner 2003, 387–93 and Brickley and Ives 2008, 54–6, table A1.

70 Stuart-Macadam 1989.

71 Ortner and Ericksen 1997; Ortner, Kimmerle and Diez 1999, Ortner et al. 2001; Lewis 2004; Brickley and Ives 2006, 2008; Melikian and Waldron 2003.

72 Schultz 1989; Carli-Thiele 1995. On histological features of scurvy in non-adults, see Brickley and Ives 2008, 65–7, table 4.6.

Table 3.3 Macroscopic and radiological features required for a diagnosis of scurvy in non-adults

Bones affected	Macroscopic features	Radiological features
Cranium	Abnormal porosity (sphenoid, mandible, maxilla and orbits) New bone formation (orbits and vault)	
Ribs	Fracture of bone adjacent to costochondral junction Enlargement of ribs adjacent to costochondral junction (scorbutic rosary)	
Scapulae	Abnormal porosity of cortex (supraspinous and infraspinous areas)	
Long bones	New bone formation (commonly towards ends)	Irregularity and thinning of the cortex White line of Frankel or dense metaphyseal line Radiolucent or 'scurvy' line Wimberger ring Corner fractures or sign

Modified after Brickley and Ives 2008, tables 4.2 and 4.4

Two non-adult individuals (005ie and 004e) from Eleutherna exhibit skeletal lesions suggestive of scurvy.[73] The distribution of lesions in skeleton 005ie is presented in Figure 3.6. Pathological bone changes of skeleton 005ie (4 years ± 12 months) consisted of subperiosteal new bone formation in an irregular and extensive woven pattern on the orbital roofs, mainly in the anterior areas (Figure 3.7). The lesion in the right orbit is more extensive and thicker. New bone formation extends above the supraorbital ridges on both the external (2.3 × 1.7 cm) and internal (3 × 2.4 cm) surfaces of the frontal bone. Fragments of the temporal and occipital bones exhibit similar porous activity on the external surfaces. Porous activity is also visible along the medial surface of the coronoid process of the right mandible. The metaphysis of the left tibia exhibits a hematoma, subperiosteal organized, possibly of traumatic origin (Figure 3.8). Skeleton 004e, a child (4–12 years), exhibits woven bone reaction on both mandibular rami and on the occipital bone, extending onto the superior nuchal lines (Figure 3.9).

73 Bourbou 2003c, 2004, 55–6.

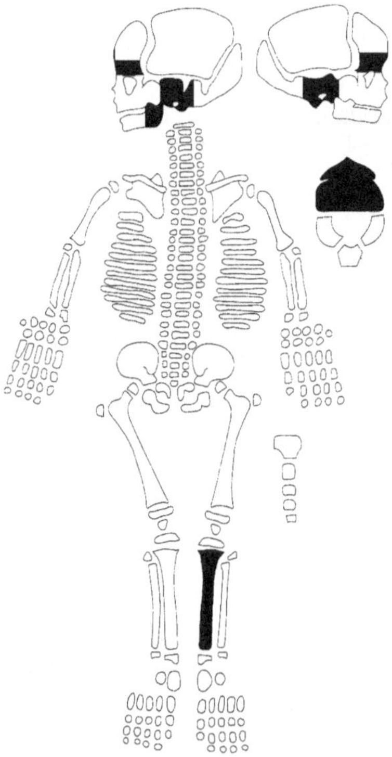

Figure 3.6 Diagram of skeleton 005ie, from Eleutherna. In black color are indicated the areas exhibiting lesions associated with scurvy

Chronic bleeding and subsequent ossification at multiple sites on the skull are associated with scurvy and are the most likely reason for the observed bone lesions, although the fragmentation of the skulls of the skeletons from Eleutherna does not allow a thorough study of the anatomical sites associated with scorbutic lesions. The mandible of skeleton 005ie is fragmentary, but evidence for abnormal porosity is present on the medial surface of the coronoid process of the mandible, where the temporalis muscle attaches. The bone reaction seen on the mandible of this individual is compatible with the type of inflammatory lesions that can occur as a result of hemorrhage induced by the stress of chewing, since the temporalis muscle is important for chewing. Regarding the hematoma, presumably of traumatic origin, observed on the tibia of skeleton 005ie, infractions (incomplete fractures) with subperiosteal hematoma are for the most part found in areas subjected to stress by the body's own weight, particularly the joints and metaphyses of the long bones of the leg, especially the femur and

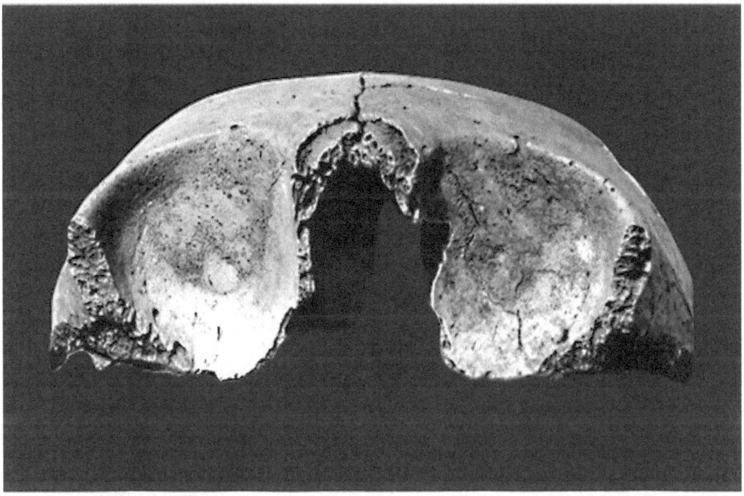

Figure 3.7 Eleutherna: Skeleton 005ie, orbital lesions associated with scurvy (photo: K. Painesi. Courtesy of Prof. P. Themelis and the Society of Messenian Archaeological Studies)

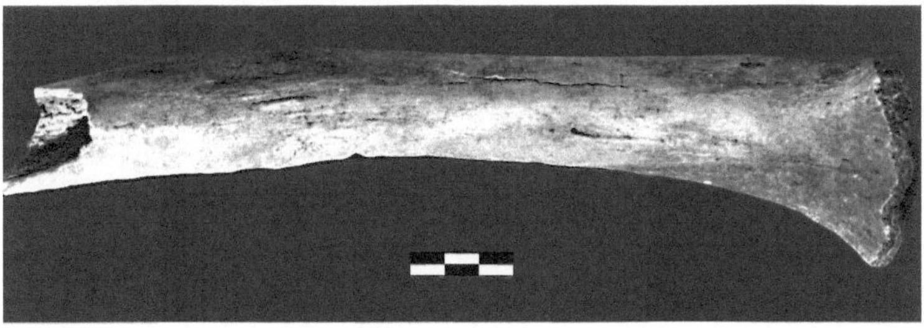

Figure 3.8 Eleutherna: Skeleton 005ie, subperiosteal hematoma on the tibial shaft associated with scurvy (photo: K. Painesi. Courtesy of Prof. P. Themelis and the Society of Messenian Archaeological Studies)

tibia.[74] In scorbutic non-adults, periosteal attachment can become so fragile that a subperiosteal hemorrhage often involves a proportionately greater area and volume. The absence of repair activities in the bone tissue along the margins of the infraction in this skeleton may indicate that there was only a short interval between the injury and the moment of death, perhaps a few hours or a few days.

74 Ortner 2003, 384.

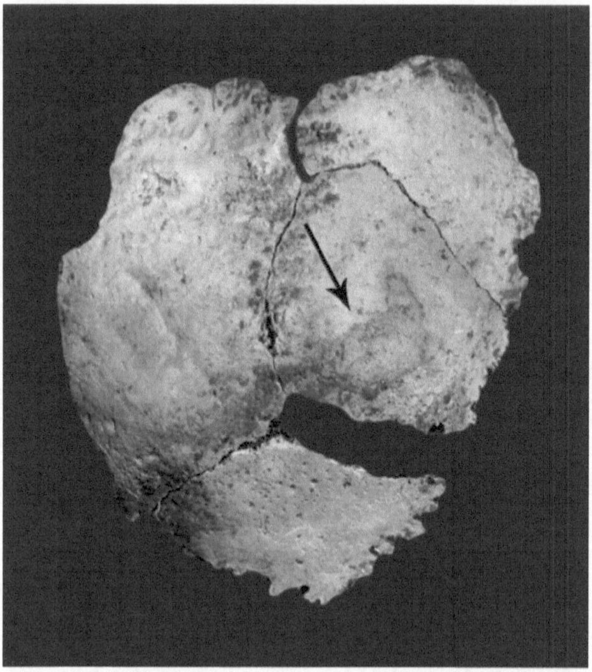

Figure 3.9 Eleutherna: Skeleton 004e, porous lesions on the occipital bone (arrow) associated with scurvy (photo: K. Painesi. Courtesy of Prof. P. Themelis and the Society of Messenian Archaeological Studies)

In any case, the process of fracture repair is known to be greatly impaired in hypovitaminosis C.

It is possible that these non-adults did not develop more extensive hemorrhage-induced subperiosteal bone formation because death, perhaps from an alternative cause, occurred relatively soon after the onset of scurvy. Vitamin C has a dual role in maintaining adequate immune function by assisting in neutralizing or destroying pathogens and by producing various protective antioxidants.[75] Children with vitamin C deficiency are especially susceptible to infections, developing otitis media, pneumonia, diphtheria and other health problems, such as digestive disturbances and general debility.[76]

A variety of pathologies can result in porous lesions of the skull, which are often attributed to anemia when accompanied by thickening of the bone marrow, to infection or to other inflammatory conditions that can stimulate an increase in

75 Jacob and Sotoudech 2002.

76 Jaffe 1972.

vasculature, as well as new bone formation. The changes observed in the orbital roofs are not typical for cribra orbitalia characteristic of anemia because they are not caused by the expansion of underlying marrow, which would be the case in anemia, and they occur in conjunction with an intact cortex.[77] In addition, there is no convincing evidence of bone deformity and/or bone changes in the skull that can be associated with rickets.

Scurvy has been thought to be rare in fruit-abundant areas, but common at high altitudes. It is uncertain whether ancient Greek, Byzantine and Arab physicians recognized scurvy as a clinical condition, since the temperate climate of the Mediterranean and Near East encourages the cultivation of vitamin C-rich fruits and vegetables.[78] Even during famines the inhabitants of Greece never lacked fresh produce and seafood.[79]

The observed scorbutic cases count for only 1.1% of the non-adult sample. If we accept that the rarity of scurvy in the paleopathological record of Greece can be explained by the temperate climate of the country and the abundance of vitamin C-rich fruits and vegetables, how can we interpret its sporadic presence? In a broader context it should be remembered that changes in subsistence patterns probably had a significant impact on the nutritional status of past populations. Sedentism and the transition to agriculture may have had benefits (greater food production) but also disadvantages, such as the adoption of diets containing a far more restricted range of plants. It has been suggested that populations could have moved from a diet of as many as 200–300 species of plant foods to one of a couple of domesticated cereals and probably only 20–50 plant foods.[80] Cereal grains (for example, wheat), which would have formed the basis of a daily diet, lack vitamin C.[81] Scurvy does not usually develop under 'normal' living conditions, but it is commonly associated with natural or man-made disasters. Impoverished living conditions and environmental stress are attested for the scorbutic cases from the late Roman/early Byzantine sites of Stymphalos and Eleutherna.[82] Populations undergoing stressful periods due to economic, political or environmental turbulence are potentially more at risk of developing the condition. The development of the condition is often associated with specific

77 Ortner and Putschar 1985, 263.

78 The Hippocratic writers of the late fifth century BC may have known of scurvy, as they mention gum lesions and leg pains; see Aufderheide and Rodríguez-Martín 1998, 312.

79 Grmek 1989, 77.

80 Cordain 1999, 23.

81 This link between the development of scurvy and the adoption of agriculture is suggested by Papathanasiou 2005 for the case she reports from the Neolithic (3500–2900 BC) site of Alepotrypa cave in Greece.

82 Bourbou 2004; Garvie-Lok 2008.

culturally derived behaviours. Weaning practices, including the introduction of cereal-based supplementary foodstuff after cessation of breastfeeding, should be taken under consideration, as metabolic conditions are often argued to coincide with weaning.[83] Finally, it is possible that sample biases, lack of systematic work on non-adult populations and misdiagnosed cases may have resulted so that only few cases have entered the paleopathological record.

Non-Specific Infections

Periostitis

Periostitis (or periosteal new bone formation) refers to the deposition of a new layer of bone under an inflamed periosteum as the result of injury or infection.[84] Non-adults are more susceptible to bone infection, due to the abundant blood supply in the red bone marrow at the ends of the long bones. Although a good blood supply is essential to maintain rapid growth in these areas, it is also a route for the transportation of foreign organisms to these sites.[85] Since diagnosis of periostitis in non-adults is rather problematic, few cases have entered the palaeopathological record.[86] Problems in diagnosis basically arise from difficulties in distinguishing between pathological change and normal growth processes, especially in infants and children, or between different pathological conditions.[87] In archaeological bones observation of the lesions' patterning (single bones or specific distribution pattern), as well as the nature of the new bone deposits, facilitates the diagnosis and interpretation of the condition.

Table 3.4 Periostitis in the non-adult sample (individuals affected)

Site	Total no.	Affected	CPR%
Eleutherna	51	2	3.9
Kefali	40	3	7.5
Stylos	16	2	12.5
Total	*107*	*7*	*6.5*

83 Bourbou and Garvie-Lok 2009.

84 Lewis 2007, 134.

85 Ulijaszek 1990.

86 Mensford et al. 1978; Grauer 1993; Anderson and Carter 1994; Ribot and Roberts 1996; Walker 1997.

87 This fact led Ribot and Roberts 1996, 71 to highlight the need of microscopical applications and agreement on the minimum requirement for scoring subperiosteal new bone formation on the long bones and skull in individuals under the age of 6 ± 2 years.

In non-adult individuals of the sample localized periostitis is observed along the shafts of one or two long bones (Tables 3.4 and 3.5). Seven non-adult individuals or 4.0% exhibited periosteal reaction. Absolute frequency rate is 4.6% or ten affected bones of 216. When comparing between time periods, five individuals (3.7%), and two individuals (5.0%) are attested for the early and middle Byzantine period respectively. Absolute frequency rate is 3.8% or seven bones of 183 for the early Byzantine sites, and 9.0% or three bones of 33 for the middle Byzantine sites.

Table 3.5 Periostitis in the non-adult sample (bones affected)

Site	Total bones	Bones affected	TPR%
Clavicle			
Kefali	24	1	4.1
Scapula			
Stylos	7	1	14.2
Humerus			
Kefali	42	2	4.7
Radius			
Kefali	26	2	7.6
Femur			
Eleutherna	61	1	1.6
Stylos	13	1	7.6
Total (femur)	*74*	*2*	*2.7*
Tibia			
Eleutherna	30	1	3.3
Stylos	13	1	7.6
Total (tibia)	*43*	*2*	*4.6*
Total	*216*	*10*	*4.6*

The loosely organized woven bone suggests that the lesions were still active at the time of death (Figure 3.10).[88] It is possible that a general ongoing infectious process affected the individuals since birth or even before, and contributed directly to their early death. Trauma is another possible diagnosis due to the localized nature of the lesion and the normal internal architecture of all of the bones.[89]

---

88 New bone layers disorganized and porous in appearance (woven bone) represent an active phase; remodeled and continuous with the original cortex (lamellar bone) indicate that the condition occurred and healed before the individual's death; a mix of both types represents a chronic and active case.

89 Anderson and Carter 1994.

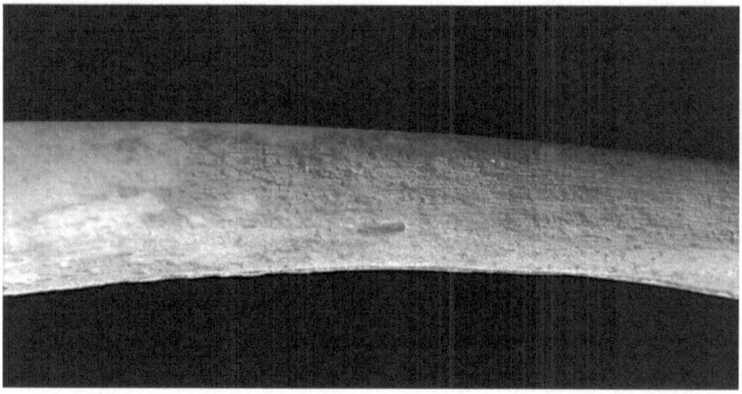

Figure 3.10 Stylos: Skeleton 003, non-specific periostitis on the left tibia

Infantile cortical hyperostosis

The specific etiology of infantile cortical hyperostosis (ICH) or Caffey's disease is still unknown, but it is most possibly related to a viral infection. Other possible etiologies include genetic defects, hypervitaminosis, trauma, arterial abnormality or an allergic reaction of collagen.[90] The condition comprises swelling, irritability and bone lesions characterized by massive deposition of layered periosteal woven bone on one or several bones in a rough and uneven contour.[91] The average age of onset is 9 weeks but cases of recurrent ICH have been reported in individuals up to 19 years of age.[92] The spontaneous healing of the condition, usually within three months, leaves no traces behind, thus hindering possible diagnosis in archaeological bones.[93]

Skeleton 007 from Stylos (7.5–8.5 years of age) exhibits porotic hyperostosis on the right parietal bone and diffuse periosteal reaction in the form of woven bone on almost all recovered bones (Figure 3.11): both mandibular rami, both radii, both ulnae, seven right and 12 left ribs, both ilia, ischia and pubic bones, both femora, both tibiae (Figures 3.12), both fibular shafts (recovered in fragments) and both calcanei. The distribution pattern of the periosteal lesions indicates infantile cortical hyperostosis as the most plausible diagnosis. Current clinical data suggest that the skeletal lesions indicative of ICH include the

90 Caffey 1978; Lewis 2007, 144.

91 Lewis 2007, 143.

92 Keipert and Campbell 1970; Swerdloff, Ozonoff and Gyepes 1970.

93 Only a few cases are reported: see Rogers and Waldron 1988; Farwell and Molleson 1993; Bagousse and Blondiaux 2001; Lewis and Gowland 2005.

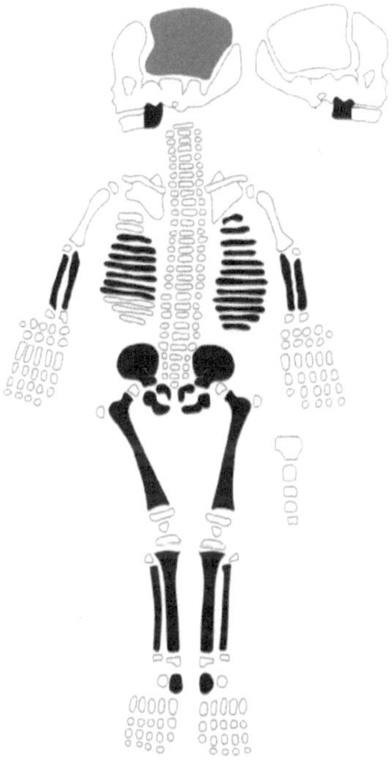

Figure 3.11 Diagram of skeleton 007, from Stylos. In black color are indicated the areas affected with periostitis; in grey color are indicated the areas with porotic hyperostosis

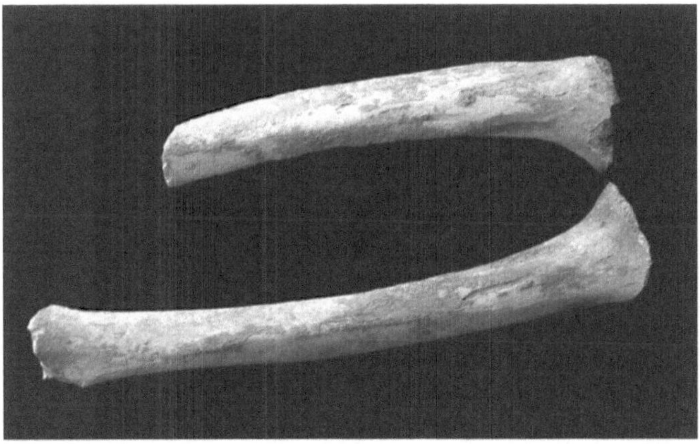

Figure 3.12 Stylos: Skeleton 007, diffuse periosteal reaction on both tibiae (photo: C. Bourbou)

mandible, clavicle and long bones.[94] Although the condition is not fatal in itself, factors such as the general immune status of the individual and nutritional and hygiene conditions may have contributed to the child's death.

Tentative diagnoses include scurvy and hypervitaminosis A. Skeletal evidence for scurvy consists of new bone formation, potentially anywhere on the skeleton; however although woven bone was present on both mandibular rami, other pathognomonic features of the condition are missing due to the fragmentary preservation of the skull, or not present. Diffuse periosteal activity is also present in cases of hypervitaminosis A along with cortical hyperostosis and usually becomes manifested no earlier than the end of the first year of life.[95]

---

[94] Couper, McPhee and Morris 2001. Lesions may be asymmetric, sparing the metaphyses and epiphyses: see Lewis 2007, 144, fig. 7.5.

[95] Resnick 1995, 3345.

Chapter 4

The Byzantine World on a Plate

Evidence from Documentary Sources

Through the process of cooking, raw products are transformed into a signifier of culture where people meet and interact.[1] Recipes surviving from the Byzantine period tell of luxurious feasts offered during imperial dinners, while a daily peasant diet relied on the basic foodstuffs. Both of these settings – an imperial banquet summoning the most prestigious and powerful elite and a traditional meal among members of a peasant family – represent the ideology, rituals and social and moral values of Byzantine society.[2] What did people eat in Byzantine times? The answer to this question has been the main subject of congresses such as the one-day meeting *Food and Cooking in Byzantium* (Museum of Byzantine Culture, Thessaloniki, 2001) and the 37th Spring Symposium of Byzantine Studies, *Eat, Drink and Be Merry (Luke 12:19): Production, Consumption and Celebration of Food and Wine in Byzantium* (University of Birmingham, 2003), and also of special volumes such as *Feast, Fast or Famine: Food and Drink in Byzantium* (Australian Association for Byzantine Studies, 2005). These congresses and publications have focused on topics such as the most frequently consumed foodstuffs, methods of preparation and cooking, and the preservation of various products in Byzantium. But were the Byzantines aware of the nutritional quality and importance of certain foodstuffs and the quantity and frequency of meals needed for a balanced diet, as suggested by Byzantine physicians in their works? Several versions of such a 'dietary calendar' exist, some of them attributed to a certain Hierophilos, which relate that specific categories of products must be consumed according to the season and climate; but it is highly speculative to argue for a widespread and firm application of such a daily regimen.[3]

---

1 Lévi-Strauss 1969.

2 For imperial dinners as a way for the emperor to disseminate political propaganda, see, e.g., Malberg 2007.

3 The dietary comments in these versions are taken from a pamphlet attributed to a certain sophist, Hierophilos, of uncertain date; the name is probably intended to hint at the Herophilos, who was a major figure in classical medicine (335–280 BC); see Romano 1999; Dalby 2003, 161–9; Koder 2007, 67–72.

Documentary evidence and artistic representations have traditionally served as the primary sources of information about the Byzantine diet. Literary sources include regulations for the taxation and sale of foods, physicians' comments on diet, travelers' tales, records of supplies purchased for troops or ships' crews and the dietary regimens at monasteries.[4] Artistic representations such as religious images, illustrations in manuscripts and the mosaics and wall paintings of churches, palaces and houses, especially during the fifth and sixth centuries AD, depict the bounty of nature and the food sources available to the Byzantines.[5] However, one must decipher and extract information from them with caution, due to the artistic conventions, stereotypes and symbolism inherent in these depictions.[6]

Briefly outlined here are the main foodstuffs consumed by the Byzantines as attested in the written sources. Oil, wine and wheat formed the basic elements of the Byzantine diet – what Braudel calls the 'essential trinity' of Mediterranean crops.[7] The grains in primary use appear to have been wheat and barley, especially wheat.[8] Another medieval grain crop was millet, whose importance seems to have varied by region and economic status.[9] Other grains traditionally grown or used include oats, rye and rice.[10] Various legumes, such as broad beans, chickpeas, peas, lentils, vetch and lupins, were also consumed.[11]

---

4 See, e.g., Koukoules 1952, 9–135; Dembinska 1985; Kaplan 1992; Mango and Dagron 1995; Kislinger 1996; Braudel 1998; Bober 1999; Flandrin and Montanari 1996; Talbot 2007.

5 Although mosaics and wall paintings provide images of earthly fruits, agricultural activities, animal husbandry, game, fish and wild fowl, they offer more information on tableware and comestibles than on Byzantine gastronomy and diet; see, e.g., Mundell Mango 2007; Vroom 2007.

6 For a thorough discussion of the use of artistic sources for studying Byzantine food, see Anagnostakis and Papamastorakis 2005, 147–72; Maguire 1987, 2005.

7 Braudel 1966, 215. For the prices of cereals and other important foodstuffs such as oil, wine, meat, cheese and fish, which not only are of interest to the researcher from a statistical point of view but have much to say on Byzantine standards of living, agricultural production and the laws of the market, see Cheynet 2005. On oil and wine, see also Koukoules 1952, 121–9; Anagnostakis 1995, 1996; Koder 2005, 26; Tsougarakis 2007; Stathakopoulos 2007b; Anagnostakis 2008.

8 See Braudel 1966; Teall 1959; Dalby 1996, 2003; Kazhdan 1997; Motsias 1998.

9 In Roman times millet had been considered a food of the poor; see Garnsey 1988; Gallant 1991. The same notion of millet as an inferior food is shared by the Byzantine physician Symeon Seth; see Teall 1959, 99. Matthaiou 1997 also argues that millet was taxed at a lower rate than other grains in Ottoman Greece.

10 Oats and rye were of minor significance, but rice became quite important in later times; Dalby 1996.

11 Vetches were commonly used as animal feed or sown to enrich soil, while lupins were eaten by both humans and animals, becoming more important as a human food when

Historical documents indicate that sheep, goats, pigs, chickens and cattle were the main domesticated animals in the Byzantine countryside, with sheep and goats predominating.[12] In addition to domesticated animals and birds, hunted and collected meat was likely included in the diet.[13] Since meat turns bad quickly, it was often processed.[14] Freezing and freeze-drying as well as smoking of food were not common in Byzantine times.[15] The use of snow and ice for preserving meat is mentioned in the *Geoponica*, but this seems to be an exception and not a practice in daily use.[16] The most effective way of preserving meat must have been a combination of drying and salting.[17] The milk of sheep and goats was predominantly used for the production of dairy products such as cheese,[18] yogurt and butter.[19] Less frequently mentioned is another dairy preparation, *trachanas*, a dried mixture of milk, cheese and roasted grain.[20]

Most of the marine species known to have been consumed in the Roman era are also mentioned in Byzantine times.[21] More than 110 names of fishes and about 30 names of other aquatic organisms are found in the Byzantine literature.

---

other crops failed; Dalby 1996; Motsias 1998.

12 Faunal remains retrieved for stable isotope analysis from the sites of Eleutherna, Sourtara and Kastella include sheep, goat, pig, dog and red deer (see below). Published analyses of animal bones from Byzantine contexts are rare; see, e.g., Nobis 1993; Mylona 2008a, in her study of the animal remains from the middle Byzantine house at Pyrgi (Hagia Anna), has identified nine different species, including donkey, cow, pig, sheep, goat, wild goat, red deer, chicken and possible hare or rabbit. Sheep outnumber goats, while pigs and cows are the next most commonly encountered animals. Mylona 1997, 2003, 2008b has also studied animal remains from the late Roman/early Byzantine (fifth to seventh centuries AD) house complex at Itanos in east Crete. Besides the great number of fish bones (see below), the sample also included mammal and bird remains.

13 Dembinska 1985; Kazhdan 1997; Dalby 2003; Motsias 1998. Koder 2005, 22 argues that no veal was consumed and that chicken was not frequently consumed.

14 Frost 1999; Anagnostakis 2005, 88–90; Grünbart 2007, 45–8.

15 Hellmann 1990; Koder 2007, 60.

16 *Geoponica* (ed. Beckh 1895), XIX.9.2; Weber 1980, 83.

17 For a brief overview of the process, see Grünbart 2007, 48.

18 Braudel 1966; Kazhdan 1997; Dalby 2003, 72–4.

19 Motsias 1998.

20 This was a travel food, prepared for consumption simply by stirring it into hot water. It was important to soldiers and shepherds; Hill and Bryer 1995.

21 A variety of fishes are portrayed as the protagonists of the satire *Psarologos* (ed. Krumbacher 1903). See also Koukoules 1952, 79–88 (on the various species) and 331–41 (on the fishing modes and devices applied); Dagron 1995; Braund 1995; Dalby 1996; Maniatis 2000; Kislinger 2005, 52. Reports on fish remains from Byzantine sites are rare. The very rich assemblage recovered at Itanos included small and large fishes of coastal varieties, belonging to members of four families: sea breams (Sparidae), parrot-fish (Scaridae), groupers/combers

Most of the information has been retrieved from medical texts, whose writers are dealing with food and nutrition. In these texts fishes are classified into categories based on their physiology (*sklirosarkoi*, *skilorosarkoi plateis*, *malakosarkoi* or *apalosarkoi* and *mesaioi*) and origin (*aigialodeis* or *aigialeioi*, *petraioi*, *pelagioi*, *thalassioi*, *potamioi* and *limnaioi*), since these are determining factors for the nutritional value of each species.[22] Preserved fish (salted or dried) and preserved fish eggs such as caviar (sturgeon eggs) and botargo (salted and pressed mullet roe) were likely to have been important; additionally, there is evidence for the use of fish sauce (*garum*).[23] However, Koder argues that *garum* was not common or popular between the early Byzantine period and the eleventh century, or even later, since the word *garon* is rarely found outside lexica and medical texts.[24]

Finally, fruits (grapes, figs, melon), vegetables (celery, lettuce, endive, cress, kohlrabi, turnips, eggplant, cabbage) and wild vegetables gathered in season were also included in the Byzantine menu.[25] Nuts (almonds, chestnuts, pistachios, walnuts, pine nuts) appear to have also formed a significant portion of the diet.[26] Known and well appreciated was honey, which also served as a basic component of various desserts.[27]

Archaeological findings and medical and hagiographical texts provide useful information on practices of feeding the newborn. The topic of the cruel separation of young mothers and their breastfeeding infants by death is often found in funerary inscriptions from the Byzantine period. An example of these is the inscription (sixth century AD ?) associated with a funerary monument found in the area of the Panathenaic Stadium, commemorating a young mother whose death left her children 'in need of milk'.[28] Magico-religious actions associated

---

(Serranidae) and picarels (Centracanthidae). Turtle and seashell remains were also included. For these remains, see Mylona 1997, 2003, 2008b; for the excavation, see Greco et al. 1998.

22 See, e.g., Chrone-Vakalopoulos and Vakalopoulos 2008; the authors provide a systematic terminology of the fishes and the various aquatic organisms attested in the Byzantine sources, and identify each species with its current scientific name.

23 Dalby 1996. For the preparation of *garum* see Koder 2005, 24–5.

24 Koder 2007, 72.

25 To make fruits available the whole year, drying was the simplest and commonest process; see Grünbart 2007, 43–4. Vegetables were consumed fresh, dried or preserved in salt and vinegar, like modern pickles; see Koukoules 1952, 88–102; Teall 1959, 98–100; Koder 1992, 1995, 2005, 23–4; Littlewood, Maguire and Wolschke-Bulmahn 2002; Dalby 2003, 74–7; Anagnostakis and Papamastorakis 2005, 158–66. A wealth of information on fruits and vegetables can be found in the Byzantine poem *Porikologos* (ed. Winterwerb 1992).

26 Motsias 1998.

27 Anagnostakis 2000; Koder 2005, 26.

28 Sironen 1997, 236, no. 195, translates the text of the inscription as follows: 'The good Athenodora of Attica, the religious wife of Thaumasius, who gave birth to little children

with mothers failing to produce milk for their newborns, such as the use of specific herbs or amulets made of *galatopetra*, are also attested.[29] Although the archaeological record has not yet revealed any examples of feeding-vessels from the Byzantine period, we can securely assume that they existed, as written sources attest attempts at artificial feeding.[30] The hagiographical text describing the Vita of St Theodore Tiron (the Recruit) relates that after the death of Theodore's mother, his father succeeded in manufacturing a breast-shaped glass vessel for feeding the infant until solid food could be introduced.[31]

Byzantine physicians included in their works chapters on the care of the newborn and especially on perinatal nutrition, conveying the eclectic knowledge of physicians of the Roman imperial period, such as Rufus and Soranus from Ephesus (first century AD), enriched with additional remarks and clarifications based on their own experience.[32] Oribasius gave detailed information concerning a child's nutrition from birth through the age of 14, focusing mainly on the first two years,[33] and Aetius of Amida and Paul of Aegina followed Oribasius' recommendations on perinatal nutrition and weaning patterns.

Although physicians advised a considerable wait between birth and the onset of nursing, breastmilk was seen as the infant's ideal food. During in-utero life the growing fetus receives all essential nutrients via placenta transfer from the mother. After birth breastmilk provides the newborn with immunological protection and a supply of nutrients, as it contains over 100 different constituents that contribute to the health, growth and development of the newborn.[34] Physicians in the past failed to recognize the nutritional and immunological importance of colostrum, which is present in the first few days after birth and is replaced by mature milk by the tenth day of breastfeeding. Due to its different color (lemony-yellow) and consistency, it was often denied to the newborn. Oribasius was specific in urging that the child ought not to be fed colostrum, which he felt

---

and nursed the infants, the soil has taken away the young mother and holds her while the little children are in need of milk.'

29 Papamichael-Koutroumpa 1977–78.

30 In Western Europe some rare examples of medieval feeding-vessels have been found; see, e.g., Coulon 1994; Crawford 1999.

31 *Vita of Theodore Tiron* (Sigalas 1925), 225. For a discussion of this testimony, see Kiousopoulou 1997, 67; Rey 2004, 373.

32 An approach to the study of perinatal nutrition and weaning patterns as attested in the sources and their relevance to the isotopic signature of chemical analysis is included in the paper by Bourbou and Garvie-Lok 2009; see also Rey 2004.

33 Beaucamp 1982.

34 For example, carbohydrates in the form of lactose prevent the development of rickets, while iron and zinc are essential for growth. See the thorough discussion in Lewis 2007, 97–9.

to be harmful. He argued that immediately after birth the newborn must be fed with clear honey of high quality, followed by drops of a lukewarm solution of honey and water (*hydromel*) to be given slowly over the subsequent four days, and he advised against feeding a newborn other foods, including butter, which he thought was too heavy for the stomach of the newborn.[35] After this period nursing could commence, with the infant receiving two or three meals per day. Aetius of Amida and Paul of Aegina, following Oribasius, suggested as well that the first food given to a newborn should be honey, and afterward milk.[36] The attention that medical writers devote to the proper selection of a wet nurse suggests that often a child would not be nursed by its own mother.[37] Beaucamp's research confirms the high degree to which the medical texts reflect ordinary behavior. Her results, based on the investigation of late Antique Egyptian documents, suggest that although hiring a wet nurse was considered the ideal, this was not usually possible for the poor.[38]

Medical writers, in general, saw weaning as a fairly serious step to be approached with caution, and suggested a gradual weaning process.[39] Soranus indicated that before the age of 6 months, when a baby's body becomes firm

---

35 *Oribasius* (Raeder 1928–33), V, 5. Soranus suggested that a newborn must stay away from any kind of food for at least two days, until its body was fully recovered from the process of birth. After this interval, the baby should be given food to lick, such as *hydromel* or honey mixed with goat's milk. Soranus rejected other popular choices of butter, southernwood with butter, nosesmart or kneaded barley meal for this first food, claiming that they were too hard on the child's sensitive gastrointestinal system, *Soranos d'Ephèse* (ed. and tr. Burguière, Gourevitch and Malinas 1990), II, 11; Temkin 1991, 88. Medieval writers in Western Europe as well denied colostrum to the newborn; instead a newborn was fed with butter, the oil of sweet almonds, sugar, honey and the syrup of wines; Fildes 1986, 1995; Orme 2001 58–60, 66.

36 *Aetius of Amida* (Olivieri 1935), IV, 3; *Paul of Aegina* (Heiberg 1921 and 1924), I, 5.

37 *Oribasius* (Raeder 1928–33), V, 2–3; *Aetius of Amida* (Olivieri 1935), IV, 4–6; *Paul of Aegina* (Heiberg 1921 and 1924), I, 2–3. Soranus suggested that breastmilk should come from a wet-nurse for the first 20 days, as mother's milk was in most cases unwholesome during this period; *Soranos d'Ephèse* (ed. and tr. Burguière, Gourevitch and Malinas 1990), II, 12–14; Temkin 1991, 90–101. Although Soranus argued that after the initial 20 days a baby should ideally be nursed by its mother, he also commented that a wet-nurse was preferable in many cases to prevent exhaustion of the mother; *Soranos d'Ephèse* (ed. and tr. Burguière, Gourevitch and Malinas 1990), II, 11; Temkin 1991, 90.

38 Beaucamp 1982.

39 Medieval writers in western Europe also recommended the gradual cessation of breastfeeding by about 2 years of age; Shahar 1990. Liquid or semi-liquid foods such as animal milk, gruel or pap (a mixture of flour and bread cooked in water) might be given prior to the emergence of the first teeth, before about 6 to 9 months of age; afterwards other foods might be introduced; Fildes 1986, 1995, 101–26.

enough to tolerate solid food, an infant should be fed only milk.[40] At 6 months the first solid food could be given: crumbs of bread softened with *hydromel*, milk, sweet wine or honey with wine. Later an infant could also be given soup made of spelt, very moist porridge or an egg cooked soft enough to be sipped.[41] The introduction of solid foods at around 6 months of age did not herald an abrupt weaning process. Instead, Soranus advised a diet of breastmilk supplemented by the soft solid foods described above for at least another year. When development of the teeth allowed an infant to chew more solid foods, at around 18 to 24 months, Soranus recommended that gradual weaning of the infant should begin.[42] Oribasius was in agreement with this general time frame, treating the time before the age of 2 as the period during which the child would be nourished by milk.[43] The same notion is shared by Aetius of Amida, recommending weaning at around 20 months, and by Paul of Aegina, suggesting that a child may be brought up on milk until the age of 2 years; afterwards its diet may be changed to cereal food.[44]

Useful information about the age of weaning can also be found in the *Vitae* and miracles of saints. In the Miracles of St Thekla a child who has just been weaned is said to be old enough to walk and run, suggesting that it was at least 18 months old.[45] In the Vita of Symeon Stylites the Younger, Symeon, after his baptism at age 2, refused to nurse from his mother as she had eaten meat that had been sacrificed to idols, indicating that children could still be breastfeeding at age 2; the hagiographer also relates that when Symeon began to eat solid food his mother gave him honey on bread to eat and water to drink.[46] The Vita of St Alypios relates that the saint was taken to church by his mother at the age of 3 after his father had died, and that at this point he had already been weaned.[47] In the Vita of Michael Synkellos we see a reference to a boy who had been weaned and had reached the age of 3 years.[48] Finally, the Vita of Basil the Younger

---

40 Soranus rejected the early introduction of cereal food, commonly given as soon as 40 days after birth; *Soranos d'Ephèse* (ed. and tr. Burguière, Gourevitch and Malinas 1990), II, 21; Temkin 1991, 117.

41 *Soranos d'Ephèse* (ed. and tr. Burguière, Gourevitch and Malinas 1990), II, 21; Temkin 1991, 117.

42 *Soranos d'Ephèse* (ed. and tr. Burguière, Gourevitch and Malinas 1990), II, 21; Temkin 1991, 118–19.

43 *Oribasius* (Raeder 1928–33), V, 5.

44 *Aetius of Amida* (Olivieri 1935), book IV, 28; *Paul of Aegina* (Heiberg 1921 and 1924), book I, 5.

45 *Vita of Saint Thekla* (ed. Dagron 1978), mir. 24, p. 350.

46 *Vita of Symeon Stylites the Younger* (ed. van de Ven 1962), ch. 5–6, p. 7.

47 *Vita of Saint Alypios* (ed. Delehaye 1923), 149.

48 *Vita of Michael Synkellos* (ed. Cunningham 1991), 46.

includes a description of a woman holding in her arms a sickly child aged 4 years who was breastfeeding.[49]

Thus, the written sources suggest a weaning process that was generally quite gradual. Although physicians advised that breastmilk be withheld for a period immediately after birth, they recommended that the child should be nursed for some time. While the introduction of solid food by roughly 6 months of age was suggested, the child was not to be weaned abruptly at this time; rather, adult foods were to be introduced gradually and the child would not have been completely weaned until the age of 2, if not later. The *Vitae* and miracles of the saints suggest that this advice was heeded (or, perhaps, that it reflected common practice), as they suggest that there was a prolonged period of weaning and that nursing persisted until a child was at least 2 years of age and, in some cases, as old as 4 years.

Are We What We Eat?

Documentary evidence has been traditionally used to reconstruct past diets and weaning patterns. The study of specific pathological conditions, such as dental diseases or metabolic disorders, has also been used to indicate the type and quality of diet. In recent decades the application of stable isotope analysis of human remains has provided an alternative source that has greatly contributed to the investigation of dietary patterns in past populations. Together documentary and isotopic evidence have the potential to provide a detailed portrait of diet and weaning in the past. The following sections will present basic background information on stable isotope analysis and a number of issues that must be taken under consideration in order to securely interpret the chemical signature on human remains when projected against documentary evidence.

Stable Isotope Analysis: Some Essentials

Isotopes are chemical elements with the same number of protons in their nuclei, but different numbers of neutrons.[50] They are basically the same in terms of their chemical properties, but differ slightly in weight. Carbon has two stable isotopes (^{12}C and ^{13}C), as does nitrogen (^{14}N and ^{15}N); for both elements the lighter stable isotope (^{12}C, ^{14}N) is abundant, while the heavier (^{13}C, ^{15}N) is much rarer. The relative content of the two carbon or nitrogen isotopes in a material

---

[49] *Vita of Basil the Younger* (ed.Viliskij 1911), 316.37.

[50] For more detailed information on the measurement and behavior of stable isotopes, see Hoefs 2004.

is expressed by its stable carbon isotope ratio ($\delta^{13}C$ value) or stable nitrogen isotope ratio ($\delta^{15}N$ value). These express the ratio of one isotope to another in terms of its departure in per mil (‰) from the value of an international standard, with a negative value indicating depletion in the heavier isotope relative to the standard, and a positive value indicating enrichment.[51] Typically, the $\delta^{13}C$ values of living organisms are negative and their $\delta^{15}N$ values are positive.

The stable isotopes of an element are essentially identical chemically, participating in the same reactions to produce the same molecules. However, the slight difference in their weights can cause one isotope to participate in a reaction more readily than the other, causing the stable isotope value of the products of the reaction to differ from that of the reactants. This and other mass-dependent processes cause variation in the stable isotope ratios of different substances. For living organisms this variation follows a predictable pattern, allowing aspects of diet and behavior to be inferred from the stable isotope ratios reflected in bone collagen, the structural protein of the bone tissue.[52] The main aim of most isotopic analyses is to use the carbon isotope ratio ($\delta^{13}C$) to determine the amounts of marine vs. terrestrial foods, or C_3 vs. C_4 plant foods (or animal products), as well as to obtain further information on the protein sources from the nitrogen isotope value ($\delta^{15}N$), such as the amount of animal vs. plant protein.[53]

Following the first documentation of the effects of nursing and weaning on human $\delta^{15}N$ values, stable nitrogen isotope analysis has been used to study nursing and weaning in a number of archaeological human populations.[54] This

---

51 The primary standard for carbon is a marine carbonate fossil from the PeeDee formation in South Carolina and is referred to as PDB (for PeeDee belemnite), and the standard for nitrogen is atmospheric nitrogen, which is referred to as AIR; Katzenberg 2000, 313, table 11.2.

52 Katzenberg 2000; Mays 2000; Sealy 2001.

53 See, e.g., Bocherens et al. 1991; White, Healy and Schwarcz 1993; Ubelaker, Katzenberg and Doyon 1995; Mays 1997; Richards et al. 1998; Herrscher et al. 2001; Herrscher 2003; Polet and Katzenberg 2003; Müldner and Richards 2005; Jay and Richards 2006; Richards, Fuller and Molleson 2006; Müldner and Richards 2007a, 2007b; Salamon et al. 2008; Rutgers et al. 2009; Keenleyside, Schwarcz and Panayotova 2006; Keenleyside et al. 2009; Craig et al. 2009.

54 See, e.g., Katzenberg, Saunders and Fitzgerald 1993; Katzenberg and Pfeiffer 1995; Katzenberg, Herring and Saunders 1996; Schurr 1997; Herring, Saunders and Katzenberg 1998; Wright and Schwarcz 1999; Dupras, Schwarcz and Fairgrieve 2001; Richards, Mays and Fuller 2002; Fuller, Richards and Mays 2003; Prowse et al. 2004; Schurr and Powell 2005; Williams, White and Longstaffe 2005; Fuller et al. 2006a; Fuller et al. 2006b; Richards, Fuller and Molleson 2006; Clayton, Sealy and Pfeiffer 2006; Dupras and Tocheri 2007; Jay et al. 2008.

application is possible because changes in the $\delta^{15}N$ value of an infant's diet are also reflected in its bone collagen. The most common approach to studying weaning through archaeological remains is the study of bone samples from a number of infants and children in a burial group. These samples are analyzed and their $\delta^{15}N$ values are plotted by age at death and compared to the mean value for adult females in the population. Typically, such studies show $\delta^{15}N$ values for neonates that are similar to those of adult females. The values then rise fairly rapidly to roughly one trophic level above the mean adult female value as nursing incorporates ^{15}N-enriched collagen into the bones. After a given age, they begin to drop again; the point at which this drop begins is taken to be the age by which weaning typically began for the population in question. Observations made on fingernail clippings of modern human mothers and their babies show how this effect leads to shifting $\delta^{15}N$ values in the tissues of infants as they are born, nurse and are weaned.[55]

Generally speaking, bone as a tissue is slow to turn over, and the bones of adults may retain the isotopic signal of an earlier diet for many years. However, bone turnover in a rapidly growing infant is considerably faster, especially in small and porous bones such as the ribs. Observations on large samples of infants from archaeological skeletal populations have led researchers such as Katzenberg, Herring and Saunders, and Richards, Mays and Fuller to suggest that the lag time between weaning and a shift in infant rib $\delta^{15}N$ value is quite brief, on the order of a few months or less.[56] Although powerful, this application of stable nitrogen isotope analysis has its limitations and requires caution; for example, the onset of a drop in $\delta^{15}N$ values must be taken as the time by which weaning had typically begun for a population, rather than a precise estimate of weaning age, and problems arise from differences between the approach taken in weaning healthy and sick infants, as the weaning pattern reflected in the deceased infants from a burial population is more likely to reflect the approach preferred for an unhealthy child.[57] Because of these issues, and because of a certain normal variation in weaning age expected for any population, it is preferable to examine a large number of infants from several sites before weaning practices in a given era can be confidently reconstructed.

---

[55] Fogel, Tuross and Owsley 1989.

[56] Katzenberg, Herring and Saunders 1996; Richards, Mays and Fuller 2002.

[57] For some discussions of these, see Katzenberg, Herring and Saunders 1996; Fuller et al. 2006a, 2006b.

The Relative Importance of Foodstuffs in the Byzantine Diet

In many cases the written sources do not identify the actual consumption of specific products in the Byzantine diet. Surveying various Byzantine texts, Koder notes that certain vegetables were a non-recommended and low-esteemed food.[58] Although elaborate recipes survive for legumes, such as chickpeas and lentils flavored with imported spices, the reliance on legumes is less clear than for grain.[59] The available data suggest that the real consumption levels of legumes were sometimes quite low.[60] Similarly, assessing the frequency of consumption of various marine species and meat, which would have varied regionally and seasonally, is problematic.[61] Some animals were sold in the markets during specific seasons, such as lamb for Easter. In general, some written sources suggest fairly regular meat consumption, while others refer to it only in association with special occasions.[62]

Differential Access to the Products

Social discrimination is marked in a number of products, targeting even basic elements of the diet, such as bread. Various types of bread existed, differing in quality. Bread of lower quality, for example, *mesos* or *mesokatharos artos*, was the bread of the poor, as was *ryparos artos*, bread made of bran or barley.[63] In a lower-status diet, one based on grain and legumes, oil would have provided the main source of fat and a considerable source of calories.[64] Dairy products had special importance in rural diets. However, cheese is also included in urban diets. While some cheeses, such as Vlach, were luxury foods, others appear to have been cheap enough to appear in lower-status diets.[65] Meat of good quality was expensive. It is reasonable to assume that the upper classes must have consumed proportionally

---

58 Koder 2007, 67–71.

59 For a thorough discussion of spices used during Byzantine times, see Dalby 2002; 2007.

60 Koder 1992.

61 Dagron 1995; Braund 1995; Maniatis 2000; Dalby 2003, 66–9.

62 Dalby 1996, 196; Kazhdan 1997, 55. For example, Koder 2005, 22, argues that meat consumption was in general restricted, and that during the summer and in hot climates it was considered dangerous to consume for it decomposed quickly. See also the publication on vegetarianism and the consumption of meat in late Antiquity and Byzantium by Parry 2005.

63 Koder 2007, 65–6.

64 Braudel 1966; Dalby 1996; Koder 2005.

65 Koder 2005, 20.

higher amounts of it, but the consumption by the average Byzantine person is in more doubt.[66]

Feasting or Fasting? Dining Habits and Fasting Rules of the Byzantine Diet

Dining and fasting habits further complicate any attempt to reconstruct the diet during the Byzantine period. What type of food really belonged to the everyday diet of the Byzantines? Direct written evidence regarding everyday meals and drinks in Byzantium barely exists, in part because people almost never wrote down commonplace or self-evident details of everyday life. Koder provides a basic description of the dining habits and everyday diet of the general population.[67] Normally there were two daily meals: *ariston* or *geuma* was the first meal of the day, sometime late in the morning or at noon; the second meal, *deipnon*, was consumed early in the evening and usually before sunset. A hot cooked meal was usually served only once a day, as *deipnon*, for reasons that range from the great amount of time required to reheat the fireplace to the high cost and shortage of fuel.[68] The basis of the everyday diet for the majority of the population was bread and soup, presumably both of low quality. Such soup included *hagiozoumin*, basically consisting of water, onions, salt, marjoram and a little oil. *Atheras* was another cheap soup, made of semolina or bulgur boiled in water or milk, with drops of oil or other cooking fat.[69] Meat and fish were highly appreciated by the Byzantines, but the high prices of good-quality products, as well as fasting restrictions, prohibited regular consumption of them in large quantities.[70]

Although we should not overestimate the adherence to fasting by the people as a whole, fasting played a significant role in daily diet, since the Byzantines had to refrain from eating specific foodstuffs, especially meat, for a considerable portion of the year.[71] The early Christians took the idea of fasting as a religious practice from Jewish tradition, and by the fourth century it had become a highly praised form of behavior, signifying the struggle for holiness and perfection. For ordinary Christians the figure of the self-mortifying ascetic was an ideal to

---

66 Koder 2005, 22; 2007, 59–61.

67 Koder 2005, 17–19; 2007, 62.

68 Materials used for fuel included various types of wood, charcoal, dried dung and scrubland; see Koder 2007, 63; Dunn 1992, 240–49.

69 Koder 2007, 70.

70 Koder 2005, 22–3; 2007, 70–71.

71 Koder 2005, 19 and 2007, 61, notes that the Byzantines had to fast for at least 144 days a year in addition to the usual fasting days of Wednesdays and Fridays. For a thorough overview of fasting rules, see Nicholas and Louvaris 2005; for meat as a target product in fasting rules, see Parry 2005, 178–86.

admire, especially for monks and, most of all, virgins. Jerome (AD 345-420), advising young women on the rules according to which virgins of the Church ought to live, urges extreme frugality in relation to food (recommending vegetables, wheaten bread and occasionally a little fish) and the avoidance of wine.[72] Given this close association of fasting and sexual abstinence in early Christian tradition, it is quite possible that there was a difference in the early Christian era between the kinds and quantities of food eaten by men and by women. Because rules of fasting specifically targeted some key animal products in the diet, they should be considered when reconstructing Byzantine diets.[73]

The Likely $\delta^{13}C$ and $\delta^{15}N$ Values of Some of the Foodstuffs in the Byzantine Diet

Most food plants consumed by the Byzantines, including wheat, barley, legumes, olives and grapes, are C_3 plants, which tend to have tissue $\delta^{13}C$ values in the -33‰ to -22‰ range, with a mean value around -26.5‰.[74] Millet, which is mentioned in the sources,[75] is among the C_4 plants, which tend to have tissue $\delta^{13}C$ values in the -20‰ to -9‰ range, with a mean value around -13‰.[76] The $\delta^{13}C$ values of meat and milk from Byzantine domesticated animals would reflect their diet, with meat somewhat enriched relative to the diet[77] and milk showing a value close to that of the diet.[78] Analyses of domesticated fauna from sites in Greece of Byzantine or slightly later date yielded average collagen $\delta^{13}C$ values of -21.5‰ to -19.6‰ for sheep and goats, -20.3‰ to -19.6‰ for pigs

---

72 Grimm 1995, 233–6.

73 See also Kislinger 1996, 199–201. Monks formed a special segment of the population, for their fasting included more days throughout the year; see Dembinska 1985; Talbot 2007.

74 Bender 1971; Smith and Epstein 1971; Deines 1980. Olive oil, which may have contributed substantially to the Byzantine diet, has low $\delta^{13}C$ values characteristic of lipids, falling in the -30‰ to -27‰ range; see Spangenberg, Macko and Hunziker 1998; Royer et al. 1999.

75 Teall 1959, 99.

76 Bender 1968, 1971; Smith and Epstein 1971; Deines 1980.

77 See, e.g., Vogel 1978; Tieszen et al. 1983; Tieszen and Boutton 1989; Hare et al. 1991.

78 Data for dairy cattle show whole milk $\delta^{13}C$ to fall within about 3‰ of the animal's fodder; see Minson, Ludlow and Troughton 1975; Tyrrell et al. 1984; Boutton et al. 1988; Metges, Kempe and Schmidt 1990. The $\delta^{13}C$ value of casein, the primary protein of milk, is typically a little higher than that of whole milk; see Nakamura et al. 1982; Kornexl et al. 1997.

and -21.4‰ to -20.2‰ for cows, indicating generally C_3-based fodder.[79] The other major source of potential $\delta^{13}C$ patterning in the Byzantine diet would have been the distinctive values of marine resources. Analysis of a number of modern Aegean food-fish species yielded an average $\delta^{13}C$ value of -17.0‰ for small, low-trophic-level fish (sardine and anchovy) and one of -15.2‰ for larger species of higher trophic level.[80]

When it comes to likely $\delta^{15}N$ values, legumes – a potentially important item in the Byzantine diet – would have had low $\delta^{15}N$ values close to 0‰.[81] The $\delta^{15}N$ values of other plants in the Byzantine diet would fall close to the $\delta^{15}N$ values of the nitrogenous compounds in the soils they grew in, which would vary according to local conditions.[82] Analyses of domesticated fauna from some Byzantine-era sites in Greece found collagen $\delta^{15}N$ values for sheep and goats ranging from 4.0‰ to 6.1‰, for cattle ranging from 3.5‰ to 6.0‰ and for pigs ranging from 3.6‰ to 6.1‰.[83] Values for the animals' meat and milk protein would have been similar.[84] Subtracting a 4‰ trophic level enrichment from these collagen values suggests low $\delta^{15}N$ values in the 0‰ to 2‰ range for plants in the animals' diets; however, extension of these estimates to the $\delta^{15}N$ value of the plants eaten by humans is problematic.[85] Analysis of a number of modern Aegean food-fish species yielded an average $\delta^{15}N$ value of 6.5‰ for small, low-

---

79 Garvie-Lok 2001; Bourbou and Richards 2007. Samples for some sites extend into the early modern period; however, no significant temporal variation in faunal stable isotope values was seen at those sites; see Garvie-Lok 2001. While average $\delta^{13}C$ values indicate feeding on C_3 resources, a few individual animals have values suggesting a minor C_4 component in their diet; see Bourbou and Richards 2007.

80 Garvie-Lok 2001. Although the impact of recent industrial pollution may have altered Aegean food web $\delta^{13}C$ values, it can still be assumed that marine resources would have contributed an enriched $\delta^{13}C$ signal to Byzantine diets.

81 This assumes that they were cultivated as part of a rotation, in part to restore the available nitrogen of the soil; if grown in soils with abundant available nitrogen, legume values can be similar to those of non-legumes; see Kohl, Shearer and Harper 1980.

82 Delwiche et al. 1979; Kohl and Shearer 1980; Virginia and Delwiche 1982; Shearer et al. 1983; Schoeninger and DeNiro 1984.

83 Garvie-Lok 2001; Bourbou and Richards 2007.

84 Steele and Daniel 1978; DeNiro and Epstein 1978; Hare et al. 1991; Kornexl et al. 1997.

85 There are a number of potential problems with this method, including the possibility that domesticates were fed stems and other waste from legume crops, which would lower their tissue $\delta^{15}N$ values, and the possibility, suggested by Bogaard et al. 2007, that the $\delta^{15}N$ of grain eaten by humans was elevated due to manuring of fields (see below).

trophic-level fish (sardine and anchovy) and one of 10.5‰ for larger species of higher trophic level (Table 4.1).[86]

Table 4.1 Likely $\delta^{13}C$ and $\delta^{15}N$ values for some items of the Byzantine diet

Dietary item	Likely $\delta^{13}C$ values	Likely $\delta^{15}N$ values
C_3 plants	-33‰ to -22‰ range	
C_4 plants	-20‰ to -9‰ range	
Olive oil	-30‰ to -27‰ range	
Sheep and goat	-21.5‰ to -19.6‰	4.0‰ to 6.1‰
Pig	-20.3‰ to -19.6‰	3.6‰ to 6.1‰
Cow	-21.4‰ to -20.2‰	3.5‰ to 6.0‰
Small, low-trophic level fishes (sardine, anchovy)	-17.0‰	6.5‰
Large species	-15.2‰	10.5‰

Isotopic Analysis in Greece

Previous Isotopic Work

In recent years, stable isotope analysis has been widely applied on Greek skeletal populations. The majority of such analyses have included prehistoric material from the Neolithic and Bronze Age periods.[87] A smaller number of studies have included material from the Classical, Hellenistic and Roman periods.[88] Stable isotope analysis in Greek populations was the topic of a special session organized by A. Papathanasiou and M.P. Richards in 2006 during the 16th

---

86 Garvie-Lok 2001. As with $\delta^{13}C$ values, the impact of recent industrial pollution (especially fertilizer-laden runoff from agricultural areas) may have altered Aegean foodweb $\delta^{15}N$. However, it is still a safe assumption that marine resources would have contributed an enriched $\delta^{15}N$ signal to Byzantine diets.

87 Richards and Hedges 1999; Papathanasiou, Larsen and Norr 2000; Papathanasiou 2001; Triantaphyllou 2001; Papathanasiou 2003; Iezzi 2005; Vika 2007; Lagia, Petroutsa and Manolis 2007; Petroutsa, Richards and Manolis 2007; Richards and Hedges 2008; Richards and Vika 2008; Triantaphyllou et al. 2008; Papathanasiou, Richards and Zachou 2009; Petroutsa et al. 2009; Petroutsa and Manolis 2010; Triantaphyllou et al. 2008, Richards and Zachou 2009; Papathanasiou forthcoming; Iezzi forthcoming; Triantaphyllou and Richards forthcoming.

88 Vika 2007; Vika, Aravantinos and Richards 2009; Vika et al. forthcoming; Lagia and Richards forthcoming.

European Meeting of the Paleopathological Association in Santorini (Greece).[89] Isotopic data show that at the majority of prehistoric sites there was a primarily C_3 terrestrial diet and no evidence for significant consumption of marine food or C_4 plants such as millet.[90] The only exceptions for marine consumption were the high-status individuals buried within Grave Circles A and B at Mycenae, where there was clear evidence for such consumption, perhaps of up to 20–25% for some individuals.[91] Vika Aravantinos and Richards[92] suggest that the increased nitrogen values in humans from Classical Thebes (some 5‰ higher $\delta^{15}N$ values than the prehistoric data) are possibly indicative of freshwater fish consumption, and found support for this idea in the documentary evidence of the era. Finally, a study that investigated the breastfeeding and weaning patterns of the Bronze Age population of Lerna suggests that weaning must have started at or before the age of 2.5 years to 3 years. Interestingly, in the same study one 4-year-old individual provided evidence for late weaning, with very positive $\delta^{13}C$ and $\delta^{15}N$ values ($\delta^{13}C$ value: -19.1‰; $\delta^{15}N$ value: 9.2‰).[93]

Isotopic Analysis of Byzantine Populations

Materials and Methods

Stable isotope analysis has proved to be a useful tool for the reconstruction of Byzantine diet and attitudes toward breastfeeding and weaning.[94] In this section all available data from nine sites in Greece are brought together in order to present as complete a picture as possible of diet and weaning patterns for the period in question.[95] Together these studies offer information on the diets and weaning

89 Papers presented at this session and additional contributions will appear in a forthcoming volume of the Occasional Wiener Laboratory Series (OWLS).

90 A case of, most likely, millet consumption is suggested for a single adult individual from Kalamaki as evidenced by the enriched $\delta^{13}C$ values; Richards and Vika 2008.

91 Richards and Hedges 1999, 2008; and see the discussion on the archaeology of fishing in the Bronze Age Aegean in Mylona 2008b, 11–12.

92 Vika, Aravantinos and Richards 2009.

93 Triantaphyllou et al. 2008.

94 Data on trace element analysis are available for the populations of Gortyn in Crete – Fornaciari, Ceccanti and Menicagli 1988; and Korytiani in Epirus – Georgakopoulou and Xirotiris 2009, 211–15; however, due to the limitations inherent in this type of analysis and since only stable isotope data will be discussed here, these studies are excluded.

95 An initial attempt to survey all available isotopic data for Byzantine populations is presented in the paper by Bourbou and Garvie-Lok forthcoming, where the isotopic data from five sites in Greece (Abdera, Kastella, Nemea, Petras and Servia) are discussed.

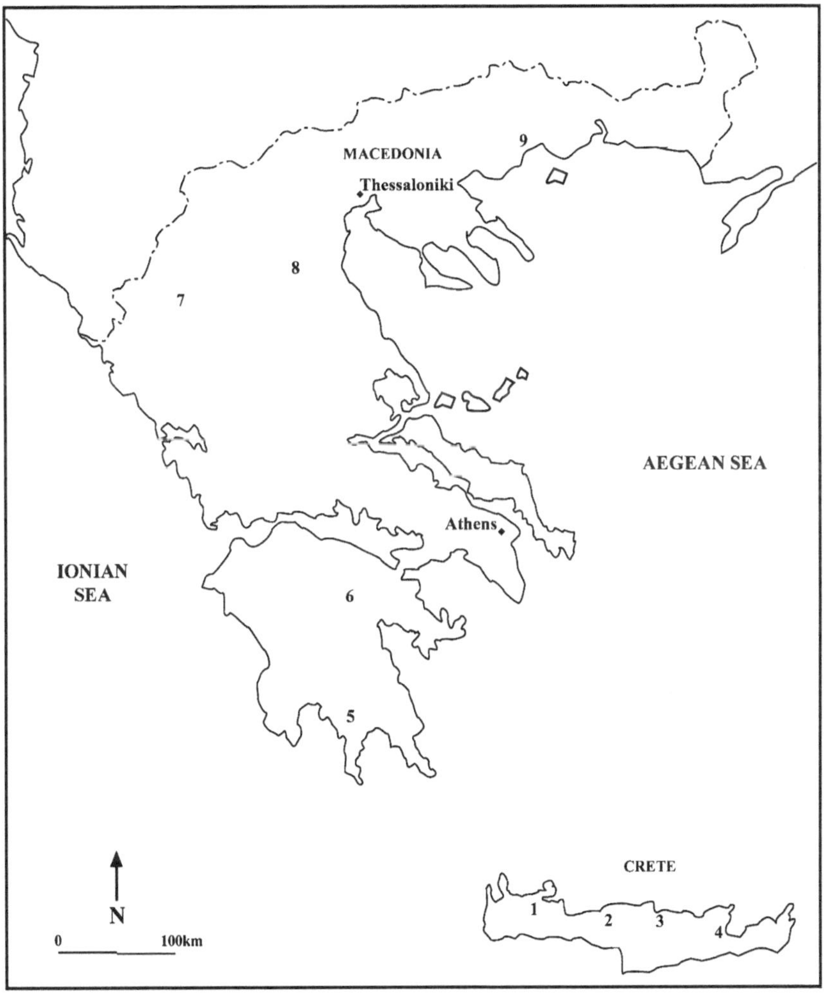

Figure 4.1 Map of sites from which bone samples are taken

Key: 1=Stylos; 2=Eleutherna; 3=Kastella; 4=Petras; 5=Messene; 6=Nemea; 7=Sourtara; 8=Servia; 9=Abdera

patterns of Byzantine communities in Greece from both inland and coastal areas, between which some variation in available resources likely existed (Table 4.2 and Figure 4.1). Garvie-Lok was the first to analyze bone collagen and carbonate from three middle Byzantine sites, as part of a wider study on diet in medieval and early modern Greece.[96] In 2004 the author, together with M.P. Richards at the University of Bradford (UK), instituted a project for stable isotope analysis of Byzantine Greek populations. This project is currently continuing at the Max Planck Institute for Evolutionary Anthropology (Germany), with the essential contribution of B.T. Fuller.

Table 4.2 Sites from which samples for stable isotope analysis have been taken

Site	Date	Type	Reference
Abdera	Sixth–ninth centuries AD and twelfth–thirteenth centuries AD	Coastal	A. Agelarakis pers. comm. 2007
Eleutherna	Sixth–seventh centuries AD	Inland	Bourbou, Fuller and Richards 2008[1]
Kastella	Eleventh century AD	Coastal	Bourbou and Richards 2007
Messene	Sixth–seventh centuries AD	Inland	Bourbou, Fuller and Richards 2008[1]
Nemea	Twelfth–thirteenth centuries AD	Inland	Garvie-Lok 2001
Petras	Twelfth–thirteenth centuries AD	Coastal	Garvie-Lok 2001
Servia	Eleventh–fifteenth centuries AD	Inland	Garvie-Lok 2001
Sourtara	Sixth–seventh centuries AD	Inland	Bourbou, Fuller and Richards 2008[1]
Stylos	Eleventh-twelfth centuries AD	Inland	Bourbou, Fuller and Richards 2008[1]

[1] Project on the investigation of Byzantine dietary patterns conducted at the Max Plank Institute (2007–09)

Samples of bone were collected mainly from ribs and long bones, and collagen was purified from these for analysis. Human bone collagen was extracted from the material recovered at Eleutherna, Kastella, Messene, Sourtara and Stylos following a modified Longin procedure,[97] as outlined in detail elsewhere,[98] with the addition of an ultrafiltration step.[99] Isotopic values for the Kastella samples were measured using a Carlo Erba elemental analyzer coupled to a ThermoFinnigan Delta Plus XL mass spectrometer at the Isotope Laboratory, Department of Archaeological Sciences, University of Bradford. Isotopic values for the samples from Eleutherna, Messene, Sourtara and Stylos were measured using a ThermoFinnigan elemental analyzer coupled to a ThermoFinnigan Delta Plus XL mass spectrometer, at the Max Planck Institute for Evolutionary Anthropology, Department of Human Evolution.

96 Garvie-Lok 2001.

97 Longin 1971.

98 Richards and Hedges 1999.

99 Brown, Nelson and Southon 1988.

For the Servia, Petras and Nemea material, the ultrafiltration step was omitted, but the material was treated with NaOH to remove contaminants.[100] Collagen preservation was assessed from sample C:N ratios, following criteria outlined by DeNiro.[101] These remains were analyzed at the Stable Isotope Laboratory of the University of Calgary (Canada), Department of Physics and Astronomy, using an NA 1500 elemental analyzer coupled to a Finnigan Mat TracerMat mass spectrometer. Stable isotope analysis of associated fauna was restricted to the available material from Eleutherna, Kastella and Sourtara.[102]

The attempted reconstruction of dietary and weaning patterns in Greek Byzantine populations was based on both indirect and direct evidence. Indirect evidence included information extracted from documentary sources, as reviewed above, and from the study of specific pathological conditions, such as dental diseases and metabolic disorders. Direct evidence included data derived from stable isotope analysis, which focused on: (1) the relative importance of animal products to the general diet; (2) the importance of marine resources and C_4 grains to the diet; (3) the possible differential access to food by gender; and (4) the reconstruction of breastfeeding and weaning patterns.

The Results of the Analysis

Table 4.3 shows the stable isotope values for the human bone samples, analyzed by the author, from the sites of Eleutherna, Kastella, Messene, Sourtara and Stylos. The adult isotopic values of the samples from these sites are graphically represented in Figure 4.2, which also includes the available data from the sites of Abdera,[103] Nemea, Petras and Servia.[104] Table 4.4 shows the isotopic values for the animal bone samples used for analysis from the sites of Eleutherna, Kastella and Sourtara. Adult and fauna values are graphically presented in Figure 4.3.[105]

---

100 Katzenberg and Weber 1999.

101 DeNiro 1985.

102 Garvie-Lok's data include all faunal samples that provided collagen, independent of time period. For example, as fish remains were not included in the faunal samples, modern Aegean fish caught in Aegean or Adriatic waters were used. The fish were purchased fresh from the Athens central market and processed for collagen extraction as appropriate.

103 A. Agelarakis pers. comm. 2007.

104 Garvie-Lok 2001.

105 Also included are stable isotope values of animal bones from Mitilini (island of Lesvos), Corinth and Athens; Garvie-Lok 2001.

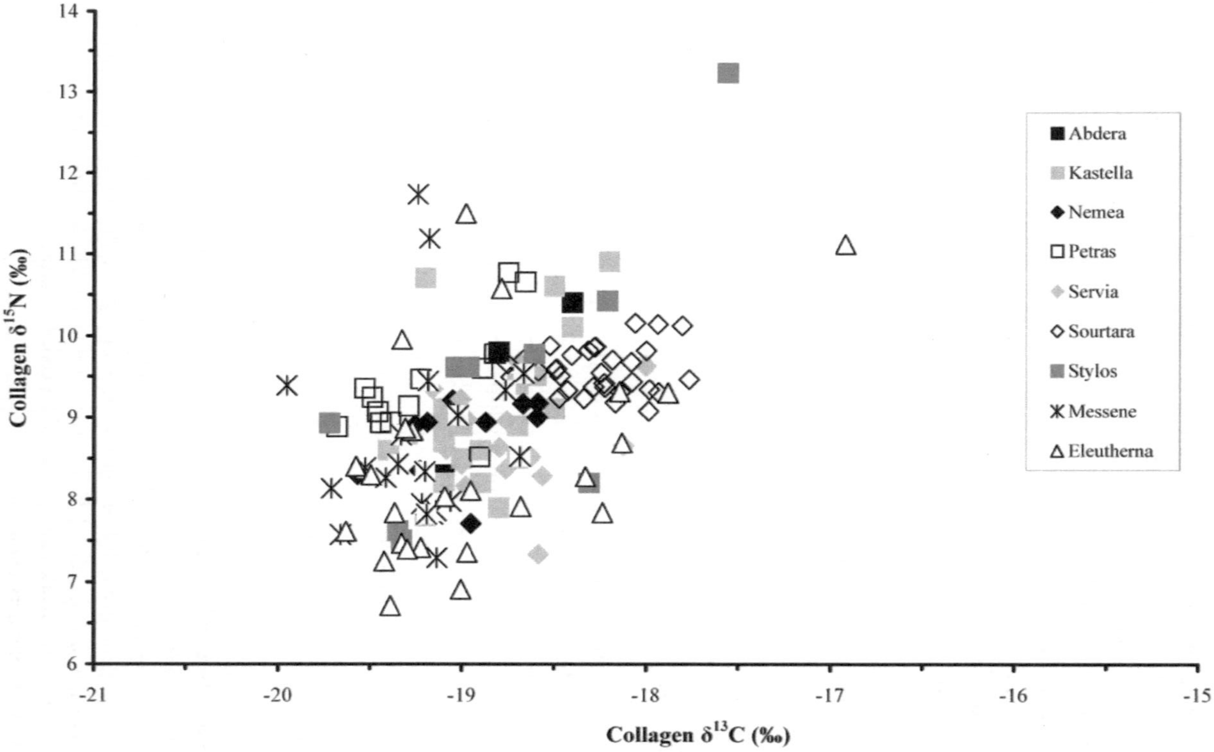

Figure 4.2 $\delta^{13}C$ and $\delta^{15}N$ values of the adult samples

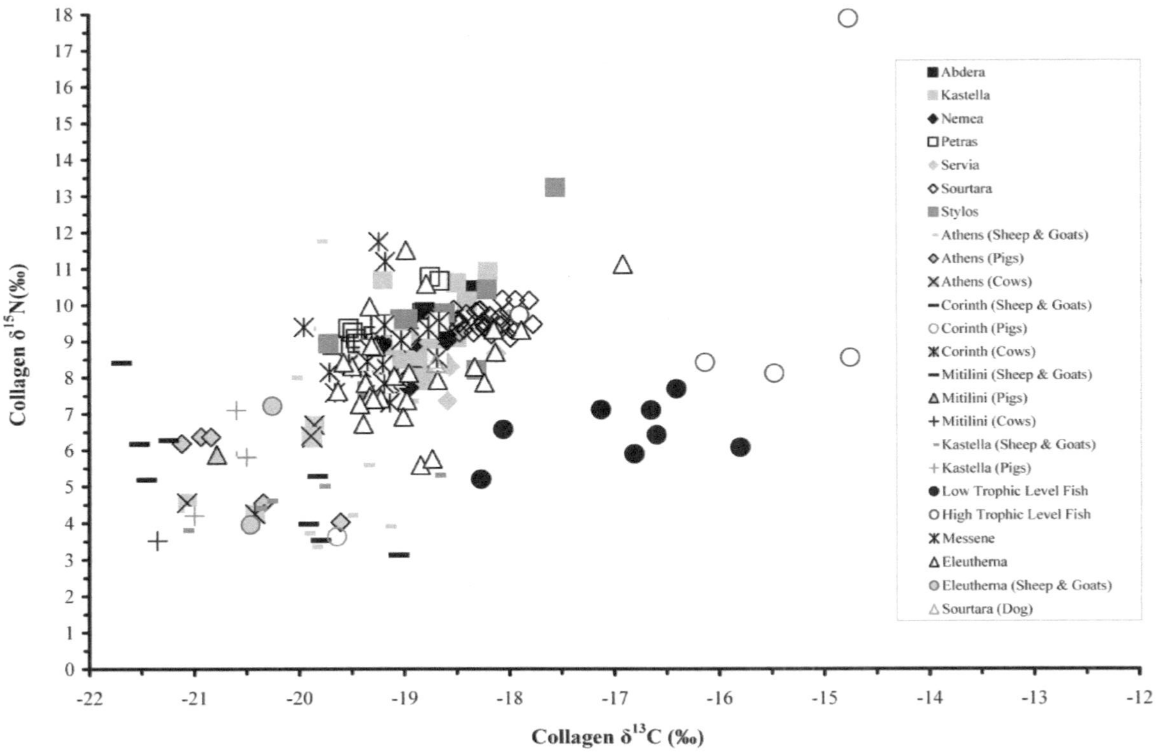

Figure 4.3 $\delta^{13}C$ and $\delta^{15}N$ values of the adult and fauna samples

Table 4.3 Stable isotope values for the human bone samples from Eleutherna, Kastella, Messene, Sourtara and Stylos

Sample no.	Skeleton no.	Burial	Sex	Age	$\delta^{13}C$	$\delta^{15}N$	C:N	%C	%N	% Yield
Eleutherna										
#39	013a	31	F	24	-18.8	5.6	3.1	43.4	16.4	1.1
#24	017b	42	M	25	-18.7	7.9	3.3	40.3	14.2	1.3
#36	011a	8	M	30	-19.3	8.8	3.3	41.3	14.5	2.6
#30	014a	34	M	35	-19.0	7.4	3.2	41.5	15.0	5.7
#41	028a	27	M	35	-18.3	8.3	3.3	39.4	13.9	1.8
#6	026a	20	M	35.2	-19.5	8.3	3.5	38.7	12.9	1.3
#7	035b	48	F	54	-19.4	6.7	3.3	40.0	14.3	1.5
#48	035a	48	F	54	-18.1	9.3	3.3	33.9	12.1	3.7
#21	019	36	F	59	-19.1	8.0	3.4	40.9	14.1	2.9
#17	016g	40	?	15 years ± 36 months	-19.0	11.5	3.6	35.7	11.7	1.4
#14	005th	18	M	17–25	-19.2	7.4	3.3	37.3	13.7	4.1
#29	021	9	F	17–25	-19.4	7.8	3.5	36.3	12.1	3.8
#32	010a	6	F	17–25	-18.8	10.6	3.4	39.3	13.5	5.1
#47	015a	33	M	17–25	-18.1	8.7	3.3	38.0	13.6	2.4
#5	005ist	18	M	25–35	-19.3	7.5	3.2	37.3	13.7	1.9
#28	036a	47	M	25–35	-19.3	8.9	3.4	40.4	13.8	1.7
#46	002b	17	M	25–35	-19.6	7.6	3.2	34.5	12.7	1.9
#23	017a	42	F	27–30	-19.3	7.4	3.0	41.1	15.8	2.0
#25	024	44	F	30–35	-18.2	7.8	3.3	40.5	14.4	5.4
#3	023a	11	F	31–35	-19.4	7.3	3.3	20.1	7.2	2.0
#16	005b	18	M	33–45	-19.0	8.1	3.2	40.7	14.7	4.9
#33	010b	6	M	33–45	-19.3	9.9	3.5	43.1	14.4	4.1
#42	007	19	M	33–45	-16.9	11.1	3.2	40.3	14.5	4.7
#31	005ke	18	M	45+	-19.6	8.4	3.6	37.6	12.2	2.1
#40	012b	32	M	45–49	-18.7	5.8	3.0	37.8	14.6	5.9
#43	006g	41	F	adult	-17.9	9.3	3.2	37.9	13.6	6.1
#45	002a	17	F	adult	-19.0	6.9	3.3	39.1	13.9	2.3
Kastella										
#1	001	4	F	c. 25	-18.7	9.4	3.3	45.2	15.8	6.2
#2	002	1	M	30–35	-18.6	9.5	3.3	46.1	16.4	6.5
#3	003	7	M	adult	-18.5	10.6	3.3	40.1	14.1	3.0
#4	004	6	M	50	-18.7	8.9	3.3	39.2	13.9	1.6
#5	009	11	M	adult	-18.2	10.9	3.3	30.2	10.8	1.4
#6	012	12	M	31	-18.9	8.2	3.3	20.0	7.1	1.6
#7	013	16	M	44	-19.1	9.0	3.3	40.0	14.2	2.2
#8	014	15	M	39	-19.1	8.8	3.4	45.5	15.7	1.0
#9	015	17	F	35–40	-19.1	9.1	3.3	47.1	16.5	3.0
#10	016	18	F	24	-19.1	8.7	3.3	42.0	14.8	3.4
#11	023	27	F	50–60	-18.9	8.6	3.3	44.7	15.8	6.5
#12	025	29	F?	adult	-19.2	7.8	3.4	40.1	13.9	2.2
#13	022	24	M	35	-19.4	8.6	3.3	44.1	15.4	4.3
#14	017	20	M	35–40	-18.4	10.1	3.4	36.8	12.8	0.5
#15	019a	21	M?	adult	-19	8.5	3.3	37.0	13.2	5.9
#S6	021	25	?	12 years ± 36 months	-19.3	8.8	3.3	37.5	13.3	2.2
#S5	020	26	?	15 years ± 36 months	-19.2	10.7	3.3	31.6	11.1	0.7

Sample no.	Skeleton no.	Burial	Sex	Age	$\delta^{13}C$	$\delta^{15}N$	C:N	%C	%N	% Yield
#S7	027	32	?	15 years ± 36 months	-18.5	9.1	3.3	32.3	11.6	3.3
#S9	026	30	?	15 years ± 36 months	-19.1	8.2	3.3	42.0	14.8	3.0
Messene										
#26	069	73	?	16	-19.1	8.0	3.4	34.9	12.0	1.2
#9	020	2(1991)	M	18	-18.7	9.5	3.4	38.7	13.4	3.9
#23	059	33	M	19	-19.1	7.3	3.4	38.0	13.2	1.8
#13	035	38	M	24	-19.2	11.7	3.5	40.2	13.3	1.4
#20	054	29	M	27	-19.3	8.8	3.4	29.1	10.0	2.0
#2	002	11	M	28	-19.2	7.9	3.4	38.0	13.2	1.7
#6	016	3	M	30	-19.2	8.3	3.4	39.3	13.5	2.6
#7	018	6	F	30	-19.2	7.8	3.3	40.0	14.1	3.3
#8	019	6	M	30	-19.2	9.4	3.4	37.3	12.9	2.2
#1	001	12	M	35	-19.2	11.2	3.6	41.3	13.5	2.7
#15	047	28	F	35	-19.4	8.3	3.4	41.2	14.2	2.4
#18	051	32	F	35	-19.5	8.4	3.5	34.8	11.7	0.9
#19	052	35	M	35	-18.7	8.5	3.2	34.6	12.5	1.6
#10	023	1(1991)	F	39	-19.1	7.9	3.3	23.2	8.2	1.9
#14	040	14	M	40	-20.0	9.4	3.6	35.9	11.6	2.5
#3	004	10	M	44	-19.0	9.0	3.3	41.4	14.6	2.0
#16	048	28	M	44	-19.4	8.4	3.6	38.6	12.6	2.4
#27	070	73	M	44	-19.2	7.8	3.4	37.8	13.1	1.1
#25	067	66	M	45	-19.7	7.6	3.4	35.8	12.4	1.7
#21	057	1(1995)	?	15 years ± 36 months	-19.7	8.1	3.5	33.2	11.1	3.3
#22	058	38	F	adult	-18.8	9.3	3.4	36.4	12.4	2.9
Sourtara										
#31	090	97	?	12 years	-17.8	10.1	3.2	38.7	14.1	4.4
#22	081	15	?	child	-18.1	9.7	3.2	40.3	14.7	2.8
#26	085	107	M	<18	-18.8	9.6	3.3	41.6	14.8	2.7
#27	086	24	F	<18	-18.3	9.2	3.2	36.1	13.1	1.0
#15	071	85	M?	c. 18	-18.4	9.3	3.2	41.5	15.0	2.7
#42	100	55	M?	24	-18.3	9.8	3.2	40.1	14.6	4.2
#1	001	78	F	31	-18.5	9.6	3.2	41.9	15.4	1.8
#5	038	37	M	35	-18.2	9.2	3.2	36.6	13.2	1.4
#6	020	63	F	35	-17.9	10.1	3.2	41.9	15.3	1.5
#17	076	93	F	35	-18.0	9.3	3.2	38.7	14.1	3.1
#4	039	95	F	39	-18.3	9.4	3.2	41.7	15.2	1.6
#9	074	25	M	42	-18.2	9.4	3.2	41.4	14.9	1.9
#18	077	89	M	44	-17.9	9.3	3.2	37.3	13.6	2.2
#7	021	22	M	c. 45	-18.2	9.5	3.2	41.9	15.2	1.9
#24	083	108	M	50	-18.2	9.7	3.3	39.1	14.0	2.6
#32	091	104	M	50	-18.5	9.2	3.2	34.9	12.6	2.0
#3	024	62	M	51	-18.4	9.8	3.2	40.1	14.7	1.3
#2	014	56	M	56	-18.1	9.4	3.2	41.9	15.1	1.1
#38	096	82	M	18–30	-18.3	9.9	3.2	43.3	15.7	3.6
#33	092	5	M	adult	-18.7	9.5	3.3	38.4	13.5	1.3
#35	093	90	?	adult	-18.0	9.8	3.2	40.7	14.9	4.1
#39	097	98	M	31–40	-17.8	9.5	3.2	42.8	15.5	5.9
#36	094	61	M	41–50	-18.1	9.3	3.2	30.8	11.2	0.8
#37	095	101	M	41–50	-18.2	9.4	3.2	41.6	15.1	3.5
#40	098	60	F	63	-18.0	9.1	3.2	40.7	14.7	2.9

Sample no.	Skeleton no.	Burial	Sex	Age	$\delta^{13}C$	$\delta^{15}N$	C:N	%C	%N	% Yield
#41	099	110	F	63	-18.3	9.9	3.3	42.2	14.9	3.9
#25	084	57	M	41–50	-18.5	9.5	3.3	42.0	15.1	2.6
Stylos										
#1	023a	1	F	30–35	-19.7	8.9	3.4	41.3	14.1	2.7
#2	003a	*	M	31–40	-19.3	7.5	3.3	41.1	14.8	3.3
#3	003a	*	F	31–40	-18.2	10.4	3.3	42.3	15.1	1.2
#4	012a	6	M	40–45	-19.0	9.6	3.3	29.6	10.6	2.0
#5	026a	*	M	31–40	-17.6	13.2	3.3	41.4	14.8	2.4
#6	001	*	F	31–40	-18.3	8.2	3.2	42.5	15.6	1.7
#7	001	*	F	31–40	-19.4	7.6	3.2	39.4	14.4	4.2
#8	007	21	M	41–50	-18.6	9.8	3.2	42.1	15.5	2.0
#9	028	22	M	51+	-19.0	9.6	3.3	35.4	12.6	1.9
#11	015	1(1990)	?	14.6–17.0 years	-20	8.3	3.4	30.1	10.4	2.5

Table 4.4 Stable isotope values for the animal bone samples from Eleutherna, Kastella and Sourtara

Species	$\delta^{13}C$	$\delta^{15}N$	C:N	%C	%N	% Yield
Eleutherna						
Sheep	-20.2	7.2	3.3	30.6	10.9	4.4
Sheep	-20.5	3.4	3.3	37.2	13.2	3.5
Kastella						
Sheep	-20.6	5.9	3.4	41.3	14.3	1.6
Red deer	-21.0	4.6	3.4	39.6	13.8	1.3
Pig	-21.0	4.2	3.4	8.6	3.0	0.5
Pig	-20.6	7.1	3.4	39.4	13.6	0.1
Pig (young)	-20.5	5.8	3.3	40.8	14.5	3.1
Goat	-18.7	5.3	3.3	37.6	13.2	1.9
Goat	-21.1	3.8	3.3	36.0	12.6	2.2
Goat	-20.3	4.6	3.3	39.5	14.0	2.1
Goat	-20.4	4.4	3.3	38.0	13.6	1.6
Goat	-19.8	5.0	3.3	37.0	13.2	4.9
Sourtara						
Dog	-18.7	8.38	3.3	34.9	12.2	2.8
Goat	-20.7	2.58	3.2	40.0	14.6	9.1

Despite possible dietary variations between inland and coastal sites, the stable isotope values of the human remains from the various sites are broadly similar (Table 4.5). Collagen shows mean $\delta^{13}C$ values ranging from -18.2 ± 0.3‰ at Sourtara to -19.2 ± 0.3‰ at Petras and mean $\delta^{15}N$ ranging from 8.2 ± 1.4‰ at Eleutherna to 9.5 ± 1.1‰ at Abdera. Bone carbonate values, while not measured from all of the sites, are also rather homogeneous, ranging from -10.7 ± 1.2‰ at Nemea to -11.2 ± 0.9‰ at Abdera (Figure 4.4).

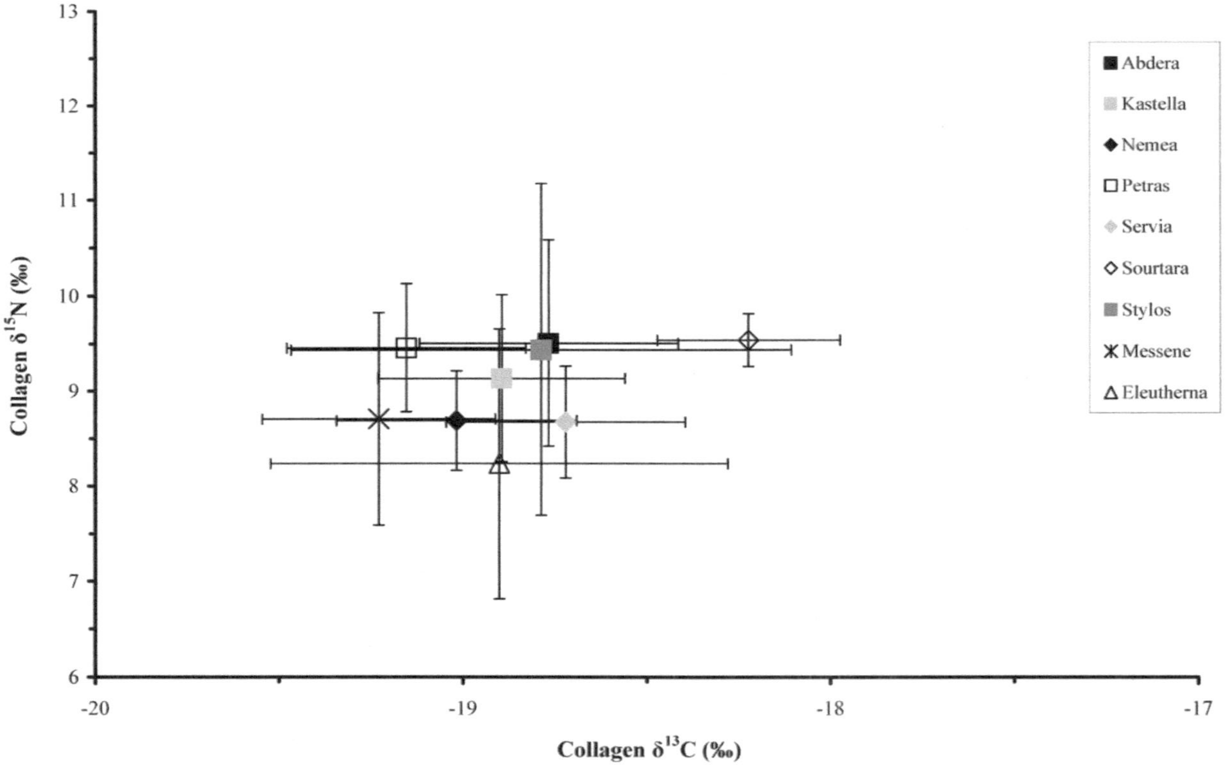

Figure 4.4 Average $\delta^{13}C$ and $\delta^{15}N$ values of the adult samples

Table 4.5 Average adult human stable isotope values by site

Site	$\delta^{13}C_{coll}$ (‰PDB)	$\delta^{15}N$ (‰AIR)	$\delta^{13}C_{carb}$ (‰PDB)
Abdera	-18.8 ± 0.4	9.5 ± 1.1	-12.8 ± 0.8
Eleutherna	-18.9 ± 0.6	8.2 ± 1.4	-
Kastella	-18.8 ± 0.3	9.1 ± 1.2	-
Messene	-19.2 ± 0.3	8.7 ± 0.9	-
Nemea	-19.0 ± 0.3	8.7 ± 0.5	-11.2 ± 0.9
Petras	-19.2 ± 0.3	9.5 ± 0.7	-12.0 ± 0.7
Servia	-18.7 ± 0.3	8.7 ± 0.6	-11.9 ± 0.6
Sourtara	-18.2 ± 0.3	9.5 ± 0.3	-
Stylos	-18.8 ± 0.7	9.4 ± 1.7	-

These human collagen values, when plotted with values for some Byzantine-era domesticated fauna and modern Aegean fish, fall in a tight cluster where $\delta^{13}C$ and $\delta^{15}N$ values are generally elevated over the domesticates (Figure 4.5). If we consider the diverse foods available to Byzantine populations, and the wide range of likely $\delta^{13}C$ and $\delta^{15}N$ values estimated above for these resources, the $\delta^{13}C$ and $\delta^{15}N$ differences between these nine human populations are relatively small. Isotopic data also demonstrate no differential access to food products by gender, although the paleopathological data and written sources attest otherwise. For example, dental pathologies affect more males than females, while a close association between fasting and sexual abstinence, targeting females, is highlighted in various sources of the early Christian tradition (see above) (Figure 4.6).

The stable isotope analysis seems to suggest the existence of a general 'Byzantine diet' that was broadly similar between communities, although it may have varied somewhat by location. Such a scenario agrees with the documentary sources, reviewed above, that suggest a fundamental reliance on a trio of staples – grain, oil and wine – that were supplemented, depending on class and other variables, by other foods. The $\delta^{13}C$ results indicate that the diet was predominately based on C_3 terrestrial foods, but there is some evidence to suggest that C_4 grains and marine protein resources were also consumed at some of the sites. The inland site of Sourtara has a range of 2‰ in $\delta^{13}C$ values but shows little change in the $\delta^{15}N$ values, which suggests that the population consumed some domesticated animals that had a C_4 component in their diet. However, substantial dependence on a C_4 grain staple, such as millet, is not indicated at any of the sites. Consumption of marine protein resources is seen at the coastal sites and for some individuals from the inland sites, and will be discussed in more detail below.

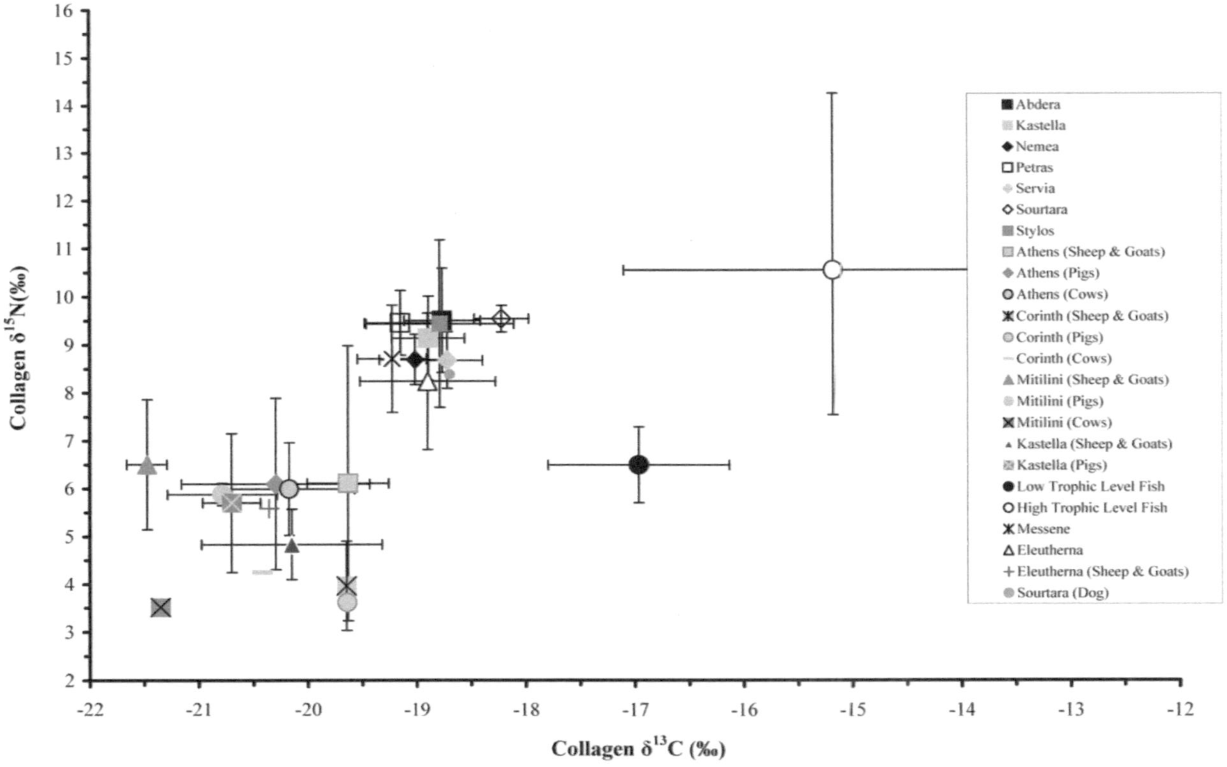

Figure 4.5 Average $\delta^{13}C$ and $\delta^{15}N$ values of the adult and fauna samples

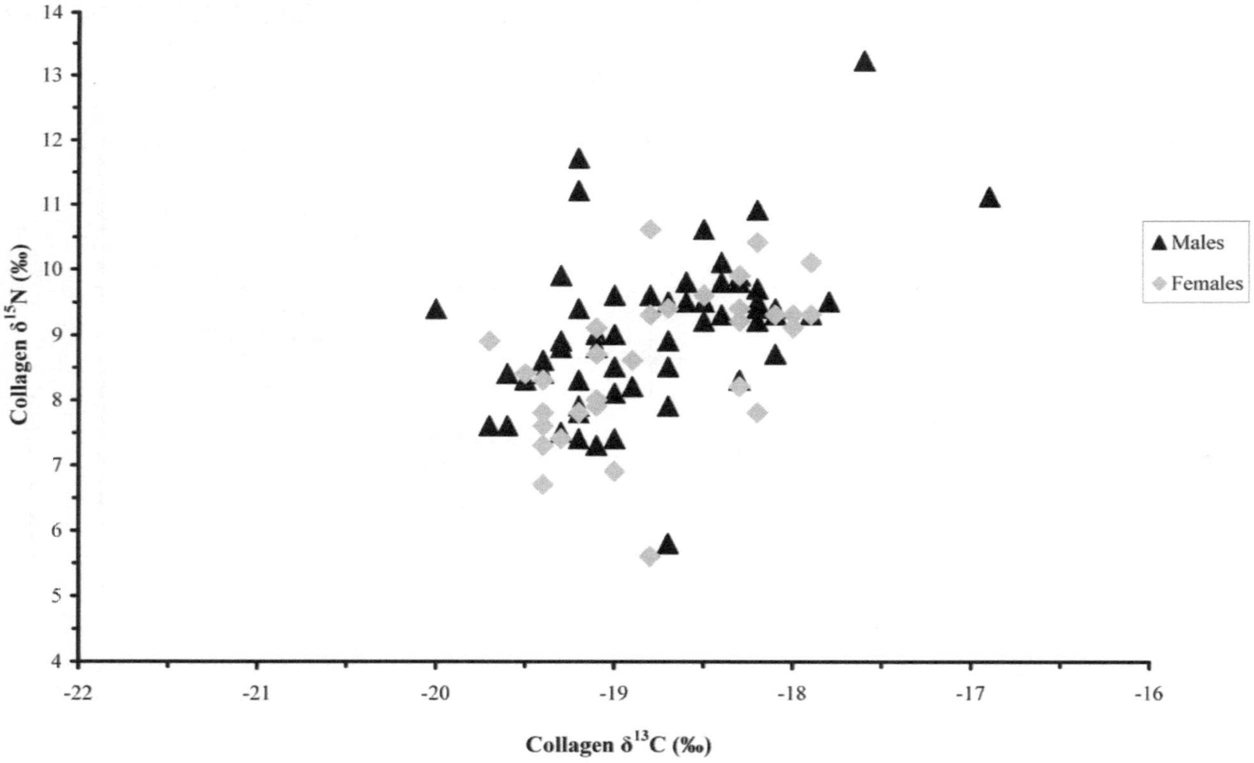

Figure 4.6 Male and female $\delta^{13}C$ and $\delta^{15}N$ values for all sites

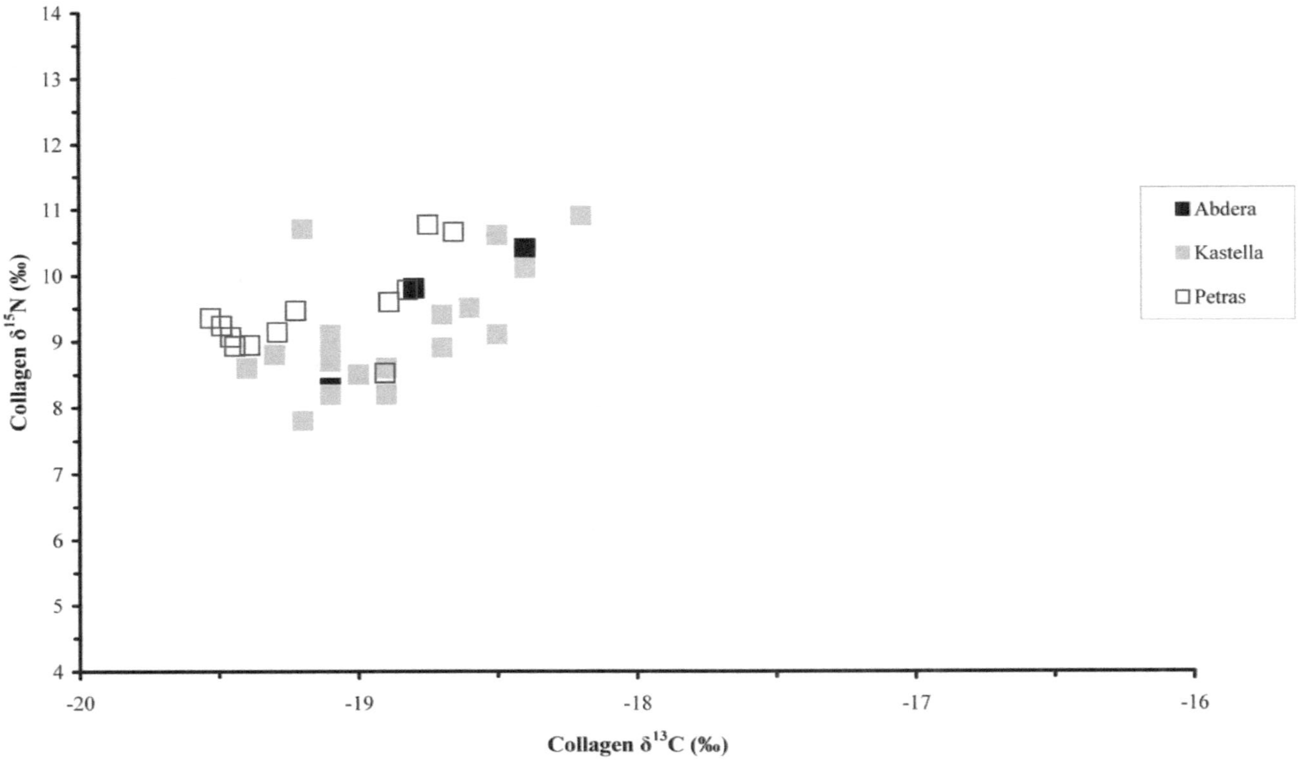

Figure 4.7 $\delta^{13}C$ and $\delta^{15}N$ values of the coastal sites of Abdera, Kastella and Petras

Variation in the consumption of resources such as C_3 and C_4 grains, animals (pigs vs. sheep and goats) and olive oil might explain the minor site-to-site differences seen in the average carbonate $\delta^{13}C$. Another potential source of variation may lie in the consumption of oily fish. The estimated bulk dairy $\delta^{13}C$ value used here is similar to the C_3 plant value and reflects the generally C_3-based diet of goats and sheep sampled to date for Byzantine sites. Within this scenario the addition of dairy foods would not be expected to shift bulk diet $\delta^{13}C$ away from the C_3 grain value.

The $\delta^{15}N$ values obtained are similar to those seen for many other European agricultural populations with respect to their substantial elevation above domesticated fauna.[106] Collagen values are ^{13}C-enriched compared to the domesticates, and ^{13}C-depleted compared to the marine resources. These results are indicative of a general diet in which most dietary protein came from domesticated fauna, with some input from marine resources. Increasing marine resource consumption causes enriched ^{13}C and ^{15}N ratios in human tissues such as hair and bone.

A closer look at the data on an individual level offers support for increased marine protein consumption at some of the sites.[107] Figure 4.7 shows data for the coastal sites of Abdera, Kastella and Petras. Here a number of individuals can be seen to stand apart from the majority, with a tendency toward the higher $\delta^{13}C$ and $\delta^{15}N$ values as expected for the consumption of marine resources. This pattern reflects some use of marine resources at these sites (a reasonable conclusion given their location), but this pattern is also evident at the inland sites (Figure 4.8). The two individuals who show evidence for the largest consumption of marine protein resources are both from inland sites. Skeleton 007 from Eleutherna has the most enriched ^{13}C value (-16.9‰) of all the individuals from the nine populations studied, as well as an elevated $\delta^{15}N$ value (11.1‰), and this indicates that a significant portion of the diet came from marine protein resources. In addition, the individual of burial 26a from Stylos displays the highest $\delta^{15}N$ value (13.2‰) of all the populations and the second most enriched ^{13}C value (-17.6‰), again indicating a diet heavily based on marine proteins.[108]

[106] Van Klinken, Richards and Hedges 2000; Privat, O'Connell and Richards 2002; Polet and Katzenberg 2003; Prowse et al. 2004; Müldner and Richards 2005; Dürrwachter et al. 2006; Jay and Richards 2006; Keenleyside, Schwarcz and Panayotova 2006; Richards, Fuller and Molleson 2006.

[107] Garvie-Lok 2001; Bourbou and Richards 2007. To eliminate the confounding effects of breastfeeding, individuals aged less than 3 years are not shown in these figures.

[108] The isotopic values and thus the diets of these individuals differ significantly from those of the other individuals in the population, and the distinction could suggest that they were migrants.

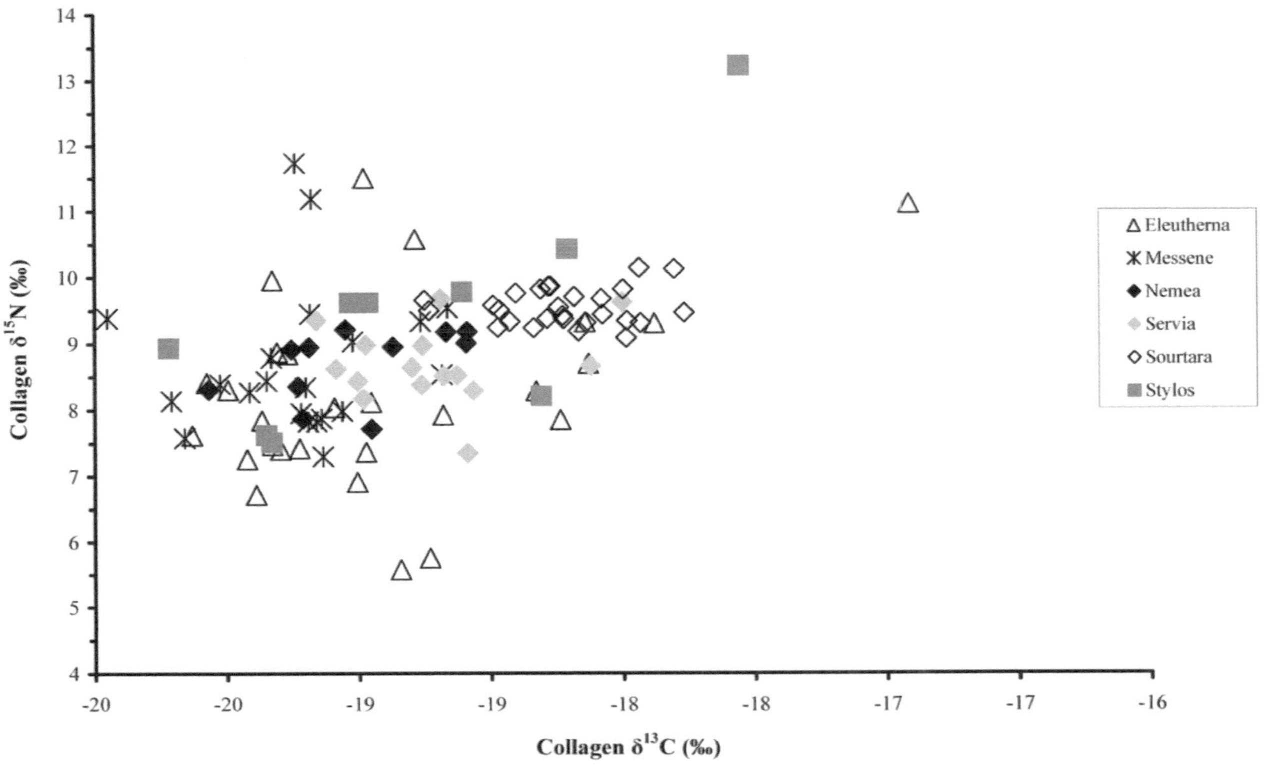

Figure 4.8 $\delta^{13}C$ and $\delta^{15}N$ values of the inland sites of Eleutherna, Messene, Nemea, Servia, Sourtara and Stylos

This finding of the consumption of marine species during the Byzantine period contrasts with previous isotopic studies of prehistoric coastal populations that found marine species contributing little or not at all to the diet.[109] The Byzantines were well aware that fish and most of the aquatic animals constituted a food source of high nutritional value, and they had perhaps developed specific fishing methods for the various species. Another possible explanation for the contrast in use of marine protein resources is that fasting rules contributed to the increased consumption of fish and aquatic species in the Byzantine era.[110] Ultimately, the major differences in time, customs and technology separating the prehistoric and Byzantine periods disallow the drawing of any direct parallels between prehistoric and Byzantine diets; but stable isotope data broadly suggest that both inland and coastal populations during the Byzantine period supplemented an essentially land-based C_3 diet with some possible C_4 and marine resources. Consumption of marine resources is possibly expected at the coastal sites, given their location, and at the inland sites freshwater fishes could have been consumed where lakes and rivers existed (as, for example, at the site of Stylos with its numerous springs of fresh water). Freshwater fishes are attested in the written sources and are known to have been consumed (see above).[111] Until more material is available, such as fish bones from the Byzantine period of Greece that can be isotopically analyzed, explanations for the consumption of fish and aquatic species in Byzantine Greece remain tentative.[112]

Although intra-site patterning of collagen values indicates that some marine exploitation occurred both at inland and coastal sites, sources other than marine protein could have contributed to some of the generally high collagen $\delta^{15}N$

[109] For example, although none of the Neolithic groups studied by Papathanasiou 2003 had a strong dependence on marine resources, the diets of the Franchthi and Kephala populations included significant amounts of such foods.

[110] For example, fasting rules allow for the consumption of fish during the Lenten period of Christmas; on the Transfiguration feast day (6 August) that is included in the fasting period for the Assumption of the Virgin Mary on August 15; and on the feast of the Annunciation (25 March) that is included in the Lenten period of Easter. In addition, the consumption of all seafood other than fish is allowed in all the fasting periods. The contribution of fasting regulations imposed by the Church are also implied as a possible factor for the increase of marine protein in later medieval diet; see, e.g., Müldner and Richards 2005, 45–6; 2007a, 695; 2007b, 168.

[111] Richards, Fuller and Hedges 2001 suggest that the application of $\delta^{34}S$ analysis has the potential to distinguish consumers of freshwater fish from consumers of terrestrial foods; see also Privat, O'Connell and Hedges 2007.

[112] Fish-bone collagen recovered from prehistoric to classical sites is currently under analysis for $\delta^{13}C$ and $\delta^{15}N$ values in an investigation of the extent of fish consumption in Greek antiquity; E. Vika pers. comm. 2009.

values seen at Byzantine sites such as Messene and Eleutherna. Recent work by Bogaard and colleagues suggests that high $\delta^{15}N$ values in some European agricultural communities may reflect elevated grain $\delta^{15}N$ due to the manuring of fields.[113] This model, however, may not apply to the Byzantine agricultural system. Although domesticates did graze on cleared fields, and would thus have deposited some manure there, they were often kept for much of the year on land remote from cultivated fields, which made their dung unavailable for fertilizer during this period.[114]

Other explanations for high $\delta^{15}N$ values at some Byzantine sites fit well with documentary evidence for the Byzantine diet. It has been suggested, for example, that high $\delta^{15}N$ values of European agricultural populations may in some cases reflect a very heavy reliance on dairy foods.[115] This scenario agrees with the importance of dairy foods in the Byzantine diet as attested in the documentary sources. Given the low cost of some dairy foods and their general availability, use of dairy foods is an attractive explanation for the generally high $\delta^{15}N$ values seen in Byzantine groups studied to date. It is also possible that high $\delta^{15}N$ values in Byzantine populations reflect consumption of dietary items of unexpectedly high $\delta^{15}N$ values, such as chickens, chicken eggs and suckling animals.[116]

Stable isotope data also provide some tentative information on weaning practices in Byzantine Greece.[117] The stable nitrogen isotope data for non-adults from Eleutherna, Kastella, Messene, Sourtara and Stylos are presented in Table 4.6. Table 4.7 presents $\delta^{15}N$ values and female mean for the samples of Nemea, Petras and Servia. The fact that the samples represent several sites complicates the interpretation of the data, as the stable $\delta^{15}N$ values for the typical adult female vary among sites, reflecting local variation in diet. The data are more easily interpreted when each non-adult value is considered in terms of its relationship to the mean adult female value for its site. This format essentially standardizes the non-adult values in terms of their elevation relative to adult female values from the same site.

113 Bogaard et al. 2007.

114 Kazhdan 1997.

115 Hedges and Reynard 2007.

116 Garvie-Lok 2001. Because foraging chickens consume many insects, their flesh and eggs show $\delta^{15}N$ values above those of herbivores; see, e.g., Schwarcz 1999.

117 See Bourbou and Garvie-Lok 2009.

Table 4.6 Non-adult $\delta^{15}N$ values and adult female mean for Eleutherna, Kastella, Messene, Sourtara and Stylos

Sample no.	Skeleton no.	Burial	Sex	Age	$\delta^{13}C$	$\delta^{15}N$	C:N	%C	%N	% Yield
Eleutherna										
#8	035d	48	?	birth–3 years	-19.3	7.7	3.3	41.5	14.7	4.4
#9	035g	48	?	birth–3 years	-19.4	6.9	3.2	40.2	14.6	3.2
#12	005ia	18	?	18 months ±6 months	-19.2	10.8	3.5	39.5	13.4	1.1
#10	005e	18	?	2 years ±8 months	-19.9	7.0	3.3	38.6	13.7	1.0
#13	005i	18	?	3 years ±12 months	-18.9	11.4	3.6	39.9	12.9	1.5
#22	020e	37	?	5 years ±16 months	-19.1	8.1	3.6	40.8	13.3	1.7
#19	016a	40	?	6 years ±24 months	-19.1	11.7	3.5	37.6	12.5	2.4
#20	020g	37	?	6 years ±24 months	-19.0	9.2	3.5	40.2	13.6	4.1
#34	006ia	41	?	6 years ±24 months	-19.1	8.1	3.2	39.8	14.4	6.7
#1	003th	13	?	4–12 years	-19.4	7.0	3.2	41.2	14.9	3.3
#2	003h	13	?	4–12 years	-20.3	7.5	3.3	36.2	12.9	0.9
#35	006th	41	?	4–12 years	-19.0	7.9	3.5	24.3	8.2	2.9
#44	002st	17	?	4–12 years	-18.2	8.0	3.3	39.7	14.1	1.9
#26	036g	47	?	8 years ±24 months	-19.0	8.3	3.4	34.2	11.7	1.7
#4	005id	18	?	9 years ±24 months	-19.3	6.7	3.3	44.4	15.8	1.3
#27	036b	47	?	9 years ±24 months	-18.7	8.7	3.3	40.4	14.5	3.2
Adult female mean=7.4 ± 1.4										
Kastella										
#S1	016b	18	?	7 years ±24 months	-19.0	8.9	3.3	40.3	14.4	5.6
#S2	016d	18	?	2 years ±8 months	-18.0	12.1	3.2	40.8	14.7	6.3
#S3	016g	18	?	0.5 months–1.5 year	-18.3	11.6	3.3	33.0	11.7	3.0
#S4	016e	18	?	10 years ±30 months	-18.8	7.9	3.2	37.2	13.4	4.0
#S8	018	22	?	4.5–5.5 years	-18.7	8.3	3.2	26.5	9.8	1.9
#S10	018e	22	?	7.5–8.5 years	-18.7	8.5	3.3	38.2	13.7	2.6
#S11	024	28	?	4 years ±12 months	-19.4	7.5	3.4	46.5	15.8	1.4
Adult female mean=8.7 ± 0.6										
Messene										
#4	005	9	?	1–3 years	-18.9	8.5	3.4	39.7	13.8	3.3

#11	026	16	?	1–3 years	-19.6	8.7	3.3	39.2	13.7	1.3
#17	050	36	?	1–3 years	-20.4	7.6	3.5	34.6	11.5	1.2
#24	060	26	?	1–3 years	-18.9	7.2	3.4	29.6	10.2	4.7
#12	032	13	?	9.5–10.5 years	-18.9	7.1	3.3	41.3	14.5	1.1
Adult female mean=8.3 ± 0.6										
Sourtara										
#19	078	91	?	Birth–3 years	-17.6	11.0	3.2	41.3	15.1	3.8
#20	079	84	?	Birth–3 years	-16.9	12.1	3.2	42.5	15.5	4.5
#21	080	81	?	Birth–3 years	-17.2	10.2	3.2	42.6	15.5	5.1
#11	051	9	?	18 months ± 6 months	-18.0	12.0	3.3	42.1	14.8	3.6
#43	102	35	?	2 years	-17.5	11.0	3.3	32.5	11.5	0.7
#29	088	12	?	3–4 years	-18.4	10.6	3.2	40.2	14.5	2.2
#25	057	44	?	3 years ± 12 months	-18.4	10.2	3.4	37.3	12.7	2.6
#30	089	79	?	4–5 years	-18.1	9.6	3.2	42.2	15.4	1.8
#23	082	4	?	5–6 years	-18.5	9.5	3.2	39.9	14.4	3.3
#14	055	20	?	6 years ± 24 months	-18.4	9.5	3.2	41.9	15.1	2.1
#16	073	30	?	6 years ± 24 months	-17.7	9.5	3.2	42.4	15.4	5.5
#28	087	2	?	8–9 years	-18.7	9.7	3.3	37.8	13.5	1.7
#34	092a	5	?	9 years	-18.5	9.6	3.2	40.7	14.1	1.5
#8	047	21	?	10 years ± 30 months	-18.5	9.9	3.3	41.6	14.9	1.9
#10	075	100	?	10 years ±30 months	-18.1	10.2	3.2	42.4	14.9	5.0
#12	049	74	?	10 years ±30 months	-18.6	9.6	3.3	41.7	14.8	2.0
Adult female mean=9.5 ± 0.4										
Stylos										
#8	012	1(1990)	?	Fetus	-19.2	10.1	3.49	39.3	13.1	2.0
#9	013	1(1990)	?	Newborn	-18.3	9.3	3.19	26.4	9.7	3.0
#4	008	26a	?	Newborn	-19.4	10.5	3.46	34.8	11.7	2.1
#2	005	16a	?	6.5–7.5 years	-19.7	8.8	3.30	27.4	9.7	3.0
#12	020	24	?	7–8 years	-19.6	10.1	3.44	42.5	14.4	1.3
#3	007	26a	?	7.5–8.5 years	-19.7	9.1	3.34	43.1	15.0	1.8
#7	011	1(1990)	?	7.5–8.5 years	-19.5	9.1	3.39	27.6	9.5	1.4
#10	014	1(1990)	?	7.5–8.5 years	-18.8	9.7	3.32	44.3	15.6	4.0
Adult female mean=8.8 ± 1.2										

Table 4.7 Non-adult $\delta^{15}N$ values and adult female mean for Nemea, Petras and Servia

Age at death	$\delta^{15}N$ (‰)
Nemea	
16–32 months	8.6
5–10 years	7.5
Adult female mean=8.5 ± 1.0	
Petras	
30–42 months	12.7
4–5 years	8.6
5.5–6.5 years	9.6
6–7 years	8.9
Adult female mean=9.2 ± 0.3	
Servia	
c. 12 months	11.3
3–7 years	9.5
8–11 years	9.2
Adult female mean=8.5 ± 0.3	

Adapted after Bourbou and Garvie-Lok 2009, table 1

*Figu*re 4.9 presents the data for the eight sites in this format. A $\delta^{15}N$ elevation is seen in the youngest individuals. Many of the non-adults aged 3 years or less at death show a substantial elevation (2‰ to 4‰) over the mean adult female value at the same site. This result is consistent with the protracted period of breastfeeding described in documentary sources reviewed above. In contrast to the general elevation seen in the youngest individuals, non-adults aged 4 years or older at death are scattered within 1‰ of the adult female mean, reflecting an essentially adult diet. The ±1‰ fluctuation in $\delta^{15}N$ around the adult female mean for these older non-adults reflects normal individual variation within each population, and is seen in adults from these sites as well. Exceptions to this are two children aged approximately 6 years from Eleutherna (skeletons 016a and 020g) that have enriched ^{15}N values, which could be a result of prolonged breastfeeding or nutritional stress.[118]

The data available from this study do not allow firm conclusions to be drawn about weaning behavior in Byzantine Greece. However, they allow us to make some tentative suggestions, and to point to directions for further research. The contrast between the elevated values seen in non-adults aged 3 years or less and the adult-like pattern seen in children aged 4 and older suggests that weaning was

[118] Fuller et al. 2005.

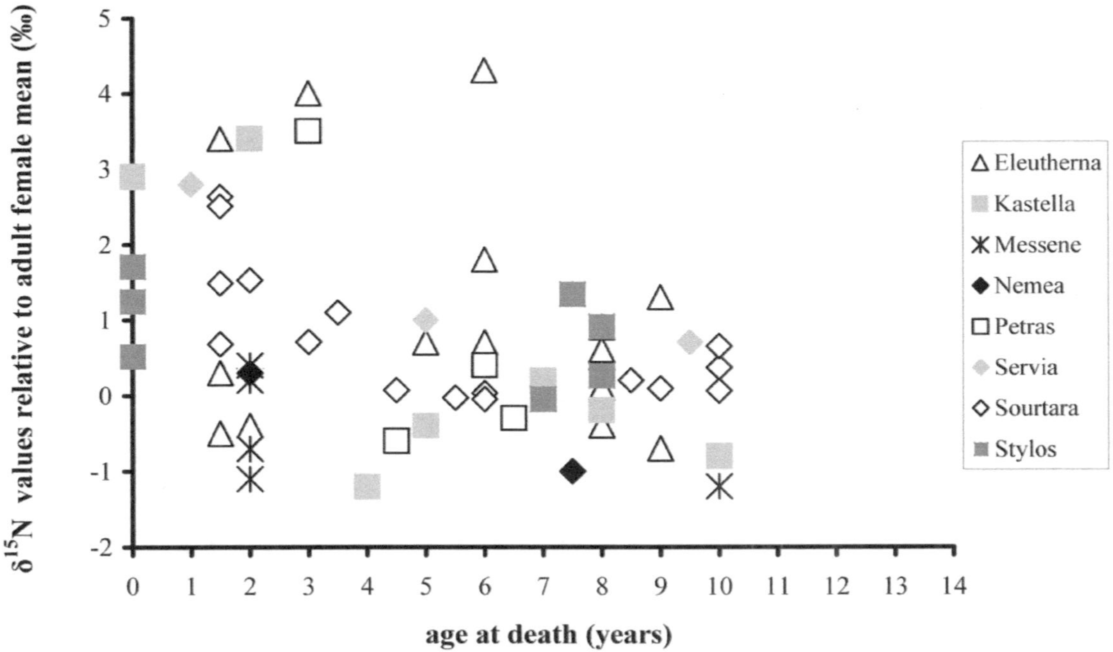

Figure 4.9 $\delta^{15}N$ non-adult values and adult female mean

complete by the fourth year. This suggestion is consistent with the documentary evidence, with the exception of the description in the Vita of Basil the Younger, and it is probably safe to conclude that the description in that Vita does not indicate that children would normally have been nursed into the fourth year.

Arriving at a more precise age of weaning than 'before 4 years of age' is not possible given the data available. Many of the non-adults aged 3 years or less at death show a substantial $\delta^{15}N$ elevation above the adult female mean for their site, suggesting that mother's milk had formed a significant portion of their diet. Due to the lag between a change in diet and a shift in bone $\delta^{15}N$ values, this result does not necessarily suggest significant nursing up to the age of 3, but does indicate that breastmilk formed a substantial part of some infants' diets well into the third year of life.

Bourbou and Garvie-Lok have also discussed the isotopic data derived from a number of Roman and late medieval sites.[119] Isotopic data for Roman populations from Isola Sacra near Rome (first to third centuries AD),[120] the Dakhleh oasis of Egypt (c. AD 250-450)[121] and Queenford Farm in Britain (late fourth to mid-sixth centuries AD)[122] are also consistent with late weaning ages. Despite wide geographic separation of these populations and presumed local cultural differences, the three studies suggest a similar weaning pattern, with some individuals nursing to the age of 3 years. Fuller and colleagues[123] have pointed out a contrast between this apparent Roman weaning pattern and that seen at the medieval British site of Wharram Percy (tenth to sixteenth centuries AD),[124] where stable isotope values suggest that children were weaned at an earlier age – between 18 months and 2 years. According to Fuller and colleagues, this contrast could reflect a stronger influence by the physician Soranus and other medical scholars among the earlier Roman populations, who appear to have followed the physicians' advice for a gradual weaning process, while later medieval populations chose to wean their children at a younger age. The Greek Byzantine data are notably consistent with the later weaning ages found among these Roman populations. Further and more extensive studies on Byzantine populations would provide additional evidence to determine whether a difference in weaning practices existed between Byzantine and medieval western European populations – with Byzantine groups having maintained traditions carried over from the Roman period.

119 Bourbou and Garvie-Lok 2009.

120 Prowse et al. 2004.

121 Dupras, Schwarcz and Fairgrieve 2001.

122 Fuller et al. 2006b.

123 Fuller et al. 2006b.

124 Richards, Mays and Fuller 2002.

The particular choice of honey and goat's milk in infant feeding, documented in the written sources, could have had serious adverse consequences on infant health.[125] Honey is often contaminated with the spores of *Clostridium botulinum*, the bacterium that secretes the toxin that causes botulism, a severe and often fatal form of food poisoning.[126] Botulinum toxin blocks the transmission of chemical signals at neuromuscular junctions; left untreated it can cause death through paralysis of the muscles of respiration.[127] In the infant, *C. botulinum* spores can colonize the intestinal tract, leading to infant botulism, an illness of varying severity whose symptoms include reduced muscle tone, difficulty suckling and sometimes respiratory problems.[128] In modern populations, most infants who develop infant botulism recover after an illness lasting several weeks or several months; in antiquity, however, recovery may have been less certain. The use of goat's milk as a dietary staple for infants can also result in serious complications. Although goat's milk is popularly seen as similar to human milk, it is relatively low in both cobalamine and folic acid (0.1 μg/l and 6 μg/l, respectively) compared to human milk (4μg/l and 52 μg/l, respectively). Infants who are fed goat's milk rather than human milk starting shortly after birth develop severe megaloblastic anemia by the age of about 3 to 5 months due to folic acid deficiency.[129] In some cases these health consequences would be visible in the osteological record. For example, the occurrence of active cribra orbitalia (see Figure 3.5 in Chapter 3) in an infant younger than 6 months suggests that the diet of the child was likely based on or supplemented with goat's milk.[130]

Weaning represents a crucial period in a child's life. The type of food introduced after cessation of breastfeeding, as well as cultural factors that influence weaning practices, can be related to the development of specific pathological conditions, and offer a plausible explanation for the clustering of deaths around the weaning age in non-adult mortality patterns. The bioarchaeological and isotopic analysis of larger non-adult samples is expected to further contribute to a better understanding of the cultural and environmental conditions in which feeding

---

125 Fairgrieve and Molto 2000.

126 Nevas et al. 2005.

127 Passmore and Eastwood 1986.

128 Arnon et al. 1979; Merenstein, Kaplan and Rosenberg 1991; Shapiro, Hatheway and Swerdlow 1998.

129 For a thorough discussion of the recommended folic acid intake and its implications, see Chanarin 1990.

130 Fairgrieve and Molto 2000 have argued that in the Roman Mediterranean, where goat's milk is known to have been given to infants, the development of this condition in such young individuals may reflect folic acid deficiency caused by a diet based on goat's milk.

practices take place, and of how these practices can enhance the maintenance of balanced health or expose a child to the risk of death.

Conclusions: Reconstructing Health and Disease Patterns in Byzantine Crete: Results and Perspectives

The investigation of daily life and living conditions in the Byzantine world is a relatively underexplored subject, taking a back seat to more visible aspects of Byzantine culture such as works of art and ecclesiastical architecture. The aim of this book has been to provide an overview of health and disease in Byzantine Crete that includes all available bioarchaeological data. Given the limited number of collections of Byzantine skeletal material that have been excavated, curated and published, a substantial quantity of evidence has been considered in this book: the evaluation of published and unpublished data compiled between 1976 and 2009 and generated by various researchers, including the author, has drawn on the evidence of 445 skeletons from six sites.

A first step in the composition of this study was the contextualization of the biological data, since neglect of the cultural context would have provided only a shallow glimpse into past human life, representing individuals as isolated vessels of suffering or healthy bodies. The combining of these pieces has created a basic framework for the study of the populations, focusing on specific aspects of Byzantine life that could contribute to the discussion of the biological data and the reconstruction of health and disease patterns. For example, natural disasters, daily hazards and conditions of sanitation are significant pieces of a larger picture that affords a better understanding of the development and buffering of various pathological conditions and the formation of mortality patterns. Examination of the qualitatively diverse biological data has produced a strong body of raw data that could facilitate future comparative studies. To this end, discussion of the biological findings includes citation of the applied methodology, definitions and diagnostic criteria for the observed pathological conditions, and photographic and radiographic aids. For the benefit of paleopathological research, estimates are provided of both the number of individuals affected by a pathological condition (crude prevalence rate) and the number of skeletal elements affected (true prevalence rate), and these are presented also in detailed tables and associated graphs.

The paleopathological basis of the present study has brought new evidence to the reconstruction of living conditions in Byzantine Crete. Through the analysis and interpretation of the mortality profiles, of the observed pathological conditions and of the data retrieved from the application of chemical analysis, the study of human remains of the populations of Byzantine Crete has offered possible answers to questions about health and disease patterns and dietary habits.

In the broadly agriculturally and pastorally based economy of Byzantine Crete, people would have been engaged in activities that contributed primarily to the household economy and to the maintenance of the most important unit of society, that of the family. For males, who by nature have a less effective immune response than females, the daily hazards encountered during the performance of demanding and hard-labor activities exposed them to the risk of temporary or permanent disability, and even to death. Females, on the other hand, were especially at risk from complications associated with pregnancy and childbirth. These conditions have enabled us to account for a clustering of deaths in the most productive age categories (from 15 to 34 years) and in some cases, where conditions were even less favorable, to account for the high number of deaths (for example, in the case of Eleutherna, where almost one-third of the population died within this age range).

The populations under study experienced a wide range of pathological conditions, which have provided valuable clues about their overall health status. Some of these conditions did not affect the normal functioning of the afflicted individual during life: these include, for example, spina bifida occulta, which even today is discovered only in the course of routine radiological examination, and button osteoma, which is one of the most common benign bone neoplasms encountered in both archaeological and modern populations. Other pathological conditions, however, prohibited their possessors from functioning satisfactorily. Such was perhaps the case of the 19-year-old individual with humerus varus, who most likely lived with a slightly disabled shoulder and arm.

The data presented here on dental, degenerative and infectious diseases, hematopoietic disorders and traumatic incidents, namely fractures, have offered an insight into the complex interaction between cultural and environmental factors, particularly in the areas of diet and subsistence, strenuous living conditions and daily hazards. Dental diseases were among the most frequently observed pathological conditions, affecting primarily middle-aged adults and male individuals. Cleaning of the teeth does not seem to have been a customary practice in the studied populations, and the types of foods that were consumed largely determined the development of specific dental diseases. Calculus, for example, the second most frequently observed pathological condition in the sample, is indicative of a more protein-rich diet, as it usually develops in the mouth in an alkaline environment.

The presence of osteoarthritis in major joints and in the vertebral column in the populations studied here has been associated with the wear and tear occasioned by everyday activities; that is, although osteoarthritis is a multifactorial condition, the primary contributing factors were determined to be age and mechanical stress. The skeletal data on degenerative joint disease demonstrates that males, particularly of younger age groups, suffered more than females. Although these sex differences in the data may be related to factors such as hormones, body size and anatomy, rather than to activity, the observed pattern may be suggestive of a more demanding lifestyle for male individuals, for whom an early onset of work could be also suspected. Schmorl's nodes, in particular, can occur idiopathically or can be associated with specific pathological conditions, but their development is most commonly the result of degenerative changes associated with ordinary stress on the vertebral column. On the basis of recent clinical studies that document a relationship between Schmorl's nodes and pain, these lesions can be expected to have adversely affected the quality of life of the populations.

For years now porotic hyperostosis and cribra orbitalia have become almost synonymous with iron-deficiency anemia in the bioarchaeological literature, and their diagnosis has been highly influenced – especially for Greek skeletal populations – by Angel's hypothesis that they reflect thalassemia genotypes as a response to endemic malaria. But multifactorial etiology is probably the most appropriate model for interpreting the causative mechanisms responsible for the development of these lesions. In the populations studied here, it is suggested that a combination of factors, including a vitamin B12-deficient diet, could account for the prevalence of porotic hyperostosis and cribra orbitalia at some sites.

Diagnoses of infectious conditions in the sample were limited to the presence of periosteal reactions, mainly on the long bones of the lower limbs (tibia and fibula), and to a possible case of actinomycosis. As actinomycosis is a chronic granulomatous, suppurative disease of humans and cattle, it could be indicative of close contact with domesticated animals, which favors the development of poor sanitary conditions. Periosteal lesions, if not of systemic hematogenous origin, could represent a bony reaction to overlying skin trauma caused by everyday activities. The predilection of male individuals to these lesions may reflect greater exposure to repeated minor trauma to their lower limbs, possibly as a consequence of gender influences on occupations.

Fractures reported in the sample reflect a lifetime of encounters with the environment and fellow humans. Middle-aged and mature males sustained the majority of the observed fractures, primarily as a consequence of falls caused by the individual's own clumsiness or accidental injuries during the performance of everyday activities. Multiple fractures on the same individual, although possibly suggestive of an exceptionally dangerous life marked by repeated traumatic events, seem unlikely to be the result of constant physical abuse, since they did not present different stages of healing. The possibility of injuries due to interpersonal violence could be suspected for the observed cranial injuries (one of them resulting in the death of the individual) and for the observed scapular fracture. None of the recorded fractures could be attributed to an underlying disease, and although complications were noted in a number of them, such as osteoarthritis or loss of the normal shape of the bone, all of the observed fractures demonstrated healing process – a clear indication that the individual survived the incident. It is suspected that the impact of each fracture played a significant role in the performance of daily activities, which could have been particularly evident if the individual was involved in manual labor. A farmer, for example, would have been less successful in performing many farming activities, due to pain, weakness and reduced range of motion.

Childhood – the most sensitive stage of the human life cycle – has merited special attention in the analysis. The study of the biological and social profile of Byzantine children highlights numerous aspects of their precarious lives, allowing a more detailed reconstruction of what it was like to be a child in Byzantine society. The investigation of non-adult mortality patterns informs us about the cultural and biological circumstances experienced by this age group, providing a reliable marker of the group's adaptability to the cultural and natural environment, and a valuable testament to the ability of the adult population to maintain good health in the most vulnerable members of the society. At those sites considered in the present study where child mortality exceeded infant mortality, as for example in Eleutherna, causes have been sought within the conditions of poor sanitation and among cultural factors that influenced weaning patterns. The presence of specific pathological conditions, such as scurvy, suggests that weaning stress played a significant role in the construction of the non-adult mortality profile.

Food, essential for the survival and maintenance of a healthy organism, has been taken up in the final chapter. The investigation of written sources, supplemented by evidence retrieved from chemical analysis, has provided a picture of Byzantine dietary habits. Documentary evidence portrays a Byzantine diet based on grain (primarily wheat and barley), oil and wine, supplemented with legumes, dairy products, meat and marine resources, but the relative importance of each foodstuff in the Byzantine diet is not always as clear.

The application of stable isotope analysis on nine Byzantine populations throughout Greece has provided new information on their dietary habits. The derived $\delta^{13}C$ and $\delta^{15}N$ values are quite tightly clustered, suggesting that all of these populations may have eaten a broadly similar diet. Carbonate $\delta^{13}C$ values, which indicate that most calories came from C_3 plants or C_3-feeding animals, are consistent with a diet based on the 'Mediterranean trinity' of wheat, oil and wine. Although substantial dependence on a C_4 grain staple, such as millet, was not indicated at any of the sites, at the inland site of Sourtara a range of 2‰ in $\delta^{13}C$ values and little change in the $\delta^{15}N$ values suggests that the population consumed some domesticated animals that had a C_4 component in their diet. Collagen $\delta^{13}C$ values are in the range usually associated with C_3 terrestrial resources, while $\delta^{15}N$ values are high relative to those of domesticated animals from Byzantine sites. The isotopic data do not support hypotheses of a general dependence on low-$\delta^{15}N$ legumes, since substantial legume consumption is inconsistent with the high collagen $\delta^{15}N$ values seen for all sites. Instead, the values suggest that significant amounts of animal protein were included in the Byzantine diet.

One unanticipated pattern offered by the stable isotope analysis is the increase in marine protein consumption, seen at the coastal sites (a reasonable expectation given their location) but also evident for some individuals at the inland sites. This pattern contrasts with previous isotopic studies on prehistoric populations, which have suggested that among coastal populations marine species contributed little if at all to the diet. Does the pattern indicate that the Byzantines were well aware that fish and most of the aquatic animals provided high nutritional value and that they had further developed specific fishing methods for the various species? Did fasting rules, where fish consumption is allowed for a considerable time throughout the year, contribute to the increased consumption of fish and aquatic species? For inland sites, the isotopic values may be indicative of a high consumption of dairy products (known from the written sources to have been generally available across classes and regions), but another possibility is that freshwater fishes (also attested in the written sources) were consumed in areas where lakes and rivers existed. Whatever the cause, the stable isotope data are broadly suggestive of inland and coastal Byzantine populations supplementing an essentially land-based C_3 diet with some possible C_4 and marine resources.

Isotopic studies conducted to date also offer insight into the diet of the very young, suggesting that Byzantine children were weaned at a relatively late age. The data available from this study affords no firm conclusions about weaning behavior in Byzantine Greece. They have allowed us, though, to make some tentative suggestions and to recommend directions for further research. The contrast between the elevated values seen in non-adults aged 3 years or less and the adult-like pattern seen in children aged 4 and older suggests that weaning was completed by the fourth year – a pattern consistent with data derived from the written sources. The study of documentary evidence on infant feeding, attesting, for example, the use of honey and goats' milk, and current clinical data have offered additional information on serious health problems, such as botulism and megaloblastic anemia, that could have resulted from the type and nutritional quality of the food introduced.

This book provides an assessment of the trends suggested by the available datasets within the biocultural context of Byzantine Crete: people experienced demanding lifestyles, where hard work was the norm both for indoor and outdoor activities; were prone to accidents – and even to violent attacks; and in some cases lived on poor diets. It is hoped that this work will also point the way for the future, encouraging the use of biological data in the tracing of past populations' health and contributing to interdisciplinary cooperation. Although this study has not exhausted the wealth of information attested in the written sources or in the archaeological record, it highlights the need for close collaboration among physical anthropologists, historians and archaeologists, since the interaction of biological and cultural data is fundamental when working with historic populations. The study of disease is an interdisciplinary task and those involved in the analysis of human skeletal remains will be better informed through familiarity with current anthropological and archaeological research agendas on a regional, national and international level. The development of a continuous and healthy dialogue between physical anthropology and archaeology will ensure that biological and cultural issues can be addressed.

Success in this collaboration will require changes in the way that physical anthropology is viewed within the field of archaeology. Most of the archaeological and anthropological work in Greece is subject to the vagaries of poorly funded projects: people working within tight budgets and on short time schedules, where post-excavation study, especially of human remains, is not always possible. Skeletons retrieved in an excavation have no less scientific value than artifacts and architectural remains. Although the latter usually monopolize the interest of researchers, the study of both the products and the producers contribute to a better reconstruction of life in the past. Human collections from historic times, including those of Byzantine Crete, are by no means less important than prehistoric ones, as historic populations offer a great advantage: the solid background of documentary evidence against which the biological data can be projected.

A hope of the author is that this book will be useful in its immediate intent, serving as a resource from which subsequent studies can extract valuable information or tackle bigger questions. For the future, an improved standardization of the methodology used in the recording, analysis, integration, interpretation and publication of data should be more easily achieved if it starts from the baseline set by current bioarchaeological studies in Greece.

Glossary

Actinomycosis: A chronic granulomatous disease of humans and cattle, that may be systemic or localized, caused by the bacterium *Actinomyces israelii* from within the oral cavity. Actinomycosis presents in three different forms depending on the location of the lesion: head/neck, abdomen and chest/lungs.

Ankylosis spondylitis: A seronegative joint disease, characterized by inflammation of the synovial joints and involvement of the tendon insertion points of bones. It usually affects the sacro-iliac joints first and then moves up the spine, which can become fused, and erosive lesions may be visible on the vertebral bodies. Spinal ligaments become inflamed and may ossify, thus fusing the spine into a characteristic "bamboo" appearance and causing decreased mobility. The condition affects males more frequently than females. Its specific cause is unknown; most people, however, have the HLA B27 antigen in their blood.

Annulus fibrosus: The tough fibrous outer zone of the intervertebral disc that normally retains the soft inner nucleus pulposus.

Appendicular: Relating to the appendages of the skeleton, namely the upper and lower limbs (arms and legs).

Botulism: A severe, often fatal form of food poisoning caused by the saprophyte *Clostridium botulinum*.

Callus: A composite mass of tissue formed at the site of a broken bone; it is composed initially of uncalcified fibrous tissue and cartilage and ultimately of bone.

Cartilage: Gristle; chondrus – a connective tissue characterized by its nonvascularity and firm consistency.

Cloaca: Cavity (pus-containing abscess) from within the bone interior.

Collagen: An important protein structural element of the body.

Colles' fracture: The distal end of the radius is broken and the fragment displaced posteriorly.

Costochondral: Relating to or joining a rib and costal cartilage.

Cribra orbitalia: The presence of many small holes on the orbital roofs.

Dental attrition: Wear on the biting surfaces of the teeth caused by normal use.

Diploic (diploë): The spongy layer of bone between the hard outer and inner layers of the flat cranial bones.

Distal: On the dental arch a location further from the median line of the jaw; on a long bone the lower end (the end farthest away from the mid-line of the body).

DNA: Abbreviation for deoxyribonucleic acid, the very long molecule that winds up to form a chromosome and that contains the complete code for the automatic construction of the body.

Eburnation: Bone sclerosis; polished joint surface that develops when a joint continues to be used after the cartilage protecting it has been destroyed.

Enamel hypoplasias: Defects on the enamel surface of the teeth in the form of horizontal lines, pits or grooves, usually more easily seen on the cheek surfaces of the incisors and canines. These defects occur only while the teeth are developing and remain as a permanent record in adulthood. Among the possible causes of enamel hypoplasias are nutritional deficiencies, fever and childhood illnesses such as measles.

Epiphysis: End part of the shaft of a long bone.

Fibrocartilage: A tough form of cartilage containing many thick bundles of collagen fibers.

Folic acid: A vitamin of the B group necessary for the synthesis of DNA and red blood cells.

Granuloma: A collection of inflammatory cells representing a chronic inflammatory process.

Hamartoma: A focal malformation that resembles a neoplasm, grossly and even microscopically, but results from faulty development in an organ.

Harris lines: Transverse lines of radiodensity at the ends of long bones. They are considered a popular indicator of physiological stress (for example, influenza, measles, surgery, starvation, vitamin deficiency, emotional stress etc.) in ancient populations, but are problematic on account of interpretation of their etiology and limitations associated with the recording of these features. Only about one-fourth of these lines in non-adults persist into adulthood.

Humerus varus: Slipped proximal epiphysis of the humerus.

Hypervitaminosis A: Excess intake of vitamin A. The condition manifests itself in diffuse periosteal reaction no earlier than the end of the first year of life.

Hypoplasias: See enamel hypoplasias.

Idiopathic: Adjective used in characterizing a disease of unknown cause.

Infantile cortical hyperostosis (or Caffey's disease): The condition affects infants in the first six months of life and is characterized by massive deposition of layered periosteal woven bone on one or more bones. Its etiology is unknown; a viral infection is suggested.

Inflammatory (inflammation): The response of living tissue to injury, featuring widening of blood vessels, with redness, heat, swelling and pain.

Intervertebral disc: A disc-shaped, fibrocartilaginous, shock-absorbing structure lying between the bodies of adjoining vertebrae in the spinal column. Each disc consists of an outer fibrous ring (annulus fibrosus) and an inner soft core (nucleus pulposus).

Kyphosis: Deformity of the spine characterized by extensive flexion.

Lamellar bone: New bone formation in a disease process; more mature, older, organized in appearance. Lamellar bone may indicate that the process was quiescent or had been overcome.

Lytic (lysis): Destruction or dissolution.

Megaloblastic anemia: Anemia characterized by high numbers of abnormally large, nucleated red blood cells, precursor cells in the bone marrow and in the blood.

Neoplasm: A new and abnormal growth of tissue that serves no function and develops at the expense of the healthy organism.

Nucleus pulposus: The pulpy (soft, spongy) core of the intervertebral disc that is surrounded by annulus fibrosus.

Osteoarthritis (OA): Degenerative disease of the synovial joints.

Osteochondritis dissecans: A form of aseptic necrosis of the epiphysis in which a fragment of cartilage and/or subchondral bone becomes detached.

Osteophyte: A bony outgrowth or protuberance.

Osteoporosis: A form of bone atrophy involving both the collagen scaffolding and mineralization; it is commonest in females after the menopause.

Parry fracture: The distal end of the ulna is broken; may indicate interpersonal violence (defense against a blow to the head by raising the forearm).

Periosteum: The thick fibrous membrane covering the entire surface of a bone except its articular cartilage.

Periostitis: Inflammation of the periosteum as a reaction to trauma or the result of certain pathological processes.

Porotic hyperostosis: Small holes on the external surface of the skull, particularly on the parietal and occipital bones.

Rickets: A metabolic disorder caused by vitamin D deficiency.

Sacralization: Fusion of the fifth lumbar vertebra with the first sacral vertebra.

Schmorl's nodes: Depression on the surface of the vertebral body, produced by the pressure introduced by the intervertebral disc.

Scoliosis: Lateral curvature of the spine.

Scurvy: A metabolic disorder caused by vitamin C deficiency.

Spina bifida occulta: A defect of the bony spinal canal usually occurring in the sacrum without protrusion of the spinal cord.

Spondylosis: Degeneration of the vertebral bodies.

Subchondral: Beneath or below the cartilage.

Sudden Infant Death Syndrome (SIDS): The sudden death of any young infant or young child, unexpected by earlier medical history, and in which a thorough postmortem examination fails to demonstrate adequate cause of death.

Subperiosteal: Under the periosteum.

Synovial joint: A mobile joint (for example, the knee joint).

Thalassemia: One of several hereditary abnormalities affecting the synthesis of globin chains of hemoglobin leading to severe anemia. It is common in the regions surrounding the Mediterranean basin.

Woven bone: New bone formation in a disease process that is immature or primary and whose appearance is porous and disorganized. Woven bone indicates that the disease process was active at the time of death.

References Cited

Primary Sources

Aboulféda. M. Reinaud and M. MacGuckin de Slane (tr.), *Abû l'Fida', Géographie d'Aboulféda*, 2 vols., Paris: Imprimerie Royale, 1848.

Aetius of Amida. A. Olivieri, *Aetii Amideni libri medicinales I–IV*, Corpus Medicorum Graecorum, Leipzig: Teubner, 1935. Olivieri, *Aetii Amideni libri medicinales V–VIII*, Corpus Medicorum Graecorum, Berlin: Akademie Verlag, 1950.

Alexander of Tralles. T. Puschmann (ed. and tr.), *Alexander von Tralles*, 2 vols, Vienna: Braumüller, 1878–79.

C. Buondelmonti. A.M. Van Spitael (ed.), *C. Buondelmonti, Descriptio insulae Crete et liber insularum, cap. XI: Creta*, Heraklion: Σύλλογος Πολιτιστικής Αναπτύξεως Ηρακλείου, 1981.

Codex Justinianus. P. Krueger and T. Mommsen (eds), *Corpus iuris civilis: Institutiones, Digesta, Codex Justinianus, Novellae*, 3 vols, Berlin: Weidmannos, 1928.

Edrisi. P.A. Jaubert (tr.), *Edrisi, Géographie d'Edrisi*, 2 vols, Paris: Imprimerie Royale, 1836–40.

Geoponica. H. Beck (ed.), *Geoponica sive Cassiani Bassi scholastici de re rustica eclogae*, Leipzig: Teubner, 1895.

Hieroclis Synecdemos. E. Honigmann (ed.), *Le Synécdemos d'Hiéroclès et l'opuscule géographique de Georges de Chypre*, Brussels: Editions de l'Institut de Philologie et d'Histoire Orientales et Slaves, 1930.

Kitâb al-Dja'rafiyya. M. Hadj-Sadok (ed.), 'Le Kitâb al-Dja'rafiyya, de Abu 'Abd Allah Mohammad ben Abi Bakr Al-Zuhrî', *Bulletin d'Etudes Orientales* 21 (1968), 1–346.

Oribasius. J. Raeder, *Oribasii collectionum medicarum reliquiae*, 5 vols, Corpus Medicorum Graecorum, Leipzig: Teubner, 1928–33.

Paul of Aegina. J. Heiberg (ed.), *Paulus Aeginita*, Corpus Medicorum Graecorum, 2 vols, Leipzig: Teubner, 1921 and 1924. F. Adams (tr.), *The Medical Works of Paulus Aeginita, the Greek Physician, Translated into English with a Copious Commentary Containing a Comprehensive View of the Knowledge Possessed by the Greeks, Romans and Arabians on All Subjects Connected with Medicine and Surgery*, London: J. Welsh; Treuttel and Würtz & Co., 1834.

Porikologos. H. Winterwerb, *Porikologos: Einleitung, kritische Ausgabe aller Versionen, Übersetzung, Textvergleiche, Glossar, kurze Betrachtungen zu den fremdsprachlichen Versionen des Werks sowie zum Opsarologos*, Cologne: Romiosini, 1992.

Psarologos. K. Krumbacher (ed.), '*Ο Ψαρολόγος*', *Das mittelgriechische Fischbuch*, Sitzungsberichte der Bayerischen Akademie der Wissenschaften, Heft 3, Munich, 1903.

Psellos. K.N. Sathas (ed.), 'Ἐπιτάφιοι λόγοι εἰς τὴν θυγατέρα Στυλιανήν. Μιχαὴλ Ψελλοῦ: Ἱστορικοὶ λόγοι ἐπιστολαὶ καὶ ἄλλα ἀνέκδοτα', *Μεσαιωνική Βιβλιοθήκη* 5 (1876), 62–87.

Ptochoprodromos. H. Eideneier (tr. and ed.), *Ptochoprodromos: Einführung, kritische Ausgabe, deutsche Übersetzung, Glossar*, Cologne: Romiosini, 1991.

Soranos d'Ephèse. P. Burguière, D. Gourevitch and Y. Malinas, *Soranos d'Ephèse. Maladies des Femmes, tome II, livre II*, Paris: Les Belles Lettres, 1990.

Vita Andreae Cretensis. A. Papadopoulos-Kerameus (ed.), 'Niketas, Vita Andreae Cretensis', *Ανάλεκτα Ιεροσολυματικής Σταχυολογίας* V (1898), 169–79.

Vita of Basil the Younger. S.G. Vilinskij (ed.), *Žitie sv. Vasilija Novogo v russkoj literature*, Zapiski Imperatorskogo novorossiskago universiteta, Istoriko-filologicheskili fakultet, vyp. 7–8, 2 vols, Odessa: Tip. 'Tekhnik', 1911.

Vita of Makarios of Pelekete. I. van den Gheyn (ed.), 'S. Macarii monasterii Pelecetes hegumeni acta graeca', *Analecta Bollandiana* 16 (1897), 140–63.

Vita of Michael Synkellos. M.B. Cunningham (ed.), *The Life of Michael the Synkellos*, Belfast: Belfast Byzantine Texts and Translations, 1991.

Vita of Symeon Stylites the Younger. P. van de Ven (ed.), *La vie ancienne de S. Syméon Stylite le Jeune*, Subsidia Hagiographica no. 32, Brussels: Société des Bollandistes, 1962.

Vita of Theodora of Thessalonike. S. Paschalides (ed.), '*Ο Βίος* τῆς ὁσιομυροβλύτιδος *Θεοδώρας* τῆς *ἐν* Θεσσαλονίκη: *Διήγηση περὶ* τῆς *μεταθέσεως* *τοῦ τιμίου λειψάνου* τῆς *ὁσίας Θεοδώρας*, Thessaloniki: Κέντρον Αγιολογικών Μελετών Ι. Μητροπόλεως Θεσσαλονίκης, 1991. A.-M. Talbot (tr.), 'Life of St. Theodora of Thessalonike', in A.M. Talbot (ed.), *Holy Women of Byzantium: Ten Saints' Lives in Translation*, Washington DC: Dumbarton Oaks Research Library and Collection, 1996, 159–237.

Vita of Saint Alypios. H. Delehaye (ed.), *Les saints stylites*, Subsidia Hagiographica no. 14, Brussels: Société des Bollandistes, 1923.

Vita of Saint Evaristos. C. van de Vorst, 'La vie de S. Evariste, higoumène à Constantinople', *Analecta Bollandiana* 41 (1923), 288–325.

Vita of Saint Ioannis Xeni. N. Tomadakis (ed.), 'Ὁ Ἅγιος Ἰωάννης ὁ Ξένος καὶ ἡ διαθήκη αὐτοῦ', *Κρητικά Χρονικά* 2 (1948), 47–72.

Vita of Saint Niconis Metanoeite. S. Lambros (ed.), 'Vita S. Niconis Metanoeite', *Νέος Ελληνομνήμων* 3 (1906), 129–228.
Vita of Saint Peter of Atroa. V. Laurent (ed.), *La vie merveilleuse de saint Pierre d'Atroa (+837)*, Subsidia Hagiographica no. 29, Brussels: Société des Bollandistes, 1956.
Vita of Saint Thekla. G. Dagron (ed.), *Vie et miracles de sainte Thècle*, Brussels: Société des Bollandistes, 1978.
Vita of Saint Theodore Tiron (the Recruit). A. Sigalas, 'Βίος καὶ ἀνατροφὴ τοῦ ἁγίου μάρτυρος Θεοδώρου,' *Επετηρίς Εταιρείας Βυζαντινών Σπουδών* 2 (1925), 220–26.

Secondary Literature

Abrahamse 1979. D. Abrahamse, 'Images of Childhood in Early Byzantine Hagiography', *Journal of Psychohistory* 6, 497–517.
Abrahamse 1984. D. Abrahamse, 'Rituals of Death in the Middle Byzantine Period', *Greek Orthodox Theological Review* 25, 125–34.
Agelarakis and Agelarakis 1989. A. Agelarakis and A. Agelarakis, 'The Paleopathological Evidence at Polystylon, Abdera', *Byzantinische Forschungen* 14, 9–25.
Albertocchi and Perna 2001. R. Albertocchi and R. Perna, 'Ceramica commune: vasi da mensa e da dispensa', in A. Di Vita (ed.), *Gortina V. 3, lo scavo del Pretorio (1980–1995)*, Monografie della Scuola Archeologica Italiana di Atene XII, Padue: Aido Ausilio Editore, 411–536.
Alexakis 2001. A. Alexakis, 'Was There Life Beyond the Life Beyond? Byzantine Ideas on Reincarnation and Final Restoration', *Dumbarton Oaks Papers* 55, 155–177.
Alexiou 2002. M. Alexiou, *The Ritual Lament in Greek Tradition*, Lanham, MA: Rowman & Littlefield.
Alt et al. 2002. K. Alt, C. Alder, C. Buitrago-Tellez, B. Lohrke, 'Infant Osteosarcoma', *International Journal of Osteoarchaeology* 12, 442–8.
Anagnostakis 1995. I. Anagnostakis, *Οίνος ο Βυζαντινός. Η άμπελος και ο οίνος στη βυζαντινή ποίηση και υμνογραφία*, Athens: Ίδρυμα Φανή Μπουτάρη.
Anagnostakis 1996. I. Anagnostakis, 'Ελλαδικά παραμύθια και ελλαδική παραμυθία στο Βυζάντιο του 10ου αι.,' in *Ελιά και Λάδι, Δ΄ Τριήμερο Εργασίας*, Καλαμάτα, 7–9 May 1993, Athens: Πολιτιστικό Ίδρυμα Ομίλου Πειραιώς, 121–50.
Anagnostakis 2000. I. Anagnostakis, 'Βυζαντινή μελωνυμία και μελίκρατος πότος. Οι αντιλήψεις για τη χρήση των μελισσοκομικών προϊόντων στο Βυζάντιο ως τον 11ο αιώνα', in *Η μέλισσα και τα προϊόντα της, ΣΤ΄ Τριήμερο Εργασίας*, Νικήτη,

12–15 September 1996, Athens: Πολιτιστικό Ίδρυμα Ομίλου Πειραιώς, 169–81.

Anagnostakis 2005. I. Anagnostakis, 'Τροφικές δηλητηριάσεις στο Βυζάντιο. Διατροφικές αντιλήψεις και συμπεριφορές (6ος–11ος αι.)', in D. Papanikola-Bakirtzi (ed.), *Πρακτικά ημερίδας Περί διατροφής στο Βυζάντιο*, Θεσσαλονίκη, 4 November 2001, Athens: ΥΠ.ΠΟ.-Τ.Α.Π.Α., 61–110.

Anagnostakis 2008. I. Anagnostakis, *Βυζαντινός οινικός πολιτισμός*, Το Βυζάντιο σήμερα 6, Athens: Ινστιτούτο Βυζαντινών Ερευνών/Εθνικό Ίδρυμα Ερευνών.

Anagnostakis and Lambropoulou 2009. I. Anagnostakis and A. Lambropoulou, 'Το άθυρμα στο Βυζάντιο. Πηγές και πρωτοβυζαντινά τεκμήρια', in K. Gougouli and D. Karakatsani (eds), *Το ελληνικό παιχνίδι. Διαδρομές στην ιστορία του*, Athens: ΜΙΕΤ-Ελληνικό και Λογοτεχνικό Αρχείο, 69–89.

Anagnostakis and Papamastorakis 2005. I. Anagnostakis and T. Papamastorakis, '"...And Radishes for Appetizers": On Banquets, Radishes and Wine', in D. Papanikola-Bakirtzi (ed.), *Πρακτικά ημερίδας Περί διατροφής στο Βυζάντιο*, Θεσσαλονίκη, 4 November 2001, Athens: ΥΠ.ΠΟ.-Τ.Α.Π.Α., 147–74.

Anderson 1996. T. Anderson, 'Cranial Weapon Injuries from Anglo-Saxon Dover', *International Journal of Osteoarchaeology* 6, 10–14.

Anderson 1997. T. Anderson, 'A Medieval Case of Bilateral Humerus Varus', *Journal of Paleopathology* 9, 143–146.

Anderson 2002. T. Anderson, 'Metaphyseal Fibrous Defects in Juveniles from Medieval Norwich', *International Journal of Osteoarchaeology* 12, 144–8.

Anderson and Carter 1994. T. Anderson and A.R. Carter, 'Short Report: Periosteal Reaction in a New Born Child from Sheppey, Kent', *International Journal of Osteoarchaeology* 4, 47–8.

Andrianakis 2006. M. Andrianakis, 'Χριστιανικά Μνημεία επαρχίας Μυλοποτάμου', in *Πρακτικά Διεθνούς Επιστημονικού Συνεδρίου, Ο Μυλοπόταμος από την αρχαιότητα ως σήμερα*, Ρέθυμνο, 24–30 October 2003, Rethymno: Ιστορική και Λαογραφική Εταιρεία Ρεθύμνου, 47–78.

Andrianakis 2008. M. Andrianakis, 'Ag. Ioannis Xenos and his Cult', in *Proceedings of an International Symposium on Routes of Faith in the Medieval Mediterranean: History, Monuments, People, Pilgrimage Perspectives*, Thessaloniki, 7–10 November 2007, Thessaloniki: European Centre of Byzantine and Post-Byzantine Monuments, 256–68.

Angel 1964a. J.L. Angel, 'Osteoporosis: Thalassemia?', *American Journal of Physical Anthropology* 22, 369–74.

Angel 1964b. J.L. Angel, 'The Reaction Area of the Femoral Neck', *Clinical Orthopedics* 32, 130–42.

Angel 1966. J.L. Angel, 'Porotic Hyperostosis, Anemias, Malarias and Marshes in the Prehistoric Mediterranean', *Science* 153, 760–63.

Angel 1967. J.L. Angel, 'Porotic Hyperostosis or Osteoporosis Symmetrica', in D.R. Brothwell and A.T. Sandison (eds), *Diseases in Antiquity: A Survey of the Diseases, Injuries and Surgery of Earlier Human Populations*, Springfield, IL: Charles C. Thomas, 378–89.

Angel 1968. J.L. Angel, 'The Bases of Paleodemography' (abstract), *American Journal of Physical Anthropology* 29, 137.

Angel 1969. J.L. Angel, 'The Bases of Paleodemography', *American Journal of Physical Anthropology* 30, 427–37.

Angel 1971. J.L. Angel, *The People of Lerna: Analysis of a Prehistoric Aegean Population*, Princeton: American School of Classical Studies at Athens.

Angel 1974. J.L. Angel, 'Patterns of Fractures from Neolithic to Modern Times', *Anthropologiai Közlmények* 18, 9–18.

Angel 1977. J.L. Angel, 'Anemias of Antiquity: Eastern Mediterranean', in E. Cockburn and A. Cockburn (eds), *Porotic Hyperostosis: An Enquiry*, Detroit: Paleopathology Association Monograph 2, 1–5.

Angel 1978. J.L. Angel, 'Porotic Hyperostosis in the Eastern Mediterranean', *Medical College of Virginia Quarterly* 14, 10–16.

Angel 1982. J.L. Angel, 'Osteoarthritis and Occupation (Ancient and Modern)', in V.V. Novotny (ed.), *Second Anthropological Congress of Ales Hrdlička*, Prague: Pragensis Universitas Carolina, 443–6.

Angel 1984. J.L. Angel, 'Health as a Crucial Factor in the Changes from Hunting to Developed Farming in the Eastern Mediterranean', in M.N. Cohen and G.J. Armelagos (eds), *Paleopathology at the Origins of Agriculture*, Orlando: Academic Press, 51–73.

Angel and Bisel 1985. J.L. Angel and S.C. Bisel, 'Health and Nutrition in Mycenean Greece: A Study in Human Skeletal Remains', in N.C. Wilkie and W.P.D. Coulson (eds), *Contributions to Aegean Archaeology*, Minneapolis: Centre for Ancient Studies, University of Minnesota, 197–209.

Antoniadis-Bibicou 1973. H. Antoniadis-Bibicou, 'Quelques notes sur l'enfant de la moyenne époque byzantine (du VIe au XII siècle), *Annales de démographie historique (enfant et société)*', Paris: La Haye, 77–83.

Antonopoulos 1986. E. Antonopoulos, 'Prolégomènes à une typologie de l'enfance de la moyenne époque byzantine (du VIe au XIIe siècle)', in J. Silva (ed.), *Historicité de l'enfance et de la jeunesse dans la production historique récente*, 271–87, Athens: Εθνικό Ἵδρυμα Ερευνών.

Argoff and Wheeler 1998. C.E. Argoff and A.H. Wheeler, 'Spinal and Radicular Pain Disorders', *Neurologic Clinics* 16, 833–49.

Armelagos 1990. G.J. Armelagos, 'Health and Disease in Prehistoric Populations', in A.C. Swedlund and G.J. Armelagos (eds), *Disease in Populations in*

Transition: Anthropological and Epidemiological Perspective, New York: Bergin and Garvey, 127–45.

Armelagos 1998. G.J. Armelagos, 'Introduction: Sex, Gender and Health Status in Prehistoric and Contemporary Populations', in A.L. Grauer and P. Stuart-Macadam (eds), *Sex and Gender in Paleopathological Perspective*, Cambridge: Cambridge University Press, 1998.

Arnon et al. 1979. S.S. Arnon, T.F. Madura, K. Damus, B. Thompson, R.M. Wood, J. Chin, 'Honey and Other Environmental Risk Factors for Infant Botulism', *Journal of Pediatrics* 94, 331–6.

Atoche-Peña, Rodríguez-Martín and Ramírez-Rodríguez 2008. P. Atoche-Peña, C. Rodríguez-Martín and A. Ramírez-Rodríguez, *Mummies and Science: World Mummies Research, Proceedings of the VIth World Congress on Mummy Studies*, Teguise (Lanzarote), 20–24 February 2007, Santa Cruz de Tenerife: Contacto Centro de Artes Gráficas.

Atti del Congresso Internazionale Creta Roman e Protobizantina 2004. *Atti del Congresso Internazionale Creta Romana e Protobizantina*, Heraklion, 23–30 September 2000, vols I, II, III–I, III–II, Padua: Aido Ausilio Editore.

Aubert 1989. J.-J. Aubert, 'Threatened Wombs: Aspects of Ancient Uterine Magic', *Greek, Roman and Byzantine Studies* 30, 421–9.

Aufderheide and Rodríguez-Martín 1998. A. Aufderheide and C. Rodríguez-Martín, *The Cambridge Encyclopedia of Human Paleopathology*, Cambridge: Cambridge University Press.

Bagousse and Blondiaux 2001. A.-L. Bagouse and J. Blondiaux, 'Hyperostoses corticales foetal et infantile à Lisieux (IVe s.): retour à Costebelle', *Centre Archaeologique du Var Revue*, 60–64.

Baker, Dupras and Tocheris 2005. B. Baker, T. Dupras and M. Tocheris, *The Osteology of Infants and Children*, College Station: Texas A&M University Press.

Bakirtzis 2003. Ch. Bakirtzis, *Βυζαντινά τσουκαλολάγηνα*, Δημοσιεύματα του Αρχαιολογικού Δελτίου αρ. 39, Athens: ΥΠ.ΠΟ.-Τ.Α.Π.Α.

Bakke 2005. O.M. Bakke, *When Children Became People. The Birth of Childhood in Early Christianity*, Minneapolis: Fortress Press.

Bandy 1970. A. Bandy, *The Greek Christian Inscriptions of Crete*, Athens: Χριστιανική Αρχαιολογική Εταιρεία.

Barber 1997. C. Barber, 'Homo Byzantinus?', in L. James (ed.), *Women, Men and Eunuchs: Gender in Byzantium*, New York: Routledge, 185–199.

Barker 1992a. D.J.P. Barker, *The Fetal and Infant Origins of Adult Disease*, London: BMJ Books.

Barker 1992b. D.J.P. Barker, 'Fetal Growth and Adult Disease', *British Journal of Obstetrics and Gynaecology* 99, 275–82.

Barker and Martyn 1992. D.J.P. Barker and C.N. Martyn, 'The Maternal and Fetal Origins of Cardiovascular Disease', *Journal of Epidemiology and Community Health* 46, 8–11.

Barker and Osmond 1986. D.J.P. Barker and C. Osmond, 'Childhood Respiratory Infection and Adult Chronic Bronchitis in England and Wales', *British Medical Journal* 239, 1271–5.

Barlow 1883. T. Barlow, 'On Cases Described as "Acute Rickets" Which Are Possibly a Combination of Scurvy and Rickets, the Scurvy Being an Essential and the Rickets a Variable', *Medico-Chirurgical Transactions* 66, 159–219.

Barnes 1994. E. Barnes, *Developmental Defects of the Axial Skeleton in Paleopathology*, Niwot: University Press of *Colorado*.

Barnes 2002. E. Barnes, 'The Dead Do Tell Tales', in *Corinth XX: Corinth the Centenary 1896–1996*, Princeton: American School of Classical Studies at Athens, 435–43.

Barnes and Ortner 1997. E. Barnes and D.J. Ortner, 'Multifocal Eosinophilic Granuloma with a Possible Trepanation in a Fourteenth Century Greek Young Individual', *International Journal of Osteoarchaeology* 7, 542–7.

Baxter 2005a. J.E. Baxter, *The Archaeology of Childhood: Children, Gender and Material Culture*, Walnut Creek, CA: AltaMira Press.

Baxter 2005b. J.E. Baxter, 'Introduction. The Archaeology of Childhood in Context', *Archaeological Papers of the American Anthropological Association* 15, 1–9.

Beaucamp 1977. J. Beaucamp, 'La situation juridique de la femme à Byzance', *Cahiers de civilisation médiévale* 20, 145–76.

Beaucamp 1982. J. Beaucamp, 'L'allaitement: mère ou nourrice?', *Jahrbuch der Österreichischen Byzantinistik* 32, 549–58.

Beaucamp 1990. J. Beaucamp, *Le statut de la femme à Byzance (4e–7e siècle), vol. i. Le droit impérial*, Paris: Ed. de Boccard.

Beaucamp 1992. J. Beaucamp, *Le statut de la femme à Byzance (4e–7e siècle), vol. ii. Les pratiques sociales*, Paris: Ed. de Boccard.

Beaucamp 2000. J. Beaucamp, 'Les femmes et l'Eglise: droit canonique, idéologie et pratiques sociales à Byzance', *KANON XVI, Mother, Nun, Deaconess, Images of Women According to Eastern Canon Law*, 87–112.

Bell and Piper 2000. L. Bell and K. Piper, 'An Introduction to Palaeohistopathology', in M. Cox and S. Mays (eds), *Human Osteology in Archaeology and Forensic Science*, London: Greenwich Medical Media, 255–73.

Bender 1968. M.M. Bender, 'Mass Spectrometric Studies of Carbon 13 Variations in Corn and Other Grasses', *Radiocarbon* 10, 468–72.

Bender 1971. M.M. Bender, 'Variations in the 13C/12C Ratios of Plants in Relation to the Pathway of Photosynthetic Carbon Dioxide Fixation', *Phytochemistry* 10, 1239–44.

Bennett 2000. D. Bennett, 'Medical Practice and Manuscripts in Byzantium', *Social History of Medicine* 13, 279–91.

Bennike 1987. P. Bennike, *Paleopathology of Danish Skeletons*, Copenhagen: Akademisk Forlag.

Bennike et al. 2005. P. Bennike, M. Lewis, H. Schutkowski, F. Valentin, 'Comparisons of Child Morbidity in Two Contrasting Medieval Cemeteries from Denmark', *American Journal of Physical Anthropology* 127, 734–46.

Berger and Trinkaus 1995. D.T Berger and E. Trinkaus, 'Patterns of Trauma among the Neanderthals', *Journal of Archaeological Science* 22, 841–52.

Bjørnholt and James 2007. B.K. Bjørnholt and L. James, 'The Man in the Street: Some Problems of Gender and Identity in Byzantine Material Culture', in M. Grünbart, E. Kislinger, A. Muthesius, D. Stathakopoulos (eds.), *Material Culture and Well-Being in Byzantium (400–1453), Proceedings of the International Conference*, Cambridge, 8–10 September 2001, Vienna: Verlag der Österreichischen Akademie der Wissenschaften, 51–56.

Bliquez 1984. L.J. Bliquez, 'Two Lists of Greek Surgical Instruments and the State of Surgery in Byzantine Times', *Dumbarton Oaks Papers* 38, 187–204.

Blom et al. 2005. D.E Blom, J.E. Buikstra, L. Keng, P.D. Tomczak, E. Shoreman, D. Stevens-Tuttle, 'Anemia and Childhood Mortality: Latitudinal Pattering along the Coast of Pre-Columbian Peru', *American Journal of Physical Anthropology* 127, 152–69.

Blondiaux et al. 2002. G. Blondiaux, J. Blondiaux, F. Secousse, A. Cotten, P.-M. Danze, R.-M. Flipo, 'Rickets and Child Abuse: The Case of a Two Year Old Girl from the 4th Century in Lisieux (Normandy)', *International Journal of Osteoarchaeology* 12, 209–15.

Bober 1999. P.P. Bober, *Art, Culture, and Cuisine: Ancient and Medieval Gastronomy*, Chicago: The University of Chicago Press.

Bocherens et al. 1991. H. Bocherens, M. Fizet, A. Mariotti, C. Olive, G. Bellon, D. Billiou, 'Application de la biogéochimie isotopique (^{13}C, ^{15}N) à la determination du régime alimentaire des populations humaines et animales durant les périodes antique et médiévale', *Archives des Sciences* 44, 329–40.

Bogaard et al. 2007. A. Bogaard, T.H.E. Heaton, P. Poulton, I. Merbach, 'The Impact of Manuring on Nitrogen Isotope Ratios in Cereals: Archaeological Implications for Reconstruction of Diet and Crop Management Practices', *Journal of Archaeological Science* 34, 335–43.

Boldsen 2007. J.L. Boldsen, 'Early Childhood Stress and Adult Age Mortality – A Study of Dental Enamel Hypoplasia in the Medieval Danish Village of Tirup', *American Journal of Physical Anthropology* 132, 59–66.

Borboudakis 1968. E. Borboudakis, 'Δοκιμαστικὴ ἀνασκαφὴ Ἁγίου Πέτρου τῶν Ἐνετῶν Ἡρακλείου', *Αρχαιολογικόν Δελτίον* 23, 427–9.

Bouras 1982–83. C. Bouras, 'Houses in Byzantium', *Δελτίον της Χριστιανικής Αρχαιολογικής Εταιρείας* 11, 1–26

Bourbou 1996. C. Bourbou, *Analysis of the Human Skeletal Remains from the Middle Byzantine Cemetery of Ambelia (Filotas, W. Macedonia, Greece)*, Unpublished skeletal report, 17th Ephorate of Prehistoric and Classical Antiquities (Hellenic Ministry of Culture).

Bourbou 2001a. C. Bourbou, 'Infant Mortality: The Complexity of It All!', *Eulimeni* II, 187–201.

Bourbou 2001b. C. Bourbou, 'A Proto-Byzantine Case of Unilateral Humerus Varus', Paper presented at the 23rd Conference of Hellenic Association of Biological Sciences, Chios, 24–27 May.

Bourbou 2003a. C. Bourbou, '*Interpreting Life and Death in Middle-Byzantine Greece (9th–13th centuries AD)*', Unpublished report, Wiener Laboratory Research Associate (ASCSA).

Bourbou 2003b. C. Bourbou, 'A Survey of Neoplastic Diseases in Ancient and Medieval Greek Populations', *Eulimeni* V, 181–8.

Bourbou 2003c. C. Bourbou, 'The Interaction between a Population and Its Environment: Probable Case of Subadult Scurvy from Early-Byzantine Greece', *Eres* 11, 105–14.

Bourbou 2004. C. Bourbou, *The People of Early Byzantine Eleutherna and Messene (6th–7th Centuries A.D.): A Bioarchaeological Approach*, Athens: University of Crete.

Bourbou 2005. C. Bourbou, 'Too Small to be Noticed? Children Mummies Reveal Their Stories', in E.R. Massa (ed.), *Proceedings of the Vth World Congress on Mummy Studies*, Turin, 2–5 September 2004, *Journal of Biological Research*, LXXX, Turin: Rubettino, 208–11.

Bourbou 2006a. C. Bourbou, 'To Live and Die in Middle Byzantine (11th century AD) Kastella, Central Crete, Greece', Invited lecture, Department of Anthropology, Adelphi University, New York, 3 May.

Bourbou 2006b. C. Bourbou, 'Infectious Conditions Observed on Greek Proto-Byzantine (6th–7th centuries AD) and Middle-Byzantine (11th century AD) Skeletal Series', in L. Buchet, C. Dauphin and I. Séguy (eds), *La paléodémographie. Mémoire d'os, mémoire d'hommes, Actes des 8e Journées Anthropologiques de Valbonne*, Valbonne, 5–7 June 2003, Antibes: Editions APDCA, 85–99.

Bourbou 2006c. C. Bourbou, 'On the Bioarchaeology of Death: Aspects of Childhood and Subadult Mortality Patterns during the Early and Middle Byzantine Times in Greece', Paper presented at the Dumbarton Oaks Spring Symposium Becoming Byzantine: Children and Childhood in Byzantium, Washington DC, 28–30 April.

Bourbou 2008. C. Bourbou, 'Fasting or feasting? Consumption of Meat, Dairy Products and Fish in Byzantium. Evidence from Chemical Analysis', Paper presented at the International Symposium on Animals and Environment in Byzantium (7th–12th c.), Athens, 6–7 June.

Bourbou 2009. C. Bourbou, 'Patterns of Trauma in a Medieval Urban Population (11th century AD) from Central Crete (Greece)', in L. Schepartz, S. Fox and C. Bourbou (eds), *New Directions in the Skeletal Biology of Greece*, OWLS vol. 1, Hesperia Supplement vol. 43, Princeton: American School of Classical Studies at Athens, 111–20.

Bourbou and Garvie-Lok 2006.C. Bourbou and S.J. Garvie-Lok, 'Breastfeeding and Weaning Patterns in Byzantine Times: Evidence from Human Remains and Written Sources', Paper presented at the Dumbarton Oaks Spring Symposium Becoming Byzantine: Children and Childhood in Byzantium, Washington DC, 28–30 April.

Bourbou and Garvie-Lok 2009. C. Bourbou and S.J. Garvie-Lock, 'Breast-Feeding and Weaning Patterns in Byzantine Times: Evidence from Human Remains and Written Sources', in A. Papaconstantinou and A.M. Talbot (eds), *Becoming Byzantine: Children and Childhood in Byzantium*, Washington DC: Dumbarton Oaks Research Library and Collection, 65–83.

Bourbou and Garvie-Lok forthcoming. C. Bourbou, and S.J. Garvie-Lok, 'All in the Cooking Pot: Invitation to a Dinner in Byzantine Greece', in M.P. Richards and A. Papathanasiou (eds), *Stable Isotope Dietary Studies of Prehistoric and Historic Greek Populations*, OWLS vol. 2, Princeton: American School of Classical Studies at Athens.

Bourbou and Richards 2007. C. Bourbou and M.P. Richards, 'The Middle-Byzantine Menu: Stable Carbon and Nitrogen Isotope Values from the Greek Site of Kastella, Crete', *International Journal of Osteoarchaeology* 17, 63–72.

Bourbou and Themelis in press. C. Bourbou and P. Themelis, 'Children Burials at Ancient Messene', *Actes du table ronde, L'enfant et la mort dans l'Antiquité*, Athens, 29–30 May 2008.

Bourbou and Tsilipakou 2009. C. Bourbou, and A. Tsilipakou, 'Investigating the Human Past of Greece during the 6th–7th centuries A.D. Patterns of Life and Death at the Site of Sourtara Galaniou Kozanis in Northern Greece', in L. Schepartz, S. Fox and C. Bourbou (eds), *New Directions in the Skeletal*

Biology of Greece, OWLS vol. 1, Hesperia Supplement vol. 43, Princeton: American School of Classical Studies at Athens, 121–36.

Bourbou, Fuller and Richards 2008. C. Bourbou, B.T. Fuller, M.P. Richards, 'The Application of Stable Isotope Ratio Analysis for Detecting Dietary Patterns in Greek Byzantine Populations (7th–13th centuries AD)', Paper presented at the 5th Hellenic Society for Archaeometry Symposium, Athens, 8–10 October.

Bourdara 1989. K.A. Bourdara, 'Η ἄσκηση τοῦ ἰατρικοῦ ἐπαγγέλματος ἀπὸ τὴν γυναίκα στὸ Βυζάντιο καὶ ἡ νομικὴ τῆς κατοχύρωση', in *Πρακτικά Α΄ Διεθνούς Συμποσίου, Ἡ καθημερινὴ ζωὴ στὸ Βυζάντιο. Τομὲς καὶ συνέχειες στὴν ἑλληνιστικὴ καὶ ρωμαϊκὴ παράδοση*, Αθήνα 15–17 September 1988. Athens: Ινστιτούτο Βυζαντινών Ερευνών/Εθνικό Ἵδρυμα Ερευνών, 121–34.

Boutton et al. 1988. T.W. Boutton, H.F. Tyrrell, B.W. Patterson, G.A. Varga, P.D. Klein, 'Carbon Kinetics of Milk Formation in Holstein Cows in Late Lactation', *Journal of Archaeological Science* 66, 2636–45.

Braudel 1966. F. Braudel, *La Méditerranée et le monde méditerranéen à l'époque de Philippe II*, 2 vols, Paris: Armand Colin.

Braudel 1998. F. Braudel, *Ιστορία της διατροφής: Προσεγγίσεις της σύγχρονης ιστοριογραφίας*, K. Tsicli-Aroni (tr.), Athens: E.M.N.E.-Μνήμων.

Braund 1995. D. Braund, 'Fish from the Black Sea: Classical Byzantium and the Greekness of Trade', in J. Wilkins, D. Harvey and M. Dobson (eds.), *Food in Antiquity*, Exeter: University of Exeter Press, 162–70.

Brickley 2006. M. Brickley, 'Rib Fractures in the Archaeological Record: A Useful Source of Sociocultural Information?', *International Journal of Osteoarchaeology* 16, 61–75.

Brickley and Ives 2006. M. Brickley and R. Ives, 'Skeletal Manifestations of Infantile Scurvy', *American Journal of Physical Anthropology* 129, 163–72.

Brickley and Ives 2008. M. Brickley and R. Ives, *The Bioarchaeology of Metabolic Bone Disease*, Oxford: Academic Press.

Brickley and Smith 2006. M. Brickley and M. Smith, 'Culturally Determined Patterns of Violence: Biological Anthropological Investigations at a Historic Urban Cemetery', *American Anthropologist* 108, 163–77.

Bridges 1992. P.S. Bridges, 'Prehistoric Arthritis in the Americas', *Annual Review of Anthropology* 21, 67–91.

Bridges 1996. P.S. Bridges, 'Warfare and Mortality at Koger's Island, Alabama', *International Journal of Osteoarchaeology* 6, 66–75.

Brisson, Congourdeau and Solère 2008. L. Brisson, M.-H. Congourdeau and J.-L. Solère (eds), *L'embyron: formation et animation. Antiquité grecque et latine, traditions hebraique, chrétienne et islamique*, Histoire des doctrines de l'Antiquité classique, 38, Paris: Librairie Philosophique J. Vrin.

Brokalakis 2004. G. Brokalakis, *Πρωτοβυζαντινά γεωργικά εργαλεία: η μαρτυρία των εργαλείων από την Ελεύθερνα*, Master thesis, University of Crete.

Brooks and Suchey 1990. S.T. Brooks and J.M. Suchey, 'Skeletal Age Determination Based on the Os Pubis: A Comparison of the Acsádi-Nemeskéri and Suchey-Brooks Methods', *Journal of Human Evolution* 5, 227–38.

Brothwell 1981. D.R. Brothwell, *Digging up Bones*, New York: Cornell University Press.

Brower 1990. A.C. Brower, *Radiología Articular. Arthritis en Blanco y Negro*, Madrid: Marban.

Brown 1998. P. Brown, *Ο κόσμος της ύστερης αρχαιότητας 150–750 μ.Χ.*, E. Stabogli (tr.), Athens: Εκδ. Αλεξάνδρεια.

Brown 2000. K. Brown, 'Ancient DNA Applications in Human Osteoarchaeology: Achievements, Problems and Potential', in M. Cox and S. Mays (eds), *Human Osteology in Archaeology and Forensic Science*, London: Greenwich Medical Media, 455–73.

Brown, Nelson and Southon 1988. T.A. Brown, D.E. Nelson and J.R. Southon, 'Improved Collagen Extraction by Modified Longin Method', *Radiocarbon* 30, 171–7.

Bryer 2002. A. Bryer, 2002. 'The Means of Agricultural Production: Muscle and Tools', in A. Laiou (ed.), *The Economic History of Byzantium: From the Seventh through the Fifteenth Century*, Washington DC: Dumbarton Oaks Research Library and Collection, 101–13.

Buchet and Sodini 1984. J.L. Buchet and J.-P. Sodini, 'Les tombes', in J.-P. Sodini, K. Kolokotsas (eds), *Aliki II. La Basilique Double*, Athens: Ecole française d'Athènes, 213–43.

Buckler 1948. G. Buckler, 'Byzantine Education: An Introduction to East Roman Civilization', in N. Baynes and H. Moss (eds), *Byzantium*, Oxford: Clarendon, 200–220.

Buckley 2000. H. Buckley, 'Subadult Health and Disease in Prehistoric Tonga, Polynesia', *American Journal of Physical Anthropology* 113, 481–505.

Buckley and Tayles 2003. H. Buckley and N. Tayles, 'Skeletal Pathology in a Prehistoric Pacific Island Sample: Issues in Lesion Recording, Quantification, and Interpretation', *American Journal of Physical Anthropology* 122, 303–24.

Buikstra 2006. J.E. Buikstra, 'Preface', in J.E. Buikstra and L.A. Beck (eds), *Bioarchaeology: The Contextual Analysis of Human Remains*, Amsterdam: Academic Press, xvii–xx.

Buikstra and Lagia 2009. J.E. Buikstra and A. Lagia, 'Bioarchaeological Approaches to Aegean Archaeology', in L. Schepartz, S. Fox and C. Bourbou (eds), *New Directions in the Skeletal Biology of Greece*, OWLS vol. 1, Hesperia

Supplement vol. 43, Princeton: American School of Classical Studies at Athens, 7–29.

Buikstra and Ubelaker 1994.J.E. Buikstra and D.H. Ubelaker (eds), *Standards for Data Collection from Human Skeletal Remains*, Fayetteville. AR: Archaeological Survey Research Series 44.

Bullough 1992. P.G. Bullough, *Atlas of Orthopedic Pathology and Clinical Radiologic Correlations*, New York: Gower Medical Publishing.

Burman 1938. M.S. Burman, 'A Typical Form of Humerus Varus: Adolescent Humerus Varus', *American Journal of Roentgenology and Radium Therapy* 40, 682–8.

Caffey 1978. J. Caffey, *Pediatric X-Ray Diagnosis*, Chicago: Yearbook Medical Publishers.

Cameron 1993. A. Cameron, *The Mediterranean World in Late Antiquity, AD 395–600*, London: Routledge.

Canci, Tarli and Repetto 1991. A. Canci, S.M.B. Tarli and E. Repetto, 'Osteomyelitis of Probable Haematogenous Origin in a Bronze Age Child from Toppo Daguzzo (Basilicata, Southern Italy)', *International Journal of Osteoarchaeology* 1, 135–9.

Capasso 1989. L. Capasso, 'Paleopathology of the Bronze Age Population from the Grotta dello Scoglietto Tuscany Italy', in L. Capasso (ed.), *Advances in Paleopathology*, Journal of Paleopathology Monograph Publication no. 1, Chieti: M. Solfanelli, 21–6.

Carli-Thiele 1995. P. Carli-Thiele, 'Scurvy: Investigations on the Human Skeleton Using Macroscopic and Microscopic Radiological Methods', *Journal of Paleopathology* 7, 88.

Catling and Smyth 1976. H.W. Catling and D. Smyth, 'An Early Christian Osteotheke at Knossos', *Annual of the British School at Athens* 71, 25–39.

Chanarin 1990. I. Chanarin, *The Megaloblastic Anemias*, Oxford: Blackwell Scientific Publishers.

Cheynet 2005. J.-C. Cheynet, 'La valeur marchande des produits alimentaires dans l'Empire byzantin', in D. Papanikola-Bakirtzi (ed.), *Πρακτικά ημερίδας Περί διατροφής στο Βυζάντιο*, Θεσσαλονίκη, 4 November 2001, Athens: ΥΠ.ΠΟ.-Τ.Α.Π.Α., 147–74.

Chhem and Rülhi 2004. R.K. Chhem, and F.J. Rülhi, 'Paleoradiology: Current Status and Future Challenges', *Canadian Association of Radiologists Journal* 55, 198–9.

Chhem et al. 2004. R.K. Chhem, S.K. Venkatesh, S.-C. Wang, K.-M. Wong, F.J. Rühli, E.P.Y. Siew, K. Latinis, C. Pottier, 'Multislice Computed Tomography of Two 2000-year-old Skeletons in a Soil Matrix from Angkor, Cambodia', *Canadian Association of Radiologists Journal* 55, 235–41.

Christides 1984. V. Christides, *The Conquest of Crete by the Arabs (ca. 824): A Turning Point in the Struggle between Byzantium and Islam*, Athens: Academy of Athens.

Chrone-Vakalopoulos and Vakalopoulos 2008. M. Chrone-Vakalopoulos and A. Vakalopoulos, 'Fishes and Other Aquatic Species in Byzantine Literature Classification, Terminology and Scientific Names', *Βυζαντινά Σύμμεικτα* 18, 123–57.

Clayton, Seally and Pfeiffer 2006. F. Clayton, J. Seally and S. Pfeiffer, 'Weaning Age among Foragers at Matjes River Rock Shelter, South Africa, from Stable Nitrogen and Carbon Isotope Analyses', *American Journal of Physical Anthropology* 129, 311–17.

Cohen 1989. M.N. Cohen, *Health and the Rise of Civilization*, London: Yale University Press.

Cohen and Armelagos 1984. M.N. Cohen and G.J. Armelagos (eds), *Paleopathology at the Origins of Agriculture*, New York: Academic Press.

Coleman 1969. J.E. Coleman, 'Ileia: Excavations of a Site (Elean Pylos) near Agrapidochori', *Αρχαιολογικόν Δελτίον* 24, B1, 155–61.

Congourdeau 1993a. M.-H. Congourdeau, 'La société byzantine face aux grandes pandémies', in E. Patlagean (ed.), *Maladie et société à Byzance*, Spoleto: Centro Italiano di Studi sull' alto medioevo, 21–41.

Congourdeau 1993b. M.H. Congourdeau, 'Metrodora et son oeuvre', in E. Patlagean (ed.), *Maladie et Société à Byzance*, Spoleto: Centro Italiano di Studi sull' alto medioevo, 57–96.

Congourdeau 2004. M.-H. Congourdeau, 'Genèse d'un regard chrétien sur l'embryon', in V. Dasen (ed.), *Naissance et petite enfance dans l'Antiquité, Actes du colloque de Fribourg*, 28 November–1 December 2001, Fribourg: Academic Press, 349–62.

Connor 2004. C.L. Connor, *Women of Byzantium*, New Haven/London: Yale University Press.

Constantelos 1966–67. D.J. Constantelos, 'Physician-Priests in the Medieval Greek Church', *Greek Orthodox Theological Review* 12, 141–53.

Constantinou 2005. S. Constantinou, *Female Corporeal Performances: Reading the Body in Byzantine Passions and Lives of Holy Women*, Uppsala: Uppsala University Press.

Cordain 1999.L. Cordain, 'Cereal Grains: Humanity's Double-Edged Sword', *World Review of Nutrition and Dietetics* 84, 19–73.

Cotran, Kumar and Robbins 1994. R.S. Cotran, V. Kumar and S.L. Robbins, *Robbins Pathologic Basis of Disease*, Philadelphia: W.B. Saunders.

Coughlan and Holst 2000. J. Coughlan and M. Holst, 'Health Status', in V. Fiorato, A. Boylston and C.J. Knüsel (eds), *Blood Red Roses: The Archaeology of a Mass Grave from the Battle of Towton AD 1461*, Oxford: Oxbow Books, 60–76.

Coulon 1994. G. Coulon, *L'enfant en Gaule romaine*, Paris: Editions Errance.

Couper, McPhee and Morris 2001. R. Couper., A. McPhee and L. Morris, 'Indomethacin Treatment of Infantile Cortical Periostitis in Twins', *Journal of Paediatrics and Child Health* 37, 305–8.

Cox 2000. M. Cox, 'Ageing Adults from the Skeleton', in M. Cox and S. Mays (eds), *Human Osteology in Archaeology and Forensic Science*, London: Greenwich Medical Media, 61–81.

Craig et al. 2009. O.E. Craig, M. Biazzo, T.C. O'Connell, P. Garnsey, C. Martinez-Labarga, R. Lelli, L. Salvadei, G. Tartaglia, A. Nava, L. Reno, A. Fiammenghi, O. Rickards, L. Bondioli, 'Stable Isotopic Evidence for Diet at the Imperial Roman Coastal Site of Velia (1st and 2nd Centuries AD) in Southern Italy', *American Journal of Physical Anthropology* 139, 572–83.

Crawford 1999. S. Crawford, *Childhood in Anglo-Saxon England*, Stroud: Alan Sutton Publishing.

Crislip 2005. A.T. Crislip, *From Monastery to Hospital: Christian Monasticism and the Transformation of Health Care in Late Antiquity*, Ann Arbor: The University of Michigan Press.

Dagron 1995. G. Dagron, 'Poissons, pêcheurs et poissonniers de Constantinople', in C. Mango and G. Dagron (eds), *Constantinople and its Hinterland*, Papers from the 27th Spring Symposium of Byzantine Studies, Oxford, 2–6 April 1993, Society for the Promotion of Byzantine Studies 3, Aldershot: Ashgate, 57–73.

Dagron 2002. G. Dagron, 'The Urban Economy, Seventh–Twelfth Centuries', in A. Laiou (ed.), *The Economic History of Byzantium: From the Seventh through the Fifteenth Century*, Washington DC: Dumbarton Oaks Research Library and Collection, 393–461.

Dalby 1996. A. Dalby, *Siren Feasts: A History of Food and Gastronomy in Greece*, London: Routledge.

Dalby 2002. A. Dalby, *Dangerous Tastes: The Story of Spices*, London: British Museum Press.

Dalby 2003. A. Dalby, *Flavours of Byzantium: The Cuisine of a Legendary Empire*, Totnes: Prospect, 2003.

Dalby 2007. A. Dalby, 'Some Byzantine Aromatics', in L. Brubaker and K. Linardou (eds), *Eat, Drink and Be Merry (Luke 12:19): Food and Wine in Byzantium*, Society for the Promotion of Byzantine Studies 13, Aldershot: Ashgate, 51–57.

Danforth 1982. L.M. Danforth, *The Death Rituals of Rural Greece*, Princeton: Princeton University Press.

Dasen 2004. V. Dasen (ed.), *Naissance et petite enfance dans l'Antiquité, Actes du colloque de Fribourg,* 28 November–1 December 2001, Fribourg: Academic Press.

Davies 1956. A.G.M. Davies, 'Bilateral Humerus Varus with Report of a Case', *British Journal of Radiology* 29, 295–6.

de Beylié 1902. L.M.E. de Beylié, *L'habitation byzantine,* Grenoble-Paris: Falque & F. Perrin.

Deines 1980. P. Deines, 'The Isotopic Composition of Reduced Carbon', in P. Fritz and J.C. Fontes (eds), *Handbook of Stable Isotope Geochemistry. Volume 1: The Terrestrial Environment,* Amsterdam: Elsevier, 329–406.

Delwiche et al. 1979. C.C. Delwiche, P.J. Zinke, C.M. Johnson, R.A. Virginia, 'Nitrogen Isotope Distributions as a Presumptive Indicator of Nitrogen Fixation', *Botanical Gazette* 140, S65–9.

Dembinska 1985. M. Dembinska, 'Diet: A Comparison of Food Consumption Between Some Eastern and Western Monasteries in the 4th–12th Centuries', *Byzantion* 55, 431–62.

DeNiro 1985. M.J. DeNiro, 'Post-mortem Preservation and Alteration of in Vivo Bone Collagen Isotope Ratios in Relation to Paleodietary Reconstruction', *Nature* 317, 806–9.

DeNiro and Epstein 1978. M.J. DeNiro and S. Epstein, 'Influence of Diet on the Distribution of Carbon Isotopes in Animals', *Geochimica et Cosmochimica Acta* 42, 495–506.

Dennis 2001. G.T. Dennis, 'Death in Byzantium', *Dumbarton Oaks Papers* 55, 1–8.

Detorakis 1969–70. T.E. Detorakis, '*Ἀνέκδοτον ἐγκώμιον εἰς Ἀνδρέαν Κρήτης*', *Επετηρίς Εταιρείας Βυζαντινών Σπουδών* 37, 83–96.

Detorakis 1970–71. T.E. Detorakis, ' Ἡ πανώλης ἐν Κρήτῃ. Συμβολὴ εἰς τὴν ἱστορίαν τῶν ἐπιδημιῶν τῆς νήσου', *Επιστημονική Επετηρίς της Φιλοσοφικής Σχολής του Πανεπιστημίου Αθηνών* 21, 118–36.

Di Vita 1979–80. A. Di Vita, 'I terremoti a Gortina in età romana e protobizantina, una nota', *Annuario della Scuola Archeologica de Atene* XLI–XLII, 434–40.

Di Vita 1988. A. Di Vita, *Gortina I,* Monografie della Scuola Archeologica di Atene e delle Missioni Italiane in Oriente III, Rome: 'L'Erma' di Bretschneider.

Di Vita 1997. A. Di Vita, 'Earthquakes and Civil Life at Gortyn (Crete) in the Period between Justinian and Constant II (6th–7th century AD)', in S. Stiros and R. Jones (eds), *Archaeoseismology,* Fitch Laboratory Occasional Paper 7, Athens: British School at Athens, 45–54.

Di Vita 2000. A. Di Vita, *Gortina V. Lo scavo del Pretorio (1989–1995)*, Monografie della Scuola Archeologica Italiana di Atene XII, Padua: Aido Ausilio Editore.

Dickie 1995. M.W. Dickie, 'The Fathers of the Church and the Evil Eye', in H. Maguire (ed.), *Byzantine Magic*, Washington DC: Dumbarton Oaks Research Library and Collection, 9–34.

Djuri et al. 2006. M.P. Djuri, C.A. Roberts, Z.B. Rakoevi, D. Djondi, A.R. Lei, 'Fractures in Late Medieval Skeletal Populations from Serbia', *American Journal of Physical Anthropology* 130, 167–78.

Domett and Tayles 2006. K.M. Domett and N. Tayles, 'Adult Fracture Patterns in Prehistoric Thailand: A Biocultural Interpretation', *International Journal of Osteoarchaeology* 16, 185–99.

Dorfman and Czerniak 1998. H. Dorfman and B. Czerniak, 'Metastatic Tumors in Bone', in H. Dorfman and B. Czerniak (eds), *Bone Tumors*, St Louis: Mosby, 1009–40.

Drancourt et al. 1998. M. Drancourt, G. Aboudharam, M. Signoli, O. Dutour, D. Raoult, 'Detection of 400-year-old *Yersinia pestis* DNA in Human Dental Pulp: An Approach to the Diagnosis of Ancient Septicemia', *Proceedings of the National Academy of Sciences of the United States of America* 11, 12637–40.

Drancourt et al. 2004. M. Drancourt, V. Roux, L. Vu Dang, L. Tran-Hung, D. Castex, V. Chenal-Francisque, H. Ogata, P.-E. Fournier, E. Crubézy, D. Raoult, 'Genotyping, Orientalis-like *Yersinia pestis*, and Plague Pandemics', *Emerging Infectious Diseases* 10, 1585–92.

Drancourt et al. 2007. M. Drancourt, M. Signoli, L. Vu Dang, B. Bizot, V. Roux, S. Tzortzis, D. Raoult, '*Yersinia pestis* Orientalis in Remains of Ancient Plague Patients', *Emerging Infectious Diseases* 13, 332–3.

Duffy 1984. J. Duffy, 'Byzantine Medicine in the Sixth and Seventh Centuries: Aspects of Teaching and Practice', *Dumbarton Oaks Papers* 38, 21–7.

Duggan and Wells 1964. A. Duggan and C. Wells, 'Four Cases of Archaic Disease of the Orbit', *Eye, Ear, Nose and Throat Digest* 26, 63–8.

Dunn 1992. A. Dunn, 'The Exploitation and Control of Woodland and Scrubland in the Byzantine World', *Byzantine and Modern Greek Studies* 16, 235–98.

Dupras and Tocheri 2007. T.L. Dupras and M.W. Tocheri, 'Reconstructing Infant Weaning Histories at Roman Period Kellis, Egypt Using Stable Isotope Analysis of Dentition', *American Journal of Physical Anthropology* 134, 63–74.

Dupras, Schwarcz and Fairgrieve 2001. T.L. Dupras, H.P. Schwarcz and S.I. Fairgrieve, 'Infant Feeding and Weaning Practices in Roman Egypt', *American Journal of Physical Anthropology* 115, 204–12.

Dürrwächter et al. 2006. C. Dürrwächter, O.E. Craig, M.J. Collins, J. Burger, K.W. Alt, 'Beyond the Grave: Variability in Neolithic Diets in Southern Germany?', *Journal of Archaeological Science* 33, 39–48.

Eftychiadis 1983. A. Eftychiadis, Η άσκησις της βυζαντινής ιατρικής επιστήμης και κοινωνικαί εφαρμογαί αυτής κατά σχετικάς διατάξεις, Athens: Κ. Παρισιάνος.

Eliopoulos, Lagia and Manolis 2007. C. Eliopoulos, A. Lagia and S.K. Manolis, 'A Modern, Documented Human Skeletal Collection from Greece', *Homo* 58, 221–8.

Ellefsen et al. 1994. B.K. Ellefsen, M.A. Frierson, E.M. Raney, J.A. Ogden, 'Humerus Varus: A Complication of Neonatal, Infantile and Childhood Injury and Infection', *Journal of Paediatric Orthopedics* 14, 479–86.

Ellis 2004. S. Ellis, 'Early Byzantine Housing', in K. Dark (ed.), *Secular Buildings and the Archaeology of Everyday Life in the Byzantine Empire*, Oxford: Oxbow Books, 37–52.

El-Najjar 1977a. M.Y. El-Najjar, 'Maize, Malaria and the Anemias in the Pre-Columbian New World', *Yearbook of Physical Anthropology* 20, 329–37.

El-Najjar 1977b. M.Y. El-Najjar, 'Porotic Hyperostosis in North America: A Theory', in E. Cockburn and A. Cockburn (eds), *Porotic Hyperostosis: An Enquiry*, Detroit: Paleopathology Association Monograph 2, 9–10.

El-Najjar et al. 1979. M.Y. El-Najjar, D.J. Ryan, C.G. II Turner, B. Lozoff, 'The Etiology of Porotic Hyperostosis among the Prehistoric and Historic Anasazi Indians of Southwestern United States', *American Journal of Physical Anthropology* 44, 477–88.

Emmanouilidis 1989. N.Emmanouilidis, *Το δίκαιο της ταφής στο Βυζάντιο*, Athens: Εκδ. Α.Ν. Σάκκουλα.

Erdal 2006. Y.S. Erdal, 'A Pre-Columbian Case of Congenital Syphilis from Anatolia (Nicaea, 13th century AD)', *International Journal of Osteoarchaeology* 16, 16–33.

Eshed et al. 2002. V. Eshed, B. Latimer, C.M. Greenwald, L.M. Jellema, B.M. Rothschild, S. Wish-Baratz, I. Hershkovitz, 'Button Osteoma: Its Etiology and Pathophysiology', *American Journal of Physical Anthropology* 118, 217–30.

Eyben 1993. E. Eyben (tr. P. Daly), *Restless Youth in Ancient Rome*, London: Routledge.

Facchini et al. 2004. F. Facchini, E. Rastelli and P. Brasili, 'Cribra orbitalia and Cribra Cranii in Roman Skeletal Remains from the Ravenna Area and Rimini (I–IV century AD)', *International Journal of Osteoarchaeology* 14, 126–36.

Faccia and Williams 2008. K.J. Faccia and R.C. Williams, 'Schmorl's Nodes: Clinical Significance and Implications for the Bioarchaeological Record', *International Journal of Osteoarchaeology* 18, 28–44.

Faerman 1997. M. Faerman, 'Determing the Sex of Infanticide Victims from the Late Roman Era through Ancient DNA Analysis, Paper presented at the TAG Conference, University of Bournemouth, 16–18 December.

Faerman 1999. M. Faerman, 'Ancient DNA Diagnosis of Bone Pathology in Infancy and Early Childhood', *American Journal of Physical Anthropology* 28, 125.

Faerman et al. 2000. M. Faerman, A. Nebel, D. Filon, M.G. Thomas, N. Bradman, B.D. Ragsdale, M. Schultz, A. Oppenheim, 'From a Dry Bone to a Genetic Portrait: A Case Study of Sickle Cell Anaemia', *American Journal of Physical Anthropology* 111, 153–63.

Fairgrieve and Molto 2000. S. Fairgrieve and J.E. Molto, 'Cribra Orbitalia in Two Temporally Disjunct Population Samples from the Dakhleh Oasis, Egypt', *American Journal of Physical Anthropology* 111, 319–31.

Farwell and Molleson 1993. D.E. Farwell and T.I. Molleson, *Excavations at Poundbury 1966–80, vol. 2: The Cemeteries*, Dorchester: Dorset Natural History and Archaeological Society.

Fazekas and Kósa 1978. I.G. Fazekas and F. Kósa, *Forensic Fetal Osteology*, Budapest: Akadémiai Kiadò.

Ferencz and Józsa 1992. M. Ferencz and L. Józsa, 'Congenital Syphilis on a Medieval Skeleton', *Anthropologie* 30, 95–8.

Fildes 1986. V.A. Fildes, *Breasts, Bottles and Babies: A History of Infant Feeding*, Edinburgh: Edinburgh University Press.

Fildes 1995. V.A. Fildes, 'The Culture and Biology of Breastfeeding: An Historical Review of Western Europe', in P. Stuart-Macadam and K.A. Dettwyler (eds), *Breastfeeding: Biocultural Perspectives*, New York: Adline de Gruyter, 101–26.

Filon et al. 1995. D. Filon, M. Faerman, P. Smith, A. Oppenheim, 'Sequence Analysis Reveals a β-thalassaemia Mutation in the DNA of Skeletal Remains from the Archaeological Site of Akhziv, Israel', *Nature Genetics* 9, 365–8.

Fiolitaki 2010. A. Fiolitaki, 'Ανασκαφική έρευνα στη θέση "Κεφάλα" Βρυσών Αποκορώνου', in M. Andrianakis, I. Tzahili (eds), *Πρακτικά της 1ης Συνάντησης για το Αρχαιολογικό Έργο Κρήτης*, Ρέθυμνο 28–30 Νοεμβρίου 2008, Rethymno: Πανεπιστήμιο Κρήτης-ΥΠ.ΠΟ.Τ, 745–53.

Flandrin and Montanari 1996. J.-L. Flandrin and M. Montanari (eds), *Food: Culinary History from Antiquity to the Present*, New York: Columbia University Press.

Fogel, Tuross and Owsley 1989. M.L. Fogel, N. Tuross and D. Owsley, 'Nitrogen Isotope Tracers of Human Lactation in Modern and Archaeological Populations', *Carnegie Institution Year Book* 88, 111–17.

Forbes 1995. R.J. Forbes, *Studies in Ancient Technology*, vol. 3, Leiden: Brill.

Fornaciari and Marchetti 1986. G. Fornaciari and A. Marchetti, 'Intact Smallpox Virus Particles in an Italian Mummy of Sixteenth Century', *Lancet* 2, 625.

Fornaciari, Ceccanti and Menicagli 1988. G. Fornaciari, B. Ceccanti and Menicagli, 'Recerca degli elementi guida della nutrizione e di alcuni metalli pesanti mediante spettroscopia ad assorbimento atomico', in A. di Vita (ed.), *Gortina I*, Rome: 'L' Erma' di Bretschneider, 403–16.

Forrester and Brown 1990. D.M. Forrester and J.C. Brown, *Radiología de las Enfermedades Articulares*, Barcelona: Salvat.

Fraenkel 1929. E. Fraenkel, 'Infantiler Skorbut (Möller-Barlowsche Krankheit)', in *Handbuch der Speziellen Pathologischen Anatomie und Histologie*, vol. 9, Berlin: Springer, 222–39.

Frend and Johnston 1967. W.H.C. Frend and D.E. Johnston, 'The Byzantine Basilica Church at Knossos, (Knossos Survey 36)', *Annual of the British School at Athens* 57, 186–238.

Frost 1999. F. Frost, 'Sausage and Meat Preservation in Antiquity', *Greek, Roman and Byzantine Studies* 40, 241–52.

Fulghum-Heintz 2003. M. Fulghum-Heintz, 'Magic, Medicine and Prayer', in I. Kalavrezou (ed.), *Byzantine Women and Their World*, Cambridge: Harvard University Art Museums, 275–81.

Fuller et al. 2005. B.T. Fuller, J.L. Fuller, N.E. Sage, D.A Harris, T.C. O'Connell, R.E.M. Hedges, 'Nitrogen Balance and δ^{15}N: Why You Are Not What You Eat During Nutritional Stress, *Rapid Communications in Mass Spectrometry* 19, 2497–506.

Fuller et al. 2006a. B.T. Fuller, T.I. Molleson, D.A. Harris, L.T. Gilmour, R.E.M. Hedges, 'Isotopic Evidence for Breastfeeding and Possible Adult Dietary Differences from Late/Sub-Roman Britain', *American Journal of Physical Anthropology* 129, 45–54.

Fuller et al. 2006b. B.T. Fuller, J.L. Fuller, D.A. Harris, R.E.M. Hedges, 'Detection of Breastfeeding and Weaning in Modern Human Infants with Carbon and Nitrogen Stable Isotope Ratios', *American Journal of Physical Anthropology* 129, 279–93.

Fuller, Richards and Mays 2003. B.T. Fuller, M.P. Richards and S.A. Mays, 'Stable Carbon and Nitrogen Isotopes Variations in Tooth Dentine Serial Sections from Wharram Percy', *Journal of Archaeological Science* 30, 1673–84.

Gallant 1991. T.W. Gallant, *Risk and Survival in Ancient Greece: Reconstructing the Rural Domestic Economy*, Stanford: Stanford University Press.

Galloway 1999. A. Galloway, *Broken Bones: Anthropological Analysis of Blunt Force Trauma*, Springfield, IL: Charles C. Thomas.

Garland 1988. L. Garland, 'The Life and Ideology of Byzantine Women', *Byzantion* 58, 361–93.

Garland 1999. L. Garland, *Byzantine Empresses: Women and Power in Byzantium, A.D. 527–1204*, London: Routledge.

Garland 2006. L. Garland, *Byzantine Women: Varieties of Experience 800–1200*, Aldershot: Ashgate.

Garnsey 1988. P. Garnsey, *Famine and Food Supply in the Graeco-Roman World: Responses to Risk and Crisis*, Cambridge: Cambridge University Press.

Garrison 1921. F.H. Garrison, *An Introduction to the History of Medicine*, Philadelphia: W.B. Saunders.

Garvie-Lok 2001. S.J. Garvie-Lok, *Loaves and Fishes: A Stable Isotope Reconstruction of Diet in Medieval Greece*, PhD diss., University of Calgary.

Garvie-Lok 2008. S.J. Garvie-Lok, 'Weaning Pains: Assessing Juvenile Scurvy in a Late Roman Greek Population', Paper presented at the 109th Annual Meeting of the Archaeological Institute of America, Chicago, 3–5 January.

Georgakopoulou and Xirotiris 2009. C. Georgakopoulou and N. Xirotiris, 'Anthropological Research on a Byzantine Population from Korytiani, West Greece', in L. Schepartz, S. Fox and C. Bourbou (eds), *New Directions in the Skeletal Biology of Greece*, OWLS vol. 1, Hesperia Supplement vol. 43, Princeton: American School of Classical Studies at Athens, 193–221.

Gerland 1915. E. Gerland, 'Das Wohnhaus in Byzantiner', *Der Burwart* 16, 10–19.

Gernaey et al. 1999. A.M. Gernaey, D.E. Minnikin, M.S. Copley, R.A. Dixon, J.C. Middleton, C.A. Roberts, 'Mycolic Acids and Ancient DNA Confirm an Osteological Diagnosis of Tuberculosis', *Tuberculosis* 84, 259–65.

Gilbert and Mielke 1985. R.I. Gilbert and J.M. Mielke (eds), *The Analysis of Prehistoric Diets*, Orlando: Academic Press.

Giorgi 2002. E. Giorgi, 'Indagini archeologiche nell' area del "quartiere byzantino" di Gortina: prima relazione preliminare (campagna 2002)', *Annuario della Scuola Archeologica di Atene*, LXXX, 898–906.

Gladykowska-Rzeczycka and Krenz 1995. J.J. Gladykowska-Rzeczycka and M. Krenz, 'Extensive Change within a Subadult Skeleton from a Medieval Cemetery of Sloboszewo, Mogilno District, Poland', *Journal of Paleopathology* 7, 177–84.

Goldstein 2006. L. Goldstein, 'Mortuary Analysis and Bioarchaeology', in J.E. Buikstra and L.A. Beck (eds), *Bioarchaeology: The Contextual Analysis of Human Remains*, Amsterdam: Academic Press, 375–87.

Goodman 1991. A.H. Goodman, 'Stress, Adaptation and Enamel Developmental Defects', in D.J. Ortner and A.C. Aufderheide (eds), *Human Paleopathology: Current Syntheses and Future Options*, Washington DC: Smithsonian Institution Press, 280–90.

Goodman and Rose 1990. A.H. Goodman and J.C. Rose, 'Assessment of Systemic Physiological Perturbations from Dental Enamel Hypoplasias and Associated Histological Structures', *Yearbook of Physical Anthropology* 33, 59–110.

Goodman et al. 1988. A.H. Goodman, R. Brooke Thomas, A.C. Swedlund, G. Armelagos, 'Biocultural Perspectives on Stress in Prehistoric, Historical and Contemporary Population Research', *Yearbook of Physical Anthropology* 31, 169–202.

Gordon and Buikstra 1981. C.C. Gordon and J.E. Buikstra, 'Soil pH, Bone Preservation and Sampling Bias at Mortuary Sites', *American Antiquity* 48, 566–71.

Grauer 1993. A.L. Grauer, 'Patterns of Anemia and Infection from Medieval York, England', *American Journal of Physical Anthropology* 91, 203–13.

Grauer and Roberts 1996. A. Grauer and C.A. Roberts, 'Paleoepidemiology, Healing, and Possible Treatment of Trauma in the Medieval Cemetery Population of St Helen-on-the-Walls, York, England', *American Journal of Physical Anthropology* 100, 531–44.

Greco et al. 1998. E. Greco, Th. Kalpaxis, A. Schnapp, D. Vivieers, 'Travaux menés en collaboration avec l'Ecole française en 1997', *Bulletin de Correspondance Hellénique* 122, 585–602.

Greenfield 1988. R.P.H. Greenfield, *Traditions in Belief in Late Byzantine Demonology*, Amsterdam: Adolf M. Hakkert.

Greenspan and Remagen 1998. A. Greenspan and W. Remagen, 'Metastases', in Greenspan and W. Remagen (eds), *Differential Diagnosis of Tumors and Tumor-like Lesions of Bones and Joints*, Philadelphia: W.B. Saunders, 367–87.

Grimm 1995. V. Grimm, 'Fasting Women in Judaism and Christianity in Late Antiquity', in J. Wilkins, D. Harvey and M. Dobson (eds), *Food in Antiquity*, Exeter: Exeter University Press, 225–40.

Grmek 1989. M. Grmek, *Diseases in the Ancient Greek World*, Baltimore and London: Johns Hopkins University Press.

Grünbart 2007. M. Grünbart, 'Store in a Cool and Dry Place: Perishable Goods and their Preservation in Byzantium', in L. Brubaker and K. Linardou (eds), *Eat, Drink and Be Merry (Luke 12:19): Food and Wine in Byzantium*, Society for the Promotion of Byzantine Studies 13, Aldershot: Ashgate, 39–49.

Grünbart and Stathakopoulos 2002. M. Grünbart and D. Stathakopoulos, 'Sticks and Stones: Byzantine Material Culture', *Byzantine and Modern Greek Studies* 26, 298–327.

Guardasole 2004a. A. Guardasole, 'Alexandre de Tralles et les remèdes naturels', in F. Collard and E. Samama (eds), *Mires, physiciens, barbiers et charlatans. Les marges de la médecine de l Antiquité aux débuts de l' époque moderne*, Langres: D. Guéniot, 81–99.

Guardasole 2004b. A. Guardasole, 'Sur l'*editio princeps* d'Alexandre de Tralles', in V. Boudon-Millot and G. Cobolet (eds), *Lire les médecins grecs à la Renaissance. Aux origines de l'édition médicale*, Actes du colloque international de Paris, 19–20 September 2003, Paris: De Boccard, 323–37.

Guardasole 2004c. A. Guardasole, 'L'héritage de Galien dans l'œuvre d'Alexandre de Tralles', in J. Jouanna and J. Leclant (eds), *La médecine grecque antique, Cahiers de la Villa 'Kérylos'*, no. 15, Paris: Académie des Inscriptions et Belles Lettres, 211–26.

Guardasole 2006. A. Guardasole, 'Alessandro di Tralle', in A. Garzya (ed.), *Medici bizantini, Oribasio di Pergamo, Aezio d'Amida, Alessandro di Tralle, Paolo d'Egina, Leone medico*, Turin: UTET, 555–679.

Guatelli-Steinberg and Lukacs 1999. D. Guatelli-Steinberg and J.R. Lukacs, 'Interpreting Sex Differences in Enamel Hypoplasia in Human and Non-Human Primates: Developmental, Environmental, and Cultural Considerations', *Yearbook of Physical Anthropology* 42, 73–126.

Guilland 1953. R. Guilland, 'La vie scolaire à Byzance', *Bulletin de l'Association Guillaume Budé* 1, 63–83.

Guy, Masset and Baud 1997. H. Guy, C. Masset and C.-A. Baud, 'Infant Taphonomy', *International Journal of Osteoarchaeology* 7, 221–9.

Haas et al. 2000. C.J. Haas, A. Zink, E. Molńar, U. Szeimies, U. Reischl, A. Marcsik, Y. Ardagna, O. Dutour, G. Pálfi, A. Nerlich, 'Molecular Evidence for Different Stages of Tuberculosis in Ancient Bones from Hungary', *American Journal of Physical Anthropology* 113, 293–304.

Hannsson and Ross 1983. T. Hannsson and B. Ross, 'The Amount of Bone Mineral and Schmorl's Nodes in Lumbar Vertebrae', *Spine* 8, 266–71.

Hanson 1995. A.E. Hanson, 'Uterine Amulets and Greek Uterine Medicine', *Medicina nei secoli* 7, 281–300.

Hapiot 2002. L. Hapiot, *L'endémie palustre dans le monde egéen ancien, du paléolithique à l'époque géometrique*, PhD diss., Université de Paris.

Hapiot 2003. L. Hapiot, 'Malaria and Porotic Hyperostosis in the Aegean World from Paleolithic to the Geometric Period', *Paleopathology Association Newsletter* 122, 11–14.

Hare et al. 1991. P.E. Hare, M.L. Fogel, T.W. Stafford Jr, A.D. Mitchell, T.C. Hoering, 'The Isotopic Composition of Carbon and Nitrogen in Individual Amino Acids Isolated from Modern and Fossil Proteins', *Journal of Archaeological Science* 18, 277–92.

Harstad 1986. J.J. Harstad, 'Saints, Drugs and Surgery: Byzantine Therapeutics for Breast Diseases', *Pharmacy in History* 28, 175–80.

Hayes 2001. J.W. Hayes, 'Early Christian Pottery from Knossos: The 1978–1981 Finds from the Knossos Medical Faculty Site', *British School at Athens* 96, 431–54.

Hedges and Reynard 2007. R.E.M. Hedges and L.M. Reynard, 'Nitrogen Isotopes and the Trophic Level of Humans in Archaeology', *Journal of Archaeological Science* 34, 1240–51.

Hellman 1990. U. Hellmann, *Künstiche Kälte: Die Gestichte der Kühlung im Haushalt*, Werkbund-Archiv 21, Giessen: Anabas-Verlag.

Helms 1989. C.A. Helms, *Fundamentals of Skeletal Radiology*, Philadelphia: W.B. Sanders.

Hennessy 2008. C. Hennessy, *Images of Children in Byzantium*, Farnham: Ashgate.

Herrin 1993. J. Herrin, 'In Search of Byzantine Women: Three Avenues of Approach', in A. Cameron and A. Kuhrt (eds), *Images of Women in Antiquity*, New York: Routledge, 167–89.

Herrin 2001. J. Herrin, *Women in Purple: Three Byzantine Empresses*, London: Weidenfeld & Nicolson.

Herring, Saunders and Boyce 1994. D. Herring, S. Saunders and G. Boyce, 'Bones and the Burial Registers: Infant Mortality in a 19th Century Cemetery from Upper Canada', *Council for Northeast Historical Archaeology Journal* 20, 54–70.

Herring, Saunders and Katzenberg 1998. D.A. Herring, S.R. Saunders and M.A. Katzenberg, 'Investigating the Weaning Process in Past Populations', *American Journal of Physical Anthropology* 105, 425–39.

Herrscher 2003. E. Herrscher, 'Alimentation d'une population historique: Analyse des données isotopiques de la nécropole Saint-Laurent de Grenoble (XIIIe–XVe siècle, France)', *Bulletins et Mémoires de la Société d'Anthropologie de Paris* 3–4, 145–320.

Herrscher et al. 2001. E. Herrscher, H. Bocherens, F. Valentin, R. Colardelle, Comportements alimentaires au Moyen Age à Grenoble: application de la biogéochemie isotopique à la nécropole Saint-Laurent (XIIIe–XVe s., Isère, France), *Comptes-rendus de l'Académie des Sciences* (série III, Sciences de la vie), 324, 479–487.

Hill and Bryer 1995. S. Hill and A. Bryer, 'Byzantine Porridge: Tracta, Trachanás and Tarhana', in J. Wilkins, D. Harvey and M. Dobson (eds), *Food in Antiquity*, Exeter: University of Exeter Press, 44–54.

Hillson 1986. S. Hillson, *Teeth*, Cambridge: Cambridge University Press.

Hillson 1996. S. Hillson, *Dental Anthropology*, Cambridge: Cambridge University Press.

Hodges 1980. R.E. Hodges, 'Vitamin C', in R.B. Alfin-Slater and D. Kritchevsky (eds), *Nutrition and the Adult*, New York: Plenum Press.

Hoefs 2004. J. Hoefs, *Stable Isotope Geochemistry*, Berlin: Springer-Verlag.

Holst et al. 2001. M. Holst, L. Isaac, A. Boylston, C.A. Roberts, *Hull Magistrates' Court (HMC 94): Draft Report on the Human Skeletal Remains*, Unpublished report, Bradford: University of Bradford.

Hope and Marshall 2000. V.M. Hope and E. Marshall, *Death and Disease in the Ancient City*, London and New York: Routledge.

Horden 2004. P. Horden, 'The Christian Hospital in Late Antiquity: Break or Bridge?', in F. Steger and K. P. Jankrift (eds), *Gesundheit–Krankheit: Kulturtransfer medizinischen Wissens von der Spätantike bis in die frühe Neuzeit*, Cologne: Böhlau-Verlag, 77–99.

Horden 2005. P. Horden, 'The Earliest Hospitals in Byzantium, Western Europe and Islam', *Journal of Interdisciplinary History* 35, 361–89.

Horden and Purcell 2000. P. Horden and N. Purcell, *The Corrupting Sea: A Study of Mediterranean History*, London: Blackwell.

Hummel 1999. C. Hummel, *Das Kind und seine Krankheiten in der griechischen Medizin: von Aretaios bis Johannes Aktouarios (1. bis 14. Jahrhundert)*, Frankfurt am Main: Peter Lang.

Hurwitz 1992. S. Hurwitz, *Lilith, the First Eve: Historical and Psychological Aspects of the Dark Feminine*, Einsiedeln: Daimon Verlag.

Hutchinson 1996. D.L. Hutchinson, 'Brief Encounters: Tatham Mound and the Evidence for Spanish and Native American Confrontation', *International Journal of Osteoarchaeology* 6, 51–65.

Iezzi 2005. C.A. Iezzi, *Regional Differences in the Health Status of Late Bronze Age Mycenaean Populations from East Lokris, Greece*, PhD diss., State University of New York at Buffalo.

Iezzi forthcoming. C.A. Iezzi, 'East Lokris Mycenaean Subsistence: The Isotopic and Osteological Evidence', in M.P. Richards and A. Papathanasiou (eds), *Stable Isotope Dietary Studies of Prehistoric and Historic Greek Populations*, OWLS vol. 2, Princeton: American School of Classical Studies in Athens.

Ingvarsson-Sundström 2003. A. Ingvarsson-Sundström, *Children Lost and Found: A Bioarchaeological Study of Middle Helladic Children in Asine with a Comparison to Lerna*, PhD diss., Uppsala Univeristy.

Jacob and Sotoudech 2002. R.A. Jacob and G. Sotoudech, 'Vitamin C Function and Status in Chronic Disease', *Nutrition in Clinical Care* 5, 66–74.

Jacobi and Danford 2002. K. Jacobi and M. Danford, 'Analysis of Interobserver Error Scoring Patterns in Porotic Hyperostosis and Cribra Orbitalia', *International Journal of Osteoarchaeology* 12, 248–58.

Jaffe 1972. H.L. Jaffe, Metabolic, *Degenerative and Inflammatory Diseases of Bone and Joint*, Philadelphia: Lea & Febiger.

Jay and Richards 2006. M. Jay and M.P. Richards, 'Diet in the Iron Age Cemetery Population at Wetwang Slack, East Yorkshire, UK: Carbon and Nitrogen Stable Isotope Evidence', *Journal of Archaeological Science* 33, 653–62.

Jay et al. 2008. M. Jay, B.T. Fuller, M.P Richards, C.J. Knüsel, S.S. King, 'Iron Age Breastfeeding Practices in Britain: Isotopic Evidence from Wetwang Slack, East Yorkshire', *American Journal of Physical Anthropology* 136, 327–37.

Jiménez-Brobeil, Al Oumaoui and du Souich 2007. S.A. Jiménez-Brobeil, I. Al Oumaoui and P. du Souich, 'Childhood Trauma in Several Populations from the Iberian Peninsula', *International Journal of Osteoarchaeology* 17, 189–98.

Jones and Ubelaker 2001. E. Jones and D. Ubelaker, 'Demographic Analysis of the Voegtly Cemetery Sample, Pittsburgh, Pennsylvania', *American Journal of Physical Anthropology*, Supplement 32, 86.

Jouanna 1996. J. Jouanna, *Hippocrate, Airs, Eaux, Lieux*, Paris: Les Belles Lettres.

Judd 2002. M.A. Judd, 'Ancient Injury Recidivism: An Example from the Kerma Period of Ancient Nubia', *International Journal of Osteoarchaeology* 12, 89–106.

Judd 2004. M.A. Judd, 'Trauma in the City of Kerma: Ancient Versus Modern Injury Patterns', *International Journal of Osteoarchaeology* 14, 34–51.

Judd 2008. M.A. Judd, 'The Parry Problem', *Journal of Archaeological Science* 35, 1658–66.

Judd and Roberts 1999. M.A. Judd and C.A. Roberts, 'Fracture Trauma in a Medieval British Farming Village', *American Journal of Physical Anthropology* 109, 229–43.

Jurmain 1978. R.D. Jurmain, 'Paleoepidemiology of Degenerative Joint Disease', *Medical College of Virginia Quarterly* 14, 45–46.

Jurmain 1999. R.D. Jurmain, *Stories from the Skeleton: Behavioural Reconstruction in Human Osteology*, Amsterdam: Gordon & Breach.

Jurmain 2001. R. Jurmain, 'Paleoepidemiological Patterns of Trauma in a Prehistoric Population from Central California', *American Journal of Physical Anthropology* 115, 13–23.

Jurmain and Bellifemine 1997. R. Jurmain and V.I. Bellifemine, 'Patterns of Cranial Trauma in a Prehistoric Population from Central California', *International Journal of Osteoarchaeology* 7, 43–50.

Kaestle and Horsburgh 2002. F.A. Kaestle and K.A. Horsburgh, 'Ancient DNA in Anthropology: Methods, Applications and Ethics', *Yearbook of Physical Anthropology* 45, 92–130.

Kalavrezou 2003. I. Kalavrezou, *Byzantine Women and their World*, New Haven: Yale University Press.

Kalogeras 2000. N. Kalogeras, *Byzantine Childhood Education and Its Social Role from the Sixth Century until the End of Iconoclasm*, PhD diss., The University of Chicago.

Kalogeras 2001. N. Kalogeras, 'What Do They Think about Children? Perceptions of Childhood in Early Byzantine Literature', *Byzantine and Modern Greek Studies* 25, 2–19.

Kalokyris 1955. K.D. Kalokyris, 'Συμπληρωματικὴ ἀνασκαφὴ βασιλικῆς Πανόρμου Κρήτης', *Πρακτικά της εν Αθήναις Αρχαιολογικής Εταιρείας*, 321–6.

Kalpaxis 2008. Th. Kalpaxis, 'Παρατηρήσεις στην αρχιτεκτονική της Βυζαντινής οικίας', in Th. Kalpaxis (ed.), *Ελεύθερνα. Τομέας II. 3. Βυζαντινό Σπίτι στην Αγία Άννα*, Rethymno: Πανεπιστήμιο Κρήτης, 13–23.

Kamp 2001. K. Kamp, 'Where Have All the Children Gone? The Archaeology of Childhood', *Journal of Archaeological Method and Theory* 8, 1–34.

Kaplan 1992. M. Kaplan, *Les hommes et la terre à Byzance du VIe au Xie siècle. Propriété et exploitation du sol*, Paris: Publications de la Sorbonne.

Karpozilos 1989. A. Karpozilos, 'Περὶ ἀποπάτων, βόθρων καὶ ὑπονόμων', in *Πρακτικά του Α' Διεθνούς Συμποσίου, Ἡ καθημερινὴ ζωὴ στὸ Βυζάντιο. Τομὲς καὶ συνέχειες στὴν ἑλληνιστικὴ καὶ ρωμαϊκὴ παράδοση*, Αθήνα, 15–17 September 1988, Athens: Ινστιτούτο Βυζαντινών Ερευνών/Εθνικό Ίδρυμα Ερευνών, 335–52.

Katz and Suchey 1986. D. Katz and J.M. Suchey, 'Age Determination of the Male Os Pubis', *American Journal of Physical Anthropology*, 69, 427–35.

Katzenberg 2000. M.A. Katzenberg, 'Stable Isotope Analysis: A Tool for Studying Past Diet, Demography and Life History', in M.A. Katzenberg and S.R Saunders (eds), *Biological Anthropology of the Human Skeleton*, New York: Wiley-Liss, 305–27.

Katzenberg and Pfeiffer 1995. M.A. Katzenberg and S. Pfeiffer, 'Nitrogen Isotope Evidence for Weaning Age in a Nineteenth Century Canadian Skeletal Sample', in A. Grauer (ed.), *Bodies of Evidence*, New York: Wiley-Liss, 221–35.

Katzenberg and Weber 1999. M.A. Katzenberg and A. Weber, 'Stable Isotope Ecology and Palaeodiet in the Lake Baikal Region of Siberia', *Journal of Archaeological Science* 26, 651–9.

Katzenberg, Herring and Saunders 1996. M.A. Katzenberg, D.A. Herring and S.R. Saunders, 'Weaning and Infant Mortality: Evaluating the Skeletal Evidence', *Yearbook of Physical Anthropology* 39, 177–99.

Katzenberg, Saunders and Fitzgerald 1993. M.A. Katzenberg, S.R. Saunders and W.R. Fitzgerald, 'Age Differences in Stable Carbon and Isotope Ratios in Populations of Prehistoric Maize Horticulturists', *American Journal of Physical Anthropology* 90, 267–81.

Kazhdan 1984. A. Kazhdan, 'The Image of the Medical Doctor in Byzantine Literature of the Tenth to Twelfth Centuries', *Dumbarton Oaks Papers* 38, 43–51.

Kazhdan 1997. A. Kazhdan, 'The Peasantry', in G. Cavallo (ed.), *The Byzantines*, Chicago: University of Chicago Press, 43–73.

Kazhdan 1998. A. Kazhdan, 'Women at Home', *Dumbarton Oaks Papers* 52, 1–17.

Kazhdan and Constable 1982. A. Kazhdan and G. Constable, *People and Power in Byzantium: An Introduction to Modern Byzantine Studies*, Washington DC: Dumbarton Oaks, Center for Byzantine Studies.

Keenan 1941. M.E. Keenan, 'St. Gregory of Nazianzus and Early Byzantine Medicine', *Bulletin of the History of Medicine* 9, 8–30.

Keenan 1944. M.E. Keenan, 'St. Gregory of Nyssa and the Medical Profession', *Bulletin of the History of Medicine* 15, 150–61.

Keenleyside and Panayotova 2006. A. Keenleyside and K. Panayotova, 'Cribra Orbitalia and Porotic Hyperostosis in a Greek Colonial Population (5th to 3rd centuries BC) from the Black Sea', *International Journal of Osteoarchaeology* 16, 373–84.

Keenleyside et al. 2009. Keenleyside, H. Schwarcz, L.Stirling, N. Ben Lazreg, 'Stable Isotopic Evidence for Diet in a Roman and Late Roman Population from Leptiminus, Tunisia', *Journal of Archaeological Science* 36, 51–63.

Keenleyside, Schwarcz and Panayotova 2006. A. Keenleyside, H.P. Schwarcz and K. Panayotova, 'Stable Isotopic Evidence of Diet in a Greek Colonial Population from the Black Sea', *Journal of Archaeological Science* 33, 1205–15.

Keipert and Campbell 1970. J.A. Keipert and P.E. Campbell, 'Recurrent Hyperostosis of the Clavicles: An Undiagnosed Syndrome', *Australian Paediatric Journal* 6, 97–104.

Kessler 1971. H.L. Kessler (ed.), *Kurt Weitzmann: Studies in Classical and Byzantine Manuscript Illumination*, Chicago: The University of Chicago Press.

Kilgore, Jurmain and van Gerven 1997. L. Kilgore, R. Jurmain and D. van Gerven, 'Paleoepidemiological Patterns of Trauma in a Medieval Nubian Skeletal Population', *American Journal of Physical Anthropology* 7, 103–14.

King, Humphrey and Hillson 2005. T. King, L.T. Humphrey and S. Hillson, 'Linear Enamel Hypoplasias as Indicators of Systemic Physiological Stress: Evidence from Two Known Age-at-Death and Sex Populations from Postmedieval London', *American Journal of Physical Anthropology* 128, 547–59.

Kiousopoulou 1997. A. Kiousopoulou, *Χρόνος και ηλικίες στη Βυζαντινή κοινωνία: η κλίμακα των ηλικιών από τα αγιολογικά κείμενα της μέσης εποχής (7ος–11ος αι)*, Ιστορικό Αρχείο Ελληνικής Νεολαίας 30, Athens: Εθνικό Ίδρυμα Ερευνών.

Kislinger 1989. E. Kislinger, "Η γυναικολογία στὴν καθημερινὴ ζωὴ τοῦ Βυζαντίου', in *Πρακτικά Α΄ Διεθνούς Συμποσίου*, Ἡ *καθημερινὴ ζωὴ στὸ Βυζάντιο. Τομὲς καὶ συνέχειες στὴν ἑλληνιστική καὶ ρωμαϊκὴ παράδοση*, Αθήνα, 15–17 September 1988, Athens: Ινστιτούτο Βυζαντινών Ερευνών/Εθνικό Ίδρυμα Ερευνών, 135–45.

Kislinger 1996. E. Kislinger, 'Christians of the East: Rules and Realities of the Byzantine Diet', in J.-L. Flandrin and M. Montanari (eds), *Food: Culinary History from Antiquity to the Present*, New York: Columbia University Press, 194–206.

Kislinger 2005. E. Kislinger, 'Τρώγοντας και πίνοντας εκτός σπιτιού', in D. Papanikola-Bakirtzi (ed.), *Πρακτικά ημερίδας Περί διατροφής στο Βυζάντιο*, Θεσσαλονίκη, 4 November 2001, Athens: ΥΠ.ΠΟ.-Τ.Α.Π.Α., 47–60.

Klaus, Larsen and Tam 2009. H.D. Klaus, C.S. Larsen and M.E. Tam, 'Economic Intensification and Degenerative Joint Disease: Life and Labor on the Postcontact North Coast of Peru', *American Journal of Physical Anthropology* 139, 204–21.

Knüsel 2000. C.J. Knüsel, 'Activity Related Skeletal Change', in V. Fiorato, A. Boylston and C.J. Knüsel (eds), *Blood Red Roses: The Archaeology of a Mass Grave from the Battle of Towton AD 1461*, Oxford: Oxbow Books, 103–18.

Knüsel and Boylston 2000. C.J. Knüsel and A. Boylston, 'How Has the Towton Project Contributed to Our Knowledge of Medieval and Later Warfare?', in V. Fiorato, A. Boylston and C.J. Knüsel (eds), *Blood Red Roses: The Archaeology of a Mass Grave from the Battle of Towton AD 1461*, Oxford: Oxbow Books, 169–88.

Koder 1992. J. Koder, *Ο κηπουρός και η καθημερινή κουζίνα στο Βυζάντιο*, Όψεις της Βυζαντινής Κοινωνίας 2, Athens: Ίδρυμα Γουλανδρή Χόρν.

Koder 1995. J. Koder, 'Fresh Vegetables for the Capital', in C. Mango and G. Dagron (eds), *Constantinople and its Hinterland*, Papers from the 27th Spring Symposium of Byzantine Studies, Oxford, 2–6 April 1993, Society for the Promotion of Byzantine Studies 3, Aldershot: Ashgate, 49–56.

Koder 2005. J. Koder, 'Η καθημερινή διατροφή στο Βυζάντιο με βάση τις πηγές', in D. Papanikola-Bakirtzi (ed.), *Πρακτικά ημερίδας Περί διατροφής στο Βυζάντιο*, Θεσσαλονίκη, 4 November 2001, Athens: ΥΠ.ΠΟ.-Τ.Α.Π.Α., 17–30.

Koder 2007. J. Koder, '*Stew and Salted meat*-Opulent Normality in the Diet of Every Day?', in L. Brubaker and K. Linardou (eds), *Eat, Drink and Be Merry (Luke 12:19): Food and Wine in Byzantium,* Society for the Promotion of Byzantine Studies 13, Aldershot: Ashgate, 59–72.

Kohl and Shearer 1980. D.H. Kohl and G. Shearer, 'Isotopic Fractionation Associated with Symbiotic N2 Fixation and Uptake of NO3- by Plants', *Plant Physiology* 66, 51–56.

Kohl, Shearer and Harper 1980. D.H. Kohl, G. Shearer and J.E. Harper, 'Estimates of N_2 Fixation Based on Differences in the Natural Abundance of ^{15}N in Nodulating and Nonnodulating Isolines of Soybeans', *Plant Physiology* 66, 61–5.

Kolman et al. 1999. C.J. Kolman, A. Centurion-Lara, S.A. Lukehart, D.W. Owsley, N. Tuross, 'Identification of *Treponema pallidum* Subspecies *pallidum* in a 20-year-old Skeletal Specimen', *Journal of Infectious Diseases* 180, 2060–63.

Kornexl et al. 1997. B.E. Kornexl, T. Werner, A. Roßmann, H.-L. Schmidt, 'Measurements of Stable Isotope Abundances in Milk and Milk Ingredients – A Possible Tool for Origin Assessment and Quality Control', *Zeitschrift für Lebensmittel-Untersuchung und -Forschung A* 205, 19–24.

Koukoules 1936. Ph. Koukoules, 'Περί τήν βυζαντινήν οἰκίαν', *Επετηρίς Εταιρείας Βυζαντινών Σπουδών* 12, 76–138.

Koukoules 1948. Ph. Koukoules, *Βυζαντινῶν βίος καὶ πολιτισμός*, τομ. Α', Athens: Εκδ. Παπαζήση.

Koukoules 1949. Ph. Koukoules, *Βυζαντινῶν βίος καὶ πολιτισμός*, τομ. Β', Athens: Εκδ. Παπαζήση.

Koukoules 1951. Ph. Koukoules, *Βυζαντινῶν βίος καὶ πολιτισμός*, τομ. Δ', Athens: Εκδ. Παπαζήση.

Koukoules 1952. Ph. Koukoules, *Βυζαντινῶν βίος καὶ πολιτισμός*, τομ. Ε', Athens: Collection de l'Institut Français d' Athènes.

Kourkoutidou-Nikolaidou 1997. E. Κουρκουτίδου-Νικολαΐδου, *Από τα Ηλύσια Πεδία στο Χριστιανικό Παράδεισο*, Θεσσαλονίκη: ΥΠ.ΠΟ.-Μουσείο Βυζαντινού Πολιτισμού Θεσσαλονίκης.

Kramar, Lagier and Baud 1990. C. Kramar, R. Lagier and C.A. Baud, 'Rheumatic Disease in Neolithic and Medieval Populations of Western Switzerland', *Zeitschrift für Rheumatologie* 49, 338–45.

Kuhn et al. 2007. G. Kuhn, M. Schultz, R. Müller, F.J. Rühli, 'Diagnostic Value of Micro-CT in Comparison with Histology in the Qualitative Assessment of Historical Human Postcranial Bone Pathologies', *Homo* 58, 97–115.

Kulund 1990. D.N. Kulund, *Lesiones del Deportista* (2nd edn), Barcelona: Salvat.

Kyriakakis 1974. J. Kyriakakis, 'Byzantine Burial Customs: Care for the Deceased from Death to Prothesis', *Greek Orthodox Theological Review* 19, 37–72.

Lagia 2007. A. Lagia, 'Notions of Childhood in the Classical Polis: Evidence from the Bioarchaeological Record', in A. Cohen and J.B. Rutter (eds), *Constructions of Childhood in Ancient Greece and Italy*, Hesperia Supplement vol. 41, Princeton: American School of Classical Studies at Athens, 293–306.

Lagia and Richards forthcoming. A. Lagia and M.P. Richards, 'Diet and the *polis*: An Isotopic Study of Diet in Athens and Laurion during the Classical, Hellenistic and Early Roman Periods', in M.P. Richards and A. Papathanasiou (eds), *Stable Isotope Dietary Studies of Prehistoric and Historic Greek Populations*, OWLS vol. 2, Princeton: American School of Classical Studies in Athens.

Lagia forthcoming. A. Lagia, *A Bioarchaeological Survey of Social Structure in the Polis of Athens during the Classical, Hellenistic and Roman Times*, PhD diss., University of Chicago.

Lagia, Eliopoulos and Manolis 2007. A. Lagia, C. Eliopoulos and S.K. Manolis, 'Thalassemia: Macroscopic and Radiological Study of a Case', *International Journal of Osteoarchaeology* 17, 269–85.

Lagia, Petroutsa and Manolis 2007. A. Lagia, E.I. Petroutsa, and S.K. Manolis, 'Health and Diet during the Middle Bronze Age in the Peloponnese: The Site of Koufovouno', in C. Mee and J. Renard (eds), *Cooking Up the Past: Food and Culinary Practices in the Neolithic and Bronze Age Aegean*, Oxford: Oxbow Books, 313–28.

Laiou 1977. A.E. Laiou, *Peasant Society in the Late Byzantine Empire: A Social and Demographic Study*, Princeton: Princeton University Press.

Laiou 1981. A.E. Laiou, 'The Role of Women in Byzantine Society', *Jahrbuch der Österreichischen Byzantinistik* 31, 233–60.

Laiou 1982. A.E. Laiou, *Gender, Society and Economic Life in Byzantium*: London: Variorum Reprints.

Laiou 1985. A.E. Laiou, 'Observations on the Life and Ideology of Byzantine Women', *Byzantinische Forschungen* 9, 59–102.

Laiou 1992. A.E. Laiou, *Mariage, amour et parenté à Byzance aux XIe–XIIIe siècles*, Paris: Ed. de Boccard.

Laiou 1999. A.E. Laiou, 'Women in Byzantine Society', in L.E. Mitchell (ed.), *Women in Medieval Western European Culture*, New York: Garland Publishing, 81–94.

Laiou 2000. A.E. Laiou, 'The Evolution of the Status of Women in Marriage and Family Law', in C.G. Fürst and R. Potz (eds), *Mutter, Nonne, Diakonin. Frauenbilder im Recht der Ostkirchen/Mother, Nun, Deaconess, Images of Women According to Eastern Canon Law, Kanon XVI*. Jahrbuch der Gesellschaft für das Recht der Osterkirchen, Egling: Roman Kovar, 71–85.

Laiou 2003. A.E. Laiou, 'Η διαμόρφωση της τιμής της γης στο Βυζάντιο', in A. Avramea, A. Laiou and E. Chrysos (eds), *Βυζάντιο, κράτος και κοινωνία*, Μνήμη Ν. Οικονομίδη, Athens: Ινστιτούτο Βυζαντινών Ερευνών/Εθνικό Ίδρυμα Ερευνών.

Lambert 1993. P.M. Lambert, 'Health in Prehistoric Populations of the Santa Barbara Channel Islands', *American Antiquity* 58, 509–21.

Lambert 1997. P.M. Lambert, 'Patterns of Violence in Prehistoric Hunter Gatherer Societies of Coastal Southern California', in D.W. Frayer and D.L. Martin (eds), *Troubled Times: Violence and Warfare in the Past*, Amsterdam: Gordon & Breach, 77–109.

Langenskiold 1953. A. Langenskiold, 'Adolescent Humerus Varus', *Acta Chirurgica Scandinavica* 105, 353–63.

Larsen 1997. C.S. Larsen, *Bioarchaeology: Interpreting Behavior from the Human Skeleton*, Cambridge: Cambridge University Press.

Larsen 2006. C.S. Larsen, 'The Changing Face of Bioarchaeology: An Interdisciplinary Science', in J.E. Buikstra and L.A. Beck (eds), *Bioarchaeology: The Contextual Analysis of Human Remains*, Amsterdam: Academic Press, 359–74.

Lascaratos and Tsiamis 2002. J. Lascaratos and C. Tsiamis, 'Two Cases of Smallpox in Byzantium', *International Journal of Dermatology* 41, 792–5.

Lascaratos, Lazaris and Kreatsas 2002. J. Lascaratos, D. Lazaris and G. Kreatsas, 'A Tragic Case of Complicated Labour in Early Byzantium (404 A.D.)', *European Journal of Obstetrics & Gynecology and Reproductive Biology* 105, 80–83.

Laskaris 2000. N.J. Laskaris, *Monuments funéraires paléochrétiens (et byzantins) de Grèce*, Athens: D. Vasilopoulos.

Lassithiotakis 1969. K.E. Lassithiotakis, 'Ἐκκλησίες τῆς Δυτικῆς Κρήτης', *Κρητικά Χρονικά* 21, 459–93.

Lazos 2002. Ch. Lazos, *Παίζοντας στο χρόνο, αρχαιοελληνικά και βυζαντινά παιχνίδια 1700 π.Χ.–1500 μ.Χ.*, Athens: Εκδ. Αίολος.

Learmonth 1988. A. Learmonth, *Disease Ecology*, Oxford: Basil Blackwell.

Lee 2001. F. Lee, *Hospital of St. James and St. Mary Magdalene, Chichester: Draft Report on the Human Skeletal Remains*, Unpublished report, Bradford: University of Bradford.

Lefort 2002. J. Lefort, 'The Rural Economy, Seventh–Twelfth Centuries', in A. Laiou (ed.), *The Economic History of Byzantium: From the Seventh through the Fifteenth Century*, Washington DC: Dumbarton Oaks Research Library and Collection, 231–314.

Leloir 1980. L. Leloir, 'Attitudes des pères du désert vis-à-vis des jeunes', in A. Théodoridès, P. Naster and J. Ries (eds), *L' enfant dans les civilisations orientales*, Leuven: Peeters, 145–52.

Leven 1993. K.-H. Leven, 'Zur Kenntnis der Pocken in der arabischen Medizin, im lateinischen Mittelalter und in Byzanz', in O. Engels and P. Schreiner (eds), *Die Begegnung des Westens mit dem Osten. Kongressakten des 4. Symposions des Mediävistenverbandes in Köln 1991 aus Anlass des 1000. Todesjahres der Kaiserin Theophanu*, Sinmaringen: Jan Thornbecke Verlag, 341–54.

Leven 1997. K.-H. Leven, 'Die Geschichte der Infektionskrankheiten. Von der Antike bis ins 20', *Jahrhundert, Fortschritte in der Präventive- und Arbeitsmedizin* 6, Landsberg/Lech: EcoMed, 42–50.

Lévi-Strauss 1969. C. Lévi-Strauss, *The Raw and the Cooked: Introduction to a Science of Mythology I* (tr. J. Weightman and D. Weightman), New York: Harper & Row.

Lewis 2008. J.E. Lewis, 'Identifying Sword Marks on Bone: Criteria for Distinguishing Between Cut Marks Made by Different Classes of Blade Weapons', *Journal of Archaeological Science* 35, 2001–8.

Lewis 2000. M.E. Lewis, 'Non-Adult Paleopathology: Current Status and Future Potential', in M. Cox and S. Mays (eds), *Human Osteology in Archaeology and Forensic Science*, London: Greenwich Medical Media, 39–57.

Lewis 2002. M.E. Lewis, *Urbanization and Child Health in Medieval and Post-Medieval England*, BAR British Series 339, Oxford: Archaeopress.

Lewis 2004. M.E. Lewis, 'Endocranial Lesions in Non-Adult Skeletons: Understanding their Aetiology', *International Journal of Osteoarchaeology* 14, 82–97.

Lewis 2007. M.E. Lewis, *The Bioarchaeology of Children: Perspectives from Biological and Forensic Anthropology*, Cambridge: Cambridge University Press.

Lewis and Gowland 2005. M.E. Lewis and R.L. Gowland, 'Infantile Cortical Hyperostosis: Cases, Causes, Constraints', Paper presented at the 32nd Annual Meeting of the Paleopathology Association, 5–6 April, Milwaukee, WI.

Lewis and Gowland 2007. M.E. Lewis and R.L. Gowland, 'Brief and Precarious Lives: Infant Mortality in Four Contrasting Sites from Medieval and Post-Medieval England (AD 850–1859)', *American Journal of Physical Anthropology* 134, 117–29.

Lewis and Roberts 1997. M.E. Lewis and C.A. Roberts, 'Growing Pains: The Interpretation of Stress Indicators', *International Journal of Osteoarchaeology* 7, 581–6.

Lillehammer 1989. G. Lillehammer, 'A Child is Born: The Child's World in an Archaeological Perspective', *Norwegian Archaeological Review* 22, 89–105.

Lilley et al. 1994. S.M. Lilley, G. Stroud, D.R. Brothwell, M.H. Williamson (eds), *The Jewish Burial Ground at Jewbur*, York: Council for British Archaeology.

Littlewood, Maguire and Wolschke-Bulmahn 2002. A. Littlewood, H. Maguire and J. Wolschke-Bulmahn (eds), *Byzantine Garden Culture*, Washington DC: Dumbarton Oaks Research Library and Collection.

Longin 1971. R. Longin, 'New Method of Collagen Extraction for Radiocarbon Dating', *Nature* 230, 241–2.

Lovejoy and Heiple 1981. C.O. Lovejoy and K.G. Heiple, 'The Analysis of Fractures in Skeletal Populations with an Example from the Libben Site, Ottowa County Ohio', *American Journal of Physical Anthropology* 55, 529–41.

Lovejoy et al. 1985. C.O. Lovejoy, R.S. Meindl, T.R. Pryzbeck, R.P. Mensforth, 'Chronological Metamorphosis of the Auricular Surface of the Ilium: A New Method for the Determination of Age at Death', *American Journal of Physical Anthropology* 68, 15–28.

Lovell 1997. N.C. Lovell, 'Trauma Analysis in Paleopathology', *Yearbook of Physical Anthropology* 40, 139–70.

Lovell and Dublenko 1999. N.C. Lovell and A.A. Dublenko, 'Further Aspects of Fur Trade Life Depicted in the Skeleton', *International Journal of Osteoarchaeology* 9, 248–56.

Lucas and Gill 1947. L.S. Lucas and J.H. Gill, 'Humerus Varus Following Birth Injury to the Proximal Humeral Epiphysis', *Journal of Bone and Joint Surgery* 29, 367–9.

Lucy 1994. S. Lucy, 'Children in Early Medieval Cemeteries', *Archaeological Review from Cambridge* 13, 21–34.

Lukacs 1989. J.R. Lukacs, 'Dental Palaeopathology: Methods for Reconstructing Dietary Patterns', in M.Y. İşcan and K.A.R. Kennedy (eds), *Reconstruction of Life from the Skeleton*, New York: Wiley-Liss, 261–86.

Maat 2004. G. Maat, 'Scurvy in Adults and Youngsters: The Dutch Experience – A Review of the History and Pathology of a Disregarded Disease', *International Journal of Osteoarchaeology* 14, 77–81.

Magoulias 1964. H.J. Magoulias, 'The Lives of the Saints as Sources for the History of Byzantine Medicine in the Sixth and Seventh Centuries', *Byzantinische Zeitschrift* 57, 127–50.

Maguire 1987. H. Maguire, *Earth and Ocean: The Terrestrial World in Early Byzantine Art*, University Park: Pennsylvania State University Press.

Maguire 1995. H. Maguire (ed.), *Byzantine Magic*, Washington DC: Dumbarton Oaks Research Library and Collection.

Maguire 2005. H. Maguire, 'A Fruit Story and an Aviary: Images of Food in House, Palace and Church', in D. Papanikola-Bakirtzi (ed.), *Πρακτικά ημερίδας Περί διατροφής στο Βυζάντιο*, Θεσσαλονίκη, 4 November 2001, Athens: ΥΠ.ΠΟ.-Τ.Α.Π.Α., 133–46.

Majno 1975. G. Majno, *The Healing Hand: Man and Wound in the Ancient World*, Cambridge, MA: Harvard University Press.

Makrypoulias 2000. C.G. Makrypoulias, 'Byzantine Expeditions against the Emirate of Crete c. 825–949', *Graeco-Arabica* 7–8, 347–62.

Malberg 2007. S. Malberg, 'Dazzling Dining: Banquets as an Expression of Imperial Legitimacy', in L. Brubaker and K. Linardou (eds), *Eat, Drink and Be Merry (Luke 12:19): Food and Wine in Byzantium*, Society for the Promotion of Byzantine Studies 13, Aldershot: Ashgate, 75–91.

Malgosa et al. 2004. A. Malgosa, A. Alesan, S. Safont, M. Ballbé, M.M. Ayala, 'A Dystocic Childbirth in the Spanish Bronze Age', *International Journal of Osteoarchaeology* 14, 98–103.

Mallegni 1988. F. Mallegni, 'Analisi dei resti scheletrici umani', in A. Di Vita (ed.), *Gortina I*, Monografie della Scuola Archeologica di Atene e delle Missioni Italiane in Oriente III, Rome: 'L'Erma' di Bretschneider, 339–401.

Mango and Dagron 1995. C. Mango and G. Dagron (eds), *Constantinople and its Hinterland*, Papers from the 27th Spring Symposium of Byzantine Studies, Oxford, 2–6 April 1993, Society for the Promotion of Byzantine Studies 3, Aldershot: Ashgate.

Maniatis 2000. G. Maniatis, 'The Organizational Setup and Functioning of the Fish Market in Tenth-Century Constantinople', *Dumbarton Oaks Papers* 54, 13–42.

Margarou 2000. E.L. Margarou, *Τίτλοι και επαγγελματικά ονόματα γυναικών στο Βυζάντιο. Συμβολή στη μελέτη για τη θέση της γυναίκας στη βυζαντινή κοινωνία*, Βυζαντινά Κείμενα και Μελέται 29, Thessaloniki: Κέντρο Βυζαντινών Ερευνών.

Martin et al. 1991. D.L. Martin, A.H. Goodman, G.J. Armelagos, A.L. Magennis, *Black Mesa Anasazi Health: Reconstructing Life from Patterns of Death and Disease*, Center for Archaeological Investigations, Occasional Paper 14, Carbondale: Southern Illinois University at Carbondale.

Martín-Oval and Rodríguez-Martín 1994. M. Martín-Oval and C. Rodríguez-Martín, 'Osteochondritis Dissecans among the Guanche Population of Tenerife (Canary Islands)', Paper presented at the Xth European Meeting of Paleopathological Association, Göttingen, 29 August–3 September.

Matsaggas and Marketos 1985. A.K. Matsaggas and S.G. Marketos, 'Χειρουργική επέμβαση επί συμφύων παίδων στο Βυζάντιο κατά το 10° αιώνα', *Materia Medica Graeca* 13, 415–22.

Matthaiou 1997. A. Matthaiou, *Aspects de l'alimentation en Grèce sous la domination ottomane*, Studien zur Geschichte Südosteuropas 14, Frankfurt am Main: Peter Lang.

Mays 1997. S.A. Mays, 'Carbon Stable Isotope Ratios in Mediaeval and Later Human Skeletons from Northern England', *Journal of Archaeological Science* 24, 561–8.

Mays 2000. S.A. Mays, 'New Directions in the Analysis of Stable Isotopes in Excavated Bones and Teeth', in M. Cox and S. Mays (eds), *Human Osteology in Archaeology and Forensic Science*, London: Greenwich Medical Media, 425–38.

Mays 2005. S.A. Mays, *Guidance for Best Practice for Treatment of Human Remains Excavated from Christian Burial Grounds in England*, London: English Heritage and the Church of England.

Mays 2006. S.A. Mays, 'A Paleopathological Study of Colles' Fracture', *International Journal of Osteoarchaeology* 16, 415–28.

Mays 2008. S.A. Mays, 'A Likely Case of Scurvy from Early Bronze Britain', *International Journal of Osteoarchaeology* 18, 178–87.

Mays and Faerman 2001. S.A. Mays and M. Faerman, 'Sex Identification in Some Putative Infanticide Victims from Roman Britain Using Ancient DNA', *Journal of Archaeological Science* 28, 555–9.

Mays, Brickley and Ives 2006. S.A. Mays, M. Brickley and R. Ives, 'Skeletal Manifestations of Rickets in Infants and Young Adults in a Historic Population from England', *American Journal of Physical Anthropology* 129, 362–74.

Mays, Fysh and Taylor 2002. S.A. Mays, E. Fysh and G.M. Taylor, 'Investigation of the Link between Visceral Surface Rib Lesions and Tuberculosis in a Medieval Skeletal Series from England Using Ancient DNA', *American Journal of Physical Anthropology* 119, 27–36.

McClanan 2002. A.L. McClanan, 'Weapons to Probe the Womb: The Material Culture of Abortion and Contraception in the Early Byzantine Period', in A.L. McClanan and K. Rosoff Encarnación (eds), *The Material Culture of Sex, Procreation, and Marriage in Premodern Europe*, New York: Palgrave, 33–57.

McElroy and Townsend 1996. A. McElroy and P.K. Townsend, *Medical Anthropology in Ecological Perspective*, Boulder, CO: Westview Press.

McKenna, Ball and Gettler 2007. J.J. McKenna, H.L. Ball and L.T. Gettler, 'Mother–Infant Co-Sleeping, Breastfeeding and Sudden Infant Death Syndrome (SIDS): What Biological Anthropology Has Discovered about Normal Infant Sleep and Pediatric Sleep Medicine', *Yearbook of Physical Anthropology* 45, 133–61.

McLaren 1990. A. McLaren, *A History of Contraception from Antiquity to the Present Day*, Cambridge, MA: Basic Blackwell.

Meindl and Lovejoy 1985. R.S. Meindl and C.O. Lovejoy, 'Ectocranial Suture Closure: A Revised Method for the Determination of Skeletal Age at Death Based on the Lateral-Anterior Sutures', *American Journal of Physical Anthropology* 68, 57–66.

Meindl and Lovejoy 1989. R.S. Meindl and C.O. Lovejoy, 'Age Changes in the Pelvis: Implications for Paleodemography', in M.Y. İşcan (ed.) *Age Markers in the Human Skeleton*, Springfield, IL: Charles C. Thomas, 137–68.

Melikian and Waldron 2003. M. Melikian and T. Waldron, 'An Examination of Skulls from Two British Sites for Possible Evidence of Scurvy', *International Journal of Osteoarchaeology* 13, 207–12.

Mensford et al. 1978. R.P. Mensford, C.O. Lovejoy, J.W. Lallo, G.J. Armelagos, 'The Role of Constitutional Factors, Diet, and Infectious Disease in the Etiology of Porotic Hyperostosis and Periosteal Reactions in Prehistoric Infants and Children', *Medical Anthropology* 2, 1–59.

Merbs 1983. C.F. Merbs, *Patterns of Activity-Induced Pathology in a Canadian Inuit Population*, Archaeological Survey of Canada Paper no. 119, Ottawa: National Museums of Canada.

Merbs 1989. C.F. Merbs, 'Trauma', in M.Y. İşcan and K.A.R. Kennedy (eds), *Reconstruction of Life from the Skeleton*, New York: Wiley Liss, 161–89.

Merbs and Vestergaard 1985. C.F. Merbs and E.M. Vestergaard, 'The Paleopathology of Sundown, a Prehistoric Site Near Prescott, Arizona', in C.F. Merbs and R.J. Miller (eds), *Health and Disease in the Prehistoric Southwest*, Anthropological Research Papers no. 34, Tempe: Arizona State University, 85–103.

Merenstein, Kaplan and Rosenberg 1991. G.B. Merenstein, D.W. Kaplan and A.A. Rosenberg, *Silver, Kempe Bruyn and Fulginiti's Handbook of Pediatrics*, Norwalk, CT: Appleton-Century-Crofts and Fleschner Pub.

Metges, Kempe and Schmidt 1990. C. Metges, K. Kempe and H.-L. Schmidt, 'Dependence of the Carbon-isotope Contents of Breath Carbon Dioxide, Milk, Serum and Rumen Fermentation Products on the $\delta^{13}C$ Value of Food in Dairy Cows', *British Journal of Nutrition* 63, 187–96.

Meyer 2005. M. Meyer, 'On the Hypothetical Model of Childbearing in the Octateuchs', *Δελτίον της Χριστιανικής Αρχαιολογικής Εταιρείας* 26, 311–18.

Miller 1996. T. Miller, 'The Care of Orphans in the Byzantine Empire', in C. Itnyre (ed.), *Medieval Family Roles: A Book of Essays*, New York: Garland, 121–36.

Miller 2003. T. Miller, *The Orphans of Byzantium*, Washington DC: Catholic University of America Press.

Minson, Ludlow and Troughton 1975. D.J. Minson, M.M. Ludlow and J.H. Troughton, 'Differences in Natural Carbon Isotope Ratios of Milk and Hair from Cattle Grazing Tropical and Temperate Pastures', *Nature* 256, 602.

Mitchell, Nagar and Ellenblum 2006. P.D Mitchell, Y. Nagar and R. Ellenblum, 'Weapon Injuries in the 12th Century Crusader Garrison of Vadum Iacob Castle, Galilee', *International Journal of Osteoarchaeology* 16, 145–55.

Moffatt 1977. A. Moffatt, 'Schooling in the Iconoclast Centuries', in A. Bryer and J. Herrin (eds), *Iconoclasm*, Birmingham: Centre for Byzantine Studies, University of Birmingham, 85–92.

Moffatt 1986. A. Moffatt, 'The Byzantine Child', *Social Research* 53, 705–23.

Mogle and Zias 1995. P. Mogle and I. Zias, 'Trephination as a Possible Treatment for Scurvy in a Middle Bronze Age (ca 2000 BC) Skeleton', *International Journal of Osteoarchaeology* 5, 77–81.

Møller-Christensen and Sadison 1963. V. Møller-Christensen and A.T. Sadison, 'Usura Orbitae (Cribra Orbitalia) in the Collection of Crania in the Anatomy Department of the University of Glasgow', *Pathological Microbiology* 26, 175–83.

Molleson and Cox 1993. T. Molleson and M. Cox, *The Spitafields Project, vol. 2. The Anthropology: The Middling Sort*, CBA Research Report no. 86, London: Council for British Archaeology.

Moore and Scott 1997. J. Moore and E. Scott (eds.), *Invisible People and Processes: Writing Gender and Childhood into European Archaeology*, London: Leicester University Press.

Morrisson and Sodini 2002. C. Morrisson and J.-P. Sodini, 'The Sixth-Century Economy', in A. Laiou (ed.), *The Economic History of Byzantium: From the Seventh through the Fifteenth Century*, Washington DC: Dumbarton Oaks Research Library and Collection, 171–217.

Morse 1978. D. Morse, *Ancient Disease in the Midwest*, State Museum Reports of Investigations no.15, Springfield: Illinois State Museum.

Motsias 1998. Ch. Motsias, *Τι έτρωγαν οι Βυζαντινοί*, Athens: Εκδ. Κάκτος.

Müldner and Richards 2005. G. Müldner and M.P. Richards, 'Fast or Feast: Reconstructing Diet in Later Medieval England by Stable Isotope Analysis', *Journal of Archaeological Science* 32, 39–48.

Müldner and Richards 2007a. G. Müldner and M.P. Richards, 'Stable Isotope Evidence for 1500 Years of Human Diet at the City of York, UK', *American Journal of Physical Anthropology* 133, 682–97.

Müldner and Richards 2007b. G. Müldner and M.P. Richards, 'Diet and Diversity at Later Medieval Fishergate: The Isotopic Evidence', *American Journal of Physical Anthropology* 134, 162–74.

Mulhern 2002. D. Mulhern, 'Probable Case of Binder Syndrome in a Skeleton from Quarai, New Mexico', *American Journal of Physical Anthropology* 118, 371–7.

Mundell Mango 2007. M. Mundell Mango, 'From "Glittering Sideboard" to Table: Silver in the Well-Appointed *triclinium*', in L. Brubaker and K. Linardou (eds), *Eat, Drink and Be Merry (Luke 12:19): Food and Wine in Byzantium*, Society for the Promotion of Byzantine Studies 13, Aldershot: Ashgate, 127–61.

Musgrave 1976. J.H. Musgrave, 'Anthropological Assessment', in H.W. Catling and D. Smyth, An Early Christian Osteotheke at Knossos, *Annual of the British School at Athens* 71, 25–47.

Mylona 1997. D. Mylona, 'Etudes zooarchaeologiques', in E. Greco, Th. Kalpaxis, A. Schnapp, D. Vivieers, 'Travaux menés en collaboration avec l'Ecole française en 1996', *Bulletin de Correspondance Hellénique* 121, 809–24.

Mylona 2003. D. Mylona, 'Fishing in Late Antiquity', in E. Kotzabopoulou, Y. Hamilakis, P. Halstead, C. Gamble, P. Elefanti (eds), *Zooarchaeology in Greece: Recent Advances*, BSA Studies 9, London: British School at Athens, 103–10.

Mylona 2008a. D. Mylona, 'Τα οστά ζώων από το Βυζαντινό σπίτι στην Αγία Άννα, Πυργί', in Th. Kalpaxis (ed.), Ελεύθερνα. Τομέας II. 3, Βυζαντινό σπίτι στην Αγία Άννα, Rethymno: Πανεπιστήμιο Κρήτης, 335–48.

Mylona 2008b. D. Mylona, *Fish-Eating in Greece from the Fifth Century B.C. to the Seventh Century A.D. A Story of Impoverished Fishermen or Luxurious Fish Banquets?*, BAR International Series 1754, Oxford: Archaeopress.

Nakamura et al. 1982. K. Nakamura, D.A. Schoeller, F.J. Winkler, H.L. Schmidt, 'Geographical Variations in the Carbon Isotopic Composition of the Diet and Hair in Contemporary Man', *Biomedical Mass Spectrometry* 9, 390–94.

Nelson 1997. S.M. Nelson, *Gender in Archaeology: Analyzing Power and Prestige*, Walnut Creek, CA: Altamira Press.

Néraudau 1984. J.-P. Néraudau, *Etre enfant à Rome*, Paris: Les Belles Lettres.

Nerlich et al. 1997. A. Nerlich, C.J. Haas, A. Zink, U. Szeimies, H.G. Hagedom, 'Molecular Evidence for Tuberculosis in Ancient Egyptian Mummy', *Lancet* 350, 1404.

Nevas et al. 2005. M. Nevas, M. Lindström, K. Hautamäki, S. Puoskari, H. Korkeala, 'Prevalence and Diversity of *Clostridium botulinum* Types A, B, E and F in Honey Produced in the Nordic Countries', *International Journal of Food Microbiology* 105, 145–51.

Neves, Barros and Costa 1999. W. Neves, A.M. Barros and M.A. Costa, 'Incidence and Distribution of Postcranial Fractures in the Prehistoric Population of San Pedro de Atacama, Northern Chile', *American Journal of Physical Anthropology* 109, 253–8.

Nicholas and Louvaris 2005. A. Nicholas and J. Louvaris, 'Fast and Abstintence in Byzantium', in W. Mayer and S. Trzcionka (eds), *Feast, Fast or Famine: Food and Drink in Byzantium*, Byzantina Australiensia 15, Brisbane: Australian Association for Byzantine Studies, 189–98.

Nikolaou 1993. K. Nikolaou, *Η θέση της γυναίκας στη Βυζαντινή κοινωνία*, 'Οψεις της Βυζαντινής Κοινωνίας 6, Athens: 'Ιδρυμα Γουλανδρή-Χόρν.

Nikolaou 2005. K. Nikolaou, *Η γυναίκα στη μέση Βυζαντινή εποχή*, Μονογραφίες 6, Athens: Ινστιτούτο Βυζαντινών Ερευνών/ Εθνικό 'Ιδρυμα Ερευνών.

Nobis 1993. G. Nobis, 'Zur antiken Wild-und Hausterfauna Kretas-nach Studien an Tierresten aus den archaologischen Grabungen Poros bei Iraklion und Eleutherna bei Arkadi', *Tier und Museum* 3/4, 109–20.

Nutton 1984. V. Nutton, 'From Galen to Alexander: Aspects of Medicine and Medical Practice in Late Antiquity', *Dumbarton Oaks Papers* 38, 1–14.

Nutton 2004. V. Nutton, *Ancient Medicine*, London: Routledge.

Ogden, Pinhasi and White 2007. A.R. Ogden, R. Pinhasi and W.J. White, 'Gross Enamel Hypoplasia in Molars from Subadults in a 16th–18th Century London Graveyard', *American Journal of Physical Anthropology* 133, 957–66.

Ogden, Weil and Hempton 1976. J.A. Ogden, U.H. Weil and R.F. Hempton, 'Developmental Humerus Varus', *Clinical Orthopaedics* 116, 158–66.

Oikonomides 1990. N. Oikonomides, 'The Contents of the Byzantine House from the Eleventh to the Fifteenth Century', *Dumbarton Oaks Papers* 44, 205–14.

Oikonomou 1988. A. Oikonomou, 'Lampes paléochrétiennes d'Argos', *Bulletin de Correspondance Hellénique* 12, 481–502.

Orlandos 1937. A. Orlandos, 'Τα παλάτια και τα σπίτια του Μυστρά', *Αρχείον των Βυζαντινών Μνημείων της Ελλάδος* 3, 1–114.

Orme 2001. N. Orme, *Medieval Children*, New Haven and London: Yale University Press.

Ortner 1968. D.J. Ortner, 'Description and Classification of Degenerative Bone Changes in the Distal Surfaces of the Humerus', *American Journal of Physical Anthropology* 28, 139–56.

Ortner 1984. D.J. Ortner, 'Bone Lesions in a Probable Case of Scurvy from Metlatavic, Alaska', *MASCA Journal* 3, 79–81.

Ortner 1998. D.J. Ortner, 'Male-Female Immune Reactivity and its Implications for Interpreting Evidence in Human Skeletal Pathology', in A.L. Grauer and P. Stuart-Macadam (eds), *Sex and Gender in Paleopathological Perspective*, Cambridge: Cambridge University Press, 79–92.

Ortner 2003. D.J. Ortner, *Identification of Pathological Conditions in Human Skeletal Remains*, San Diego: Altamira Press.

Ortner and Bush 1993. D.J. Ortner and H. Bush, 'Destructive Lesions of the Spine in a 17th Century Child's Skeleton from Abingdon, Oxfordshire', *Journal of Paleopathology* 5, 143–52.

Ortner and Ericksen 1997. D.J. Ortner and M.F. Ericksen, 'Bone Changes in the Human Skull Probably Resulting from Scurvy in Infancy and Childhood', *International Journal of Osteoarchaeology* 7, 212–20.

Ortner and Mays 1998. D.J. Ortner and S. Mays, 'Dry-Bone Manifestations of Rickets in Infancy and Early Childhood', *International Journal of Osteoarchaeology* 8, 45–55.

Ortner and Putschar 1985. D.J. Ortner and G.J. Putschar, *Identification of Pathological Conditions in Human Skeletal Remains*, Washington DC and London: Smithsonian Institution.

Ortner et al. 2001. D.J. Ortner, W. Butler, J. Cafarella, L. Miligan, 'Evidence of Probable Scurvy in Subadults from Archaeological Sites in North America', *American Journal of Physical Anthropology* 114, 343–51.

Ortner, Kimmerle and Diez 1999. D.J. Ortner, E. Kimmerle and M. Diez, 'Probable Evidence of Scurvy in Subadults from Archaeological Sites in Peru', *American Journal of Physical Anthropology* 108, 321–31.

Paine et al. 2007. R.R. Paine, D. Mancinelli, M. Ruggieri, A. Coppa, 'Cranial Trauma in Iron Age Samnite Agriculturists, Alfedena, Italy: Implications for Biocultural and Economic Status', *American Journal of Physical Anthropology* 132, 48–58.

Pálfi et al. 1992. G. Pálfi, O. Dutour, M. Borreani, J.-P. Brun, J. Berato, 1992, 'Pre-Columbian Congenital Syphilis from the Late Antiquity in France', *International Journal of Osteoarchaeology* 2, 245–61.

Panagiotakis 1961–62. N. Panagiotakis, 'Ζητήματά τινα τῆς κατακτήσεως τῆς Κρήτης ὑπὸ τῶν Ἀράβων', *Κρητικά Χρονικά* B, 9–41.

Papaconstantinou and Talbot 2009. A. Papaconstantinou and A.-M. Talbot (eds), *Becoming Byzantine: Children and Childhood in Byzantium*, Washington DC: Dumbarton Oaks Research Library and Collection.

Papagrigorakis et al. 2006. M. Papagrigorakis, C. Yapijakis, P. Synodinos, E. Baziotopoulou-Valavani, 'DNA Examination of Ancient Dental Pulp

Incriminates Typhoid Fever as a Probable Cause of the Plague of Athens', *International Journal of Infectious Diseases* 10, 206–14.

Papamichael-Koutroumpa 1977–78. A. Papamichael-Koutroumpa, 'Γυναίκες γάλακτος εστερημέναι', *Επετηρίς Εταιρείας Βυζαντινών Σπουδών* 43, 263–77.

Papanikola-Bakirtzi 2002. D. Papanikola-Bakirtzi (ed.), *Ώρες Βυζαντίου-Έργα και Ημέρες στο Βυζάντιο. Καθημερινή ζωή στο Βυζάντιο*, Κατάλογος έκθεσης, Athens: ΥΠ.ΠΟ.

Papanikola-Bakirtzi 2005. D. Papanikola-Bakirtzi, 'Βυζαντινά επιτραπέζια σκεύη. Σχήμα-μορφή, χρήση και διακόσμηση', in D. Papanikola-Bakirtzi (ed.), *Πρακτικά ημερίδας Περί διατροφής στο Βυζάντιο*, Θεσσαλονίκη, 4 November 2001, Athens: ΥΠ.ΠΟ.-Τ.Α.Π.Α., 117–32.

Papathanasiou 2001. A. Papathanasiou, *A Bioarchaeological Analysis of Neolithic Alepotrypa Cave, Greece*, BAR International Series 961, Oxford: Archaeopress.

Papathanasiou 2003. A. Papathanasiou, 'Stable Isotope Analysis in Neolithic Greece and Possible Implications on Human Health', *International Journal of Osteoarchaeology* 13, 314–24.

Papathanasiou 2005. A. Papathanasiou, 'Health Status of the Neolithic Population of Alepotrypa Cave, Greece', *American Journal of Physical Anthropology* 126, 377–90.

Papathanasiou forthcoming. A. Papathanasiou, 'Stable Isotope Analyses in Neolithic and Bronze Age Greece: An Overview', in M.P. Richards and A. Papathanasiou (eds), *Stable Isotope Dietary Studies of Prehistoric and Historic Greek Populations*, OWLS vol. 2, Princeton: American School of Classical Studies in Athens.

Papathanasiou, Larsen and Norr 2000. A. Papathanasiou, C.S. Larsen and L. Norr, 'Bioarchaeological Inferences from a Neolithic Ossuary from Alepotrypa Cave, Diros, Greece', *International Journal of Osteoarchaeology* 10, 210–28.

Papathanasiou, Richards and Zachou 2009. A. Papathanasiou, M.P. Richards and E. Zachou, 'Bioarchaeological Analysis of the Human Osteological Material from Proskynas, Lokris', in L. Schepartz, S. Fox and C. Bourbou (eds), *New Directions in the Skeletal Biology of Greece*, OWLS vol. 1, Hesperia Supplement vol. 43, Princeton: American School of Classical Studies at Athens, 223–35.

Parrington and Roberts 1987. M. Parrington and D.G. Roberts, 'Demographic, Cultural, and Bioanthropological Aspects of a Nineteenth-Century Free Black Population in Philadelphia, Pennsylvania', in J.E. Buikstra (ed.), *A Life in Science: Papers in Honor of J. Lawrence Angel*, Scientific Papers 6, Kampsville, IL: Center for American Archaeology, 138–70.

Parry 2005. K. Parry, 'Vegetarianism in Late Antiquity and Byzantium: The Transmission of a Regimen', in W. Mayer and S. Trzcionka (eds), *Feast, Fast or Famine: Food and Drink in Byzantium*, Byzantina Australiensia 15, Brisbane: Australian Association for Byzantine Studies, 171–87.

Passmore and Eastwood 1986. R. Passmore and M.A. Eastwood, *Human Nutrition and Dietetics*, London: Churchill Livingstone.

Patlagean 1973. E. Patlagean, 'L'enfant et son avenir dans la famille byzantine (IVe–XIIe siècles)', *Annales de démographie historique (enfant et société)*, Paris: La Haye, 85–93.

Patlagean 1977. E. Patlagean, *Pauvreté économique et pauvreté sociale à Byzance, 4e–7e siècles*, Paris: La Haye.

Patlagean 1981. E. Patlagean, *Structure sociale, famille, chrétienté à Byzance IVe–XIe siècle*, London: Variorum Reprints.

Patlagean 1996. E. Patlagean, 'Families and Kinship in Byzantium', in A. Burguière (ed.), *History of the Family*, Oxford: Harvard University Press, 467–88.

Pazaras and Tsanana 1990. T. Pazaras and A. Tsanana, 'Ανασκαφικές έρευνες στη Βέροια Ν. Σύλλατον (1990)', *Αρχαιολογικό Έργο στη Μακεδονία και τη Θράκη* 4, 353–70.

Pentogalos and Lascaratos 1984. G.E. Pentogalos and J.G. Laskaratos, 'A Surgical Operation Performed on Siamese Twins during the Tenth Century in Byzantium', *Bulletin of the History of Medicine* 58, 99–102.

Perou 1964. M.L. Perou, *Cranial Hyperostosis*, Springfield, IL: Charles C. Thomas.

Perry 2005. M. Perry, 'Redefining Childhood through Bioarchaeology: Toward an Archaeological and Biological Understanding of Children in Antiquity', *Archaeological Papers of the American Anthropological Association* 15, 89–111.

Petridis 1986. P. Petridis, 'Lampes paléochrétiennes de Samos', *Bulletin de Correspondance Hellénique* 110, 583–671.

Petroutsa and Manolis 2010. E.I. Petroutsa and S.K. Manolis, 'Reconstructing Late Bronze Age Diet in Mainland Greece Using Stable Isotope Analysis', *Journal of Archaeological Science* 37, 614–20.

Petroutsa et al. 2009. E.I. Petroutsa, M.P. Richards, L. Kolonas, S.K. Manolis, 'Isotope Palaeodietary Analysis of Humans and Fauna from the Late Bronze Age Site of Voudeni, Greece', in L. Schepartz, S. Fox and C. Bourbou (eds), *New Directions in the Skeletal Biology of Greece*, OWLS vol. 1, Hesperia Supplement vol. 43, Princeton: American School of Classical Studies at Athens, 237–44.

Petroutsa, Richards and Manolis 2007. E.I. Petroutsa, M.P Richards and S.K. Manolis, 'Stable Isotope Analysis of Human Remains from the Early Helladic Site of Perahora, Corinth, Greece', in C. Mee and J. Renard (eds), *Cooking Up the Past: Food and Culinary Practices in the Neolithic and Bronze Age Aegean*, Oxford: Oxbow Books, 290–96.

Pfeiffer 2000. S. Pfeiffer, 'Palaeohistology: Health and Disease', in M.A. Katzenberg and S.R. Saunders (eds), *Biological Anthropology of the Human Skeleton*, New York: Wiley-Liss, 287–302.

Pike 1997. S. Pike, 'The Wiener Laboratory', *Paleopathology Association Newsletter* 100, 8–9.

Pirazzoli 1986. P.A. Pirazzoli, 'The Early Byzantine Tectonic Paroxysm', *Zeitschrift für Geomorphologie Supplement* 62, 31–49.

Pirazzoli 2004. P.A. Pirazzoli, 'Tremblements de terre et mouvements verticaux du sol en Crète à l'époque romaine et protobyzantine', in *Atti del Congresso Internazionale, Creta Romana e Protobizantina*, Heraklion, 23–30 September 2000. Padua: Aido Ausilio Editore, 1207–16.

Pirazzoli, Laborel and Stiros 1996. P.A. Pirazzoli, J. Laborel and S.C. Stiros, 'Earthquake Clustering in the Eastern Mediterranean during Historical Times', *Journal of Geophysical Research* 101, 6038–97.

Pitarakis 2009. B. Pitarakis, 'The Material Culture of Childhood in Byzantium', in A. Papaconstantinou and A.M. Talbot (eds), *Becoming Byzantine: Children and Childhood in Byzantium*, Washington DC: Dumbarton Oaks Research Library and Collection, 167–251.

Platakis 1950. E. Platakis, 'Οἱ σεισμοὶ τῆς Κρήτης ἀπό τῶν ἀρχαιοτάτων μέχρι τῶν καθ' ἡμᾶς χρόνων', *Κρητικά Χρονικά* 4, 463–524.

Polet and Katzenberg 2003. C. Polet and M.A. Katzenberg, 'Reconstruction of the Diet in a Mediaeval Monastic Community from the Coast of Belgium', *Journal of Archaeological Science* 30, 525–33.

Poulakou-Rebelakou 1992. E. Poulakou-Rebelakou, *Η παιδιατρική στο Βυζάντιο*, PhD diss., University of Athens.

Poulou-Papadimitriou 2002. N. Poulou-Papadimitriou, 'Βυζαντινές πόρπες: η περίπτωση της Μεσσήνης και της Ελεύθερνας', in P. Themelis and V. Konti (eds), *Πρακτικά του Διεθνούς Συμποσίου, Πρωτοβυζαντινή Μεσσήνη και Ολυμπία. Αστικός και αγροτικός χώρος στη Δυτική Πελοπόννησο*, Athens, 29–30 May 1998. Athens: Εταιρεία Μεσσηνιακών Αρχαιολογικών Σπουδών – Ινστιτούτο Βυζαντινών Ερευνών/Εθνικό Ίδρυμα Ερευνών, 125–36.

Poulou-Papadimitriou 2004a. N. Poulou-Papadimitriou, 'Η εφυαλωμένη κεραμική. Νέα στοιχεία για την εμφάνιση της εφυάλωσης στο Βυζάντιο', in P. Themelis (ed.), *Πρωτοβυζαντινή Ελεύθερνα, Τομέας Ι, τόμος Α΄*, Athens: Πανεπιστήμιο Κρήτης, 209–26.

Poulou-Papadimitriou 2004b. N. Poulou-Papadimitriou, 'Οι χάλκινες πόρπες', in P. Themelis (ed.), *Πρωτοβυζαντινή Ελεύθερνα, Τομέας I*, τόμος Α΄, Athens: Πανεπιστήμιο Κρήτης, 231–52.

Poulou-Papadimitriou 2008. N. Poulou-Papadimitriou, 'Στιγμές από την ιστορία του Ηρακλείου. Από την πρωτοβυζαντινή εποχή έως την περίοδο της οθωμανικής κυριαρχίας (7ος–19ος αι.)', in A. Ioannidou-Karetsou (ed.), *Ηράκλειο. Η άγνωστη ιστορία της αρχαίας πόλης*, Heraklion: Εκδ. 'Νέα Κρήτη', 151–201.

Powers 2005. N. Powers, 'Cranial Trauma and Treatment: A Case Study from the Medieval Cemetery of St. Mary Spital, London', *International Journal of Osteoarchaeology* 15, 1–14.

Prinzing 2009. G. Prinzing, 'Observations on the Legal Status of Children and the Stages of Childhood in Byzantium', in A. Papaconstantinou and A.-M. Talbot (eds), *Becoming Byzantine: Children and Childhood in Byzantium*, Washington DC: Dumbarton Oaks Research Library and Collection, 15–34.

Privat, O' Connell and Richards 2002. K.L. Privat, T.C. O'Connell and M.P. Richards, 'Stable Isotope Analysis of Human and Faunal Remains from the Anglo-Saxon Cemetery at Berinsfield, Oxfordshire: Dietary and Social Implications', *Journal of Archaeological Science* 29, 779–90.

Privat, O'Connell and Hedges 2007. K.L. Privat, T.C. O'Connell and R.E.M. Hedges, 'The Distinction between Freshwater- and Terrestrial-based Diets: Methodological Concerns and Archaeological Applications of Sulphur Stable Isotope Analysis', *Journal of Archaeological Science* 34, 1197–1204.

Prowse et al. 2004. T. Prowse, H.P. Schwarcz, S. Saunders, R. Macchiarelli, L. Bondioli, 'Isotopic Paleodiet Studies of Skeletons from the Imperial Roman-Age Cemetery of Isola Sacra, Rome, Italy', *Journal of Archaeological Science* 31, 259–72.

Rahmani 1981. L.H. Rahmani, 'Finds from a Sixth to Seventh Centuries Site Near Gaza, I: The Toys', *Israel Exploration Journal* 31, 72–80.

Rautman 2006. M. Rautman, *Daily Life in the Byzantine Empire*, Westport, CT: The Greenwood Press.

Reid and Dean 2000. D. Reid and D. Dean, 'The Timing of Linear Hypoplasias on Human Anterior Teeth', *American Journal of Physical Anthropology* 113, 135–41.

Reid et al. 1999. A.H. Reid, T.G. Fanning, J.V. Hultin, J.K. Taubenberger, 'Origin and Evolution of the 1918 "Spanish" Influenza Virus Hemagglutinin Gene', *Proceedings of the National Academy of Sciences of the United States of America* 96, 1651–6.

Rendini 1985. P. Rendini, 'Rapporti tra Africa e Creta nel VI–VII sec. d.C', *in Πεπραγμένα του Ε΄ Διεθνούς Κρητολογικού Συνεδρίου*, τομ. Α΄, Heraklion: Εταιρεία Κρητικών Ιστορικών Μελετών (ΕΚΙΜ), 263–77.

Resnick 1995. D. Resnick, *Diagnosis of Bone and Joint Disorders* (3rd edn), Philadelphia: W.B. Saunders.

Rethemiotakis 1992. G. Rethemiotakis, 'Το κεντρικό Μινωικό κτήριο από το Καστέλλι Πεδιάδος', *Αρχαιολογικόν Δελτίον* 47, 558–9.

Rethemiotakis 1997. G. Rethemiotakis, *A Chest-shaped Vessel and Other LM IIIC Pottery from Kastelli Pediada*, Monographs of the Danish Institute at Athens 1, Athens: Danish Institute.

Rey 2004. A.-L. Rey, 'Autour des nourissons byzantins et de leur régime', in V. Dasen (ed.), *Naissance et petite enfance dans l'Antiquité, Actes du colloque de Fribourg*, 28 November–1 December 2001, Fribourg: Academic Press, 363–75.

Rheidt 1991. K. Rheidt, *Die Byzantinische Wohnstadt. Altertümer von Pergamon XV, Die Stadtgrabung, Teil 2*, Berlin/New York: de Gruyter.

Ribot and Roberts 1996. I. Ribot and C.A. Roberts, 'A Study of Non-Specific Stress Indicators and Skeletal Growth in Two Medieval Subadult Populations', *Journal of Archaeological Science* 23, 67–79.

Ricci 1950. V. Ricci, *The Genealogy of Gynecology: History of the Development of Gynecology throughout the Ages, 2000 B.C.–1800 A.D.*, Philadelphia: Blakiston.

Richards 2000. M.P. Richards, 'Human Consumption of Plant Foods in the British Neolithic: Direct Evidence from Bone Stable Isotopes', in A. Fairbairn (ed.), *Plants in Neolithic Britain and Beyond*, Oxford: Oxbow Monograph, 123–35.

Richards and Hedges 1999. M.P. Richards and R.E.M. Hedges, 'How Chemical Analysis of Human Bones Can Tell Us the Diets of People Who Lived in the Past', in Y. Tzedakis and H. Martlew (eds), *Flavours of Their Times, Food and Drink in Minoan and Mycenaean Times*, Athens: Kapon Publishers.

Richards and Hedges 2008. M.P. Richards and R.E.M. Hedges, 'Stable Isotope Results from the Sites of Gerani, Armenoi and Mycenae', in H. Martlew, Y. Tzedakis and M. Jones (eds), *Archaeology Meets Science: Biomolecular and Site Investigations in Bronze Age Greece*, Oxford: Oxbow Books, 220–30.

Richards and Vika 2008. M.P. Richards and E. Vika, 'Stable Isotope Results from New Sites in the Peleponnese: Sykia, Kalamaki, and Spaliareka', in H. Martlew, Y. Tzedakis and M. Jones (eds), *Archaeology Meets Science: Biomolecular and Site Investigations in Bronze Age Greece*, Oxford: Oxbow Books, 231–4.

Richards et al. 1998. M.P. Richards, T.I. Molleson, J.C. Vogel, R.E.M. Hedges, 'Stable Isotope Analysis Reveals Variations in Human Diet at the Poundbury Camp Cemetery Site', *Journal of Archaeological Science* 25, 1247–52.

Richards, Fuller and Hedges 2001. M.P. Richards, B.T. Fuller and R.E.M. Hedges, 'Sulphur Isotopic Variation in Ancient Bone Collagen from Europe: Implications for Human Paleodiet, Residence Mobility, and Modern Pollutant Studies', *Earth and Planetary Science Letters* 191, 185–90.

Richards, Fuller and Molleson 2006. M.P. Richards, B.T. Fuller and T.I. Molleson, 'Stable Isotope Palaeodietary Study of Humans and Fauna from the Multi-period (Iron Age, Viking and Late Medieval) Site of Newark Bay, Orkney', *Journal of Archaeological Science* 33, 122–31.

Richards, Mays and Fuller 2002. M.P. Richards, S. Mays and B.T. Fuller, 'Stable Carbon and Nitrogen Isotope Values of Bone and Teeth Reflect Weaning Age at the Medieval Wharram Percy Site, Yorkshire, U.K.', *American Journal of Physical Anthropology* 119, 205–10.

Riddle 1994. J.M. Riddle, *Contraception and Abortion from the Ancient World to the Renaissance*, Cambridge, MA: Harvard University Press.

Robb et al. 2001. J. Robb, R. Bigazzi, L. Lazzarini, C. Scarsini, F. Sonego, 'Social "Status" and Biological "Status": A Comparison of Grave Goods and Skeletal Indicators from Pontecagno', *American Journal of Physical Anthropology* 115, 213–22.

Robbins 1975. S.L. Robbins, *Patologia Estructural Functional*, Madrid: Interamericana.

Roberts 1987. C.A. Roberts, 'Case Report no. 9', *Paleopathology Association Newsletter* 57, 14–15.

Roberts 1991. C.A. Roberts, 'Trauma and Treatment in the British Isles in the Historic Period: A Design for Multidisciplinary Research', in D.J. Ortner and A.C. Aufderheide (eds), *Human Paleopathology: Current Syntheses and Future Options*, Washington DC: Smithsonian Institution Press, 225–40.

Roberts 2009. C.A. Roberts, *Human Remains in Archaeology: A Handbook*, York: Council for British Archaeology.

Roberts and Cox 2003. C.A. Roberts and M. Cox, *Health and Disease in Britain: From Prehistory to the Present Day*, Gloucester: Sutton Publishing.

Roberts and Manchester 2005. C.A. Roberts and K. Manchester, *The Archaeology of Disease* (3rd edn), Gloucester: Sutton Publishing.

Roberts et al. 2005. C.A. Roberts, C. Bourbou, A. Lagia, S. Triantaphyllou, A. Tsaliki, 'Health and Disease in Greece: Past, Present and Future', in H. King (ed.), *Health in Antiquity*, London: Routledge, 32–58.

Robinson et al. 2003. S. Robinson, R. Nicholson, A. Pollard, T. O' Connor, 'An Evaluation of Nitrogen Porosimetry as a Technique for Predicting

Taphonomic Durability in Animal Bone', *Journal of Archaeological Science* 30, 391–403.

Rogers 2000. J. Rogers, 'The Paleopathology of Joint Disease', in M. Cox and S. Mays (eds), *Human Osteology in Archaeology and Forensic Science*, London: Greenwich Medical Media, 163–82.

Rogers and Waldron 1988. J. Rogers and T. Waldron, 'Two Possible Cases of Infantile Cortical Hyperostosis', *Paleopathololog Association Newsletter* 63, 9–12.

Rogers and Waldron 1995. J. Rogers and T. Waldron, *A Field Guide to Joint Disease in Archaeology*, Chichester: *John* Wiley.

Rogers et al. 1987. J. Rogers, T. Waldron, P. Dieppe, I. Watt, 'Arthropathies in Paleopathology: The Basis of Classification According to Most Probable Cause', *Journal of Archaeological Science* 14, 179–93.

Romano 1999. R. Romano, 'Il calendario dietetico di Ierofilo', *Atti dell'Accademia Pontaniana* 47, 197–222.

Rosser and Donovan 1983. J. Rosser and W.P. Donovan, 'The Architecture. Dark Age and Byzantine Occupation', in V.A. McDonald, W.D.E Coulson and J. Rosser (eds), *Excavations at Nichoria in Southwest Greece III*, Minneapolis: University of Minnesota Press.

Rothschild and Rothschild 1997. B.M. Rothschild and C. Rothschild, 'Congenital Syphilis in the Archaeological Record: Diagnostic Insensitivity of Osseous Lesions', *International Journal of Osteoarchaeology* 7, 39–42.

Royer et al. 1999. A. Royer, C. Gerard, N. Naulet, M. Lees, G.J. Martin, 'Stable Isotope Characterization of Olive Oils. I – Composition and Carbon-13 Profiles of Fatty Acids', *Journal of the American Oil Chemists' Society* 76, 357–63.

Russell 1986. J. Russell, 'Transformations in Early Byzantine Urban Life: The Contribution and Limitations of Archaeological Evidence', in *Proceedings of the 17th International Byzantine Congress*, Washington DC, 3–8 August 1986. New York: Major Papers, 37–154.

Russell 1995. J. Russell, 'The Archaeological Context of Magic in the Early Byzantine Period', in H. Maguire (ed.), *Byzantine Magic*, Washington DC: Dumbarton Oaks Research Library and Collection, 35–50.

Rutgers et al. 2009. L.V. Rutgers, M. van Strydonck, M. Boudin, C. van der Linde, 'Stable Isotope Data from the Early Christian Catacombs of Ancient Rome: New Insights into the Dietary Habits of Rome's Early Christians', *Journal of Archaeological Science*, 36, 1127–34.

Ryan and Milner 2006. T.M. Ryan and G.R. Milner, 'Osteological Applications of High-Resolution Computed Tomography: A Prehistoric Arrow Injury', *Journal of Archaeological Science* 33, 871–9.

Salamon et al. 2008. M. Salamon, A. Coppa, M. McCormick, M. Rubini, R. Vargiu, N. Tuross, 'The Consilience of Historical and Isotopic Approaches in Reconstructing Medieval Mediterranean Diet', *Journal of Archaeological Science* 35, 1667–72.

Salares 1991. R. Sallares, *The Ecology of Ancient Greek World*, London: Gerald Duckworth.

Salvadei, Ricci and Manzi 2001. L. Salvadei, F. Ricci and G. Manzi, 'Porotic Hyperostosis as a Marker of Health and Nutritional Conditions during Childhood: Studies at the Transition between Imperial Rome and the Early Middle Ages', *American Journal of Human Biology* 13, 709–17.

Sanders 1982. I. Sanders, Roman Crete. *An Archaeological Survey and Gazeteer of Late Hellenistic, Roman and Early Byzantine Crete*, Warminster: Aris and Phillips.

Santos and Roberts 2001. A.L. Santos and C.A. Roberts, 'A Picture of Tuberculosis in Young Portuguese People in the Early 20th Century: A Multidisciplinary Study of the Skeletal and Historical Evidence', *American Journal of Physical Anthropology* 115, 38–49.

Saradi 2006. H.G. Saradi, *The Byzantine City in the Sixth Century*, Athens: Society of Messenian Archaeological Studies.

Sarris 2007. P. Sarris, 'Bubonic Plague in Byzantium: The Evidence of Non-Literary Sources', in L.K. Little (ed.), *Plague in the End of Antiquity: The Pandemic of 541–750*, Cambridge: Cambridge University Press, 119–32.

Saunders 2000. S.R. Saunders, 'Subadult Skeletons and Growth-Related Studies', in M.A. Katzenberg and S.R. Saunders (eds), *Biological Anthropology of the Human Skeleton*, New York: Wiley-Liss, 135–61.

Saunders and Barrans 1999. S.R. Saunders and L. Barrans, 'What Can Be Done About the Infant Category in Skeletal Samples?', in R.D. Hoppa and C.M. Fitzgerald (eds), *Human Growth in the Past: Studies from Bones and Teeth*, Cambridge: Cambridge University Press, 183–209.

Savitt 1993. T. Savitt, 'Sudden Infant Death Syndrome', in K. Kipple (ed.), *The Cambridge World History of Human Disease*, Cambridge: Cambridge University Press, 1017–20.

Scarborough 1984a. J. Scarborough, 'Symposium on Byzantine Medicine. Introduction', *Dumbarton Oaks Papers* 38, ix–xvi.

Scarborough 1984b. J. Scarborough, 'Early Byzantine Pharmacology', *Dumbarton Oaks Papers* 38, 213–32.

Scarborough 2002. J. Scarborough, 'Herbs of the Field and Herbs of the Garden in Byzantine Medicinal Pharmacy', in A. Littlewood, H. Maguire and J. Wolschke-Bulmahn (eds), *Byzantine Garden Culture*, Washington DC: Dumbarton Oaks Research Library and Collection, 177–88.

Schepartz, Fox and Bourbou 2009. L. Schepartz, S. Fox and C. Bourbou (eds), *New Directions in the Skeletal Biology of Greece*, OWLS vol. 1, Hesperia Supplement vol. 43, Princeton: American School of Classical Studies at Athens.

Scheuer and Black 2000. L. Scheuer and L. Black, *Developmental Juvenile Osteology*, London: Elsevier Academic Press.

Scheuer and Black 2004. L. Scheuer and L. Black, *The Juvenile Skeleton*, London: Elsevier Academic Press.

Schmorl and Junghanns 1959. G. Schmorl and H. Junghanns, *The Human Spine in Health and Disease*, New York: Grune and Stratton.

Schoeninger and DeNiro 1984. M.J. Schoeninger and M.J. DeNiro, 'Nitrogen and Carbon Isotope Composition of Bone Collagen from Marine and Terrestrial Animals', *Geochimica et Cosmochimica Acta* 48, 625–9.

Schultz 1989. M. Schultz, 'Causes and Frequency of Diseases during Early Childhood in Bronze Age Populations', in L. Capasso (ed.), *Advances in Paleopathology*, Journal of Paleopathology Monograph Publication no. 1, Chieti: M. Solfanelli, 175–9.

Schultz 1999. M. Schultz, 'The Role of Tuberculosis in Infancy and Childhood in Prehistoric and Historic Populations', in G. Pálfi, O. Dutour, J. Deák, I. Hutás (eds), *Tuberculosis: Past and Present*, Budapest: TB Foundation, 503–7.

Schultz 2001. M. Schultz, 'Paleohistopathology of Bone: A New Approach to the Study of Ancient Diseases', *American Journal of Physical Anthropology* 44, 106–47.

Schultz, Timme and Schmidt-Schultz 2007. M. Schultz, U. Timme and T.H. Schmidt-Schultz, 'Infancy and Childhood in the Pre-Columbian North American Southwest – First Results of the Palaeopathological Investigation of the Skeletons from the Grasshopper Pueblo, Arizona', *International Journal of Osteoarchaeology* 17, 369–79.

Schurr 1997. M.R. Schurr, 'Stable Nitrogen Isotopes as Evidence for the Age of Weaning at the Angel Site: A Comparison of Isotopic and Demographic Measures of Weaning Age', *Journal of Archaeological Science* 24, 919–27.

Schurr and Powell 2005. M.R. Schurr and M.L. Powell, 'The Role of Changing Childhood Diets in the Prehistoric Evolution of Food Production: An Isotopic Assessment', *American Journal of Physical Anthropology* 128, 278–94.

Schwarcz 1999. H.P. Schwarcz, 'Some Biochemical Aspects of Carbon Isotopic Paleodiet Studies', in S. Ambrose and M.A. Katzenberg (eds), *Isotopic Aspects of Paleodiet*, Amsterdam: Kluwer.

Scott 1999. E. Scott, *The Archaeology of Infancy and Infant Death*, BAR International Series 819, Oxford: Archaeopress.

Scranton 1957. R.L. Scranton, *Medieval Architecture in the Central Area of Corinth*, Corinth vol. XVI, Princeton: American School of Classical Studies at Athens.

Sealy 2001. J. Sealy, 'Body Tissue Chemistry and Palaeodiet', in D.R. Brothwell and A.M. Pollard (eds), *Handbook of Archaeological Sciences*, Chichester: Wiley-Liss, 269–79.

Shahar 1990. S. Shahar, *Childhood in the Middle Ages*, London: Routledge.

Shapiro, Hatheway and Swerdlow 1998. R.L. Shapiro, C. Hatheway and D.L. Swerdlow, 'Botulism in the United States: A Clinical and Epidemiologic Review', *Annals of Internal Medicine* 129, 221–8.

Shearer et al. 1983. G. Shearer, D.H. Kohl, R.A. Virginia, B.A. Bryan, J.L. Skeeters, E.T. Nilsen, M.R. Sharifi, P.W. Rundel, 'Estimates of N_2-fixation from Variation in the Natural Abundance of ^{15}N in Sonoran Desert Ecosystems', *Oecologia* 56, 365–73.

Sidiropoulos 2000. K. Sidiropoulos, 'Νομισματικά ευρήματα', in P. Themelis (ed.), *Πρωτοβυζαντινή Ελεύθερνα Τομέας I*, τόμος Β', Rethymno: Πανεπιστήμιο Κρήτης, 261–87.

Sigalos 2004a. L. Sigalos, 'Middle and Late Byzantine Houses in Greece (Tenth to Fifteenth Centuries)', in K. Dark (ed.), *Secular Buildings and the Archaeology of Everyday Life in the Byzantine Empire*, Oxford: Oxbow Books, 53–81.

Sigalos 2004b. E. Sigalos, *Housing in Medieval and Post-Medieval Greece*, BAR International Series 1291, Oxford: Archaeopress.

Singer and Underwood 1962. C. Singer and E.A. Underwood, *A Short History of Medicine*, New York: Oxford University Press.

Sironen 1997. E. Sironen, *The Late Roman and Early Byzantine Inscriptions of Athens and Attica*, PhD diss., University of Helsinki.

Slaus 2000. M. Slaus, 'Biocultural Analysis of Sex Differences in Mortality Profiles and Stress Levels in the Late Medieval Population from Nova Raca, Croatia', *American Journal of Physical Anthropology* 111, 193–209.

Smith 1996. M.O. Smith, '"Parry" Fractures and Female-Directed Interpersonal Violence: Implications from the Late Archaic Period of West Tennessee', *International Journal of Osteoarchaeology* 6, 84–91.

Smith and Epstein 1971. B.N. Smith and S. Epstein, 'Two Categories of $^{12}C/^{13}C$ Ratios for Higher Plants', *Plant Physiology* 47, 380–84.

Smith and Kahila 1992. P. Smith and G. Kahila, 'Identification of Infanticide in Archaeological Sites: A Case Study from the Late Roman–Early Byzantine Periods at Ashkelon, Israel', *Journal of Archaeological Science* 19, 667–75.

Sodini 2004. J.-P. Sodini, 'La naissance de l'habitat médiéval en Méditerranée byzantine: le cas de Gortyne', in *Atti del Congresso Internazionale, Creta Romana e Protobizantina*, Heraklion, 23–30 September 2000, Padua: Aido Ausilio Editore, 669–86.

Sofaer Derevensky 2000. J.S. Soafer Derevensky, *Children and Material Culture*, London: Routldge.

Soren 2008. D. Soren, 'Malaria, Magic and Infant Burials at Lugnano in Teverina, Umbria', Paper presented at the 109th Annual Meeting of the Archaeological Institute of America, Chicago, 3–5 January.

Soren, Fenton and Birkby 1995. D. Soren, T. Fenton and W. Birkby, 'The Late Roman Infant Cemetery near Lugnano in Teverina, Italy: Some Implications', *Journal of Paleopathology* 7, 13–42.

Spanakis 1993. S. Spanakis, *Πόλεις και χωριά της Κρήτης στο πέρασμα των αιώνων: μητρώον των οικισμών*, Heraklion: Γ. Δετοράκης.

Spangenberg, Macko and Hunziker 1998. J.E. Spangenberg, S.A. Macko and J. Hunziker, 'Characterization of Olive Oil by Carbon Isotope Analysis of Individual Fatty Acids: Implications for Authentication', *Journal of Agricultural and Food Chemistry* 46, 4179–84.

Starida 2003. L. Starida, 'Μεσοβυζαντινή εφυαλωμένη κεραμική από το Ηράκλειο', in *Πρακτικά 7ου Διεθνούς Συνεδρίου Μεσαιωνικής Κεραμικής της Μεσογείου*, Θεσσαλονίκη, 11–16 October 1999, Athens: ΥΠ.ΠΟ-Τ.Α.Π.Α, 713–24.

Stathakopoulos 2002. D. Stathakopoulos, 'Rain Miracles in Late Antiquity: An Essay in Typology', *Jahrbuch der Österreichischen Byzantinistik* 52, 73–87.

Stathakopoulos 2004. D. Stathakopoulos, *Famine and Pestilence in the Late Roman and Early Byzantine Empire. A Systematic Survey of Subsistence Crises and Epidemics*, Birmingham Byzantine and Ottoman Monographs vol. 9, Aldershot: Ashgate.

Stathakopoulos 2007a. D. Stathakopoulos, 'Crime and Punishment. The Plague in the Byzantine Empire, 541–749', in L.K. Little (ed.), *Plague in the End of Antiquity: The Pandemic of 541–750*, Cambridge: Cambridge University Press, 99–118.

Stathakopoulos 2007b. D. Stathakopoulos, 'Between the Field and the Plate: How Agricultural Products Were Processed Into Food', in L. Brubaker and K. Linardou (eds), *Eat, Drink and Be Merry (Luke 12:19): Food and Wine in Byzantium*, Society for the Promotion of Byzantine Studies 13, Aldershot: Ashgate, 27–38.

Steele and Daniel 1978. K.W. Steele and R.M. Daniel, 'Fractionation of Nitrogen Isotopes by Animals: A Further Complication to the Use of Variations in the Natural Abundance of ^{15}N for Tracer Studies', *Journal of Archaeological Science* 90, 7–9.

Steinbock 1976. R.T. Steinbock, *Paleopathological Diagnosis and Interpretation: Bone Diseases in Ancient Human Populations*, Springfield, IL: Charles C. Thomas.

Stern 2001.E. M. Stern, *Roman, Byzantine and Early Medieval Glass 10 BCE–700 CE.* Ernesto Wolf Collection, New York: Hatje Cantz Publishers.

Stirland 1996. A. Stirland, 'Patterns of Trauma in a Unique Medieval Parish Cemetery', *International Journal of Osteoarchaeology* 6, 92–100.

Stockwell 1993. E. Stockwell, 'Infant Mortality', in K. Kiple (ed.) *The Cambridge World History of Human Disease*, Cambridge: Cambridge University Press, 224–9.

Stravopodi et al. 2009. E. Stravopodi, S.K. Manolis, S. Kousoulakos, V. Aleporou, M.P. Schultz, 'Porotic Hyperostosis in Neolithic Greece: New Evidence and Further Implications', in L. Schepartz, S. Fox and C. Bourbou (eds), *New Directions in the Skeletal Biology of Greece*, OWLS vol. 1, Hesperia Supplement vol. 43, Princeton: American School of Classical Studies at Athens, 257–70.

Stuart-Macadam 1989. P. Stuart-Macadam, 'Nutritional Deficiency Disease: A Survey of Scurvy, Rickets and Iron Deficiency Anemia', in M.Y. İşcan and K.A.R. Kennedy (eds), *Reconstruction of Life from the Skeleton*, New York: Wiley-Liss, 201–22.

Swerdloff, Ozonoff and Gyepes 1970. B.A. Swerdloff, M.B. Ozonoff and M.T. Gyepes, 'Late Recurrence of the Infantile Cortical Hyperostosis (Caffey's Disease)', *American Journal of Roentgenology* 108, 461–7.

Tachdjian 1972. M.O. Tachdjian, *Pediatric Orthopedic*, Philadelphia: W.B. Saunders.

Talbot 1994. A.-M. Talbot, 'Byzantine Women, Saints' Lives and Social Welfare', in E. Albu Hanawalt and C. Lindeberg (eds), *Through the Eye of The Needle: Judeo-Christian Roots of Social Welfare*, Kirksville, MO: Thomas Jefferson University Press, 105–22.

Talbot 1997. A.-M. Talbot, 'Women', in G. Cavallo (ed.), *The Byzantines*, Chicago: University of Chicago Press, 117–43.

Talbot 2001. A.-M. Talbot, *Women and Religious Life in Byzantium*, Aldershot: Ashgate.

Talbot 2007. A.-M. Talbot, 'Mealtime in Monasteries: The Culture of the Byzantine Refectory', in L. Brubaker and K. Linardou (eds), *Eat, Drink and Be Merry (Luke 12:19): Food and Wine in Byzantium*, Society for the Promotion of Byzantine Studies 13, Aldershot: Ashgate, 109–25.

Talbot 2009. A.-M. Talbot, 'The Death and Commemoration of Byzantine Children', in A. Papaconstantinou and A.M. Talbot (eds), *Becoming*

Byzantine: Children and Childhood in Byzantium, Washington DC: Dumbarton Oaks Research Library and Collection, 283–308.

Taylor 1996. G.M. Taylor, 'DNA from *Mycobacterium tuberculosis* Identified in Medieval Human Skeletal Remains Using Polymerase Chain Reaction', *Journal of Archaeological Science* 23, 789–98.

Taylor et al. 1999. G.M. Taylor, M. Goyal, A.J. Legge, R.J. Shaw, D. Young, 'Genotype Analysis of *Mycobacterium tuberculosis* from Human Skeletal Remains', *Microbiology* 145, 899–904.

Taylor et al. 2000. G.M. Taylor, S. Widdison, I.N. Brown, D. Young, T. Molleson, 'A Medieval Case of Lepromatous Leprosy from 13th–14th Century Orkney, Scotland', *Journal of Archaeological Science* 27, 1133–8.

Taylor, Rutland and Molleson 1997. G.M. Taylor, P. Rutland and T. Molleson, 'A Sensitive Polymerase Chain Reaction Method for the Detection of *Plasmodium* Species DNA in Ancient Human Remains', *Ancient Biomolecules* 1, 193–203.

Teall 1959. J.L. Teall, 'The Grain Supply of the Byzantine Empire', *Dumbarton Oaks Papers* 13, 87–140.

Temkin 1962. O. Temkin, 'Byzantine Medicine: Tradition and Empiricism', *Dumbarton Oaks Papers* 16, 97–115.

Temkin 1991. O. Temkin, *Soranus's Gynecology*, Baltimore: Johns Hopkins University Press.

Themelis 2000. P. Themelis (ed.), *Πρωτοβυζαντινή Ελεύθερνα, Τομέας I, τόμος B'*, Rethymno: Πανεπιστήμιο Κρήτης.

Themelis 2002. P. Themelis, *Αρχαία Ελεύθερνα. Ανατολικός τομέας*, Athens: ΥΠ.ΠΟ.-Τ.Α.Π.Α.

Themelis 2004. P. Themelis (ed.), *Πρωτοβυζαντινή Ελεύθερνα, Τομέας I, τόμος* A', Athens: Πανεπιστήμιο Κρήτης.

Tieszen and Boutton 1989. L. L. Tieszen and T.W. Boutton, 'Stable Carbon Isotopes in Terrestrial Ecosystem Research', in P.W. Rundel, J.R. Ehleringer and K.A. Nagy (eds), *Stable Isotopes in Ecological Research*, New York: Springer Verlag, 167–95.

Tieszen et al. 1983. L.L.Tieszen, T.W. Boutton, K.G. Tesdahl, N.A. Slade, 'Fractionation and Turnover of Stable Carbon Isotopes in Animal Tissues: Implications for δ^{13}C Analysis of Diet', *Oecologia* 57, 32–7.

Tillier et al. 2001. A.-M. Tillier, B. Arensburg, H. Duday, B. Vandermeersch, 'Brief Communication: An Early Case of Hydrocephalus: The Middle Paleolithic Qafzeh 12 Child', *American Journal of Physical Anthropology* 114, 166–70.

Todd 1920. T.W. Todd, 'Age Changes in the Pubic Bone, I: The Male White Pubis', *American Journal of Physical Anthropology* 3, 285–334.

Todd 1921. T.W. Todd, 'Age Changes in the Pubic Bone, II: The Pubis of the Male Negro-White Hybrid, III: The Pubis of the White Female, IV: The Pubis of the Female Negro-White Hybrid', *American Journal of Physical Anthropology* 4, 1–70.

Torres-Rouff and Costa Junqueira 2006. C. Torres-Rouff and M.A. Costa Junqueira, 'Interpersonal Violence in Prehistoric San Pedro de Atacama, Chile: Behavioral Implications of Environmental Stress', *American Journal of Physical Anthropology* 130, 60–70.

Touwaide 2006. A. Touwaide, 'Metrodora', in H. Cancik and H. Schneider (eds), *Brill's New Pauly: Encyclopaedia of the Ancient World*, vol. 8, Leiden and Boston: Brill, col. 836.

Triantaphyllou 2001. S. Triantaphyllou, *A Bioarchaeological Approach to Prehistoric Cemetery Populations from Central and Western Greek Macedonia*, BAR International Series 976, Oxford: Archaeopress.

Triantaphyllou and Richards forthcoming. S. Triantaphyllou and M.P. Richards, 'A Stable Isotope Analysis of Skeletal Assemblages from Prehistoric Greek Macedonia', in M.P. Richards and A. Papathanasiou (eds), *Stable Isotope Dietary Studies of Prehistoric and Historic Greek Populations*, OWLS vol. 2, Princeton: American School of Classical Studies in Athens.

Triantaphyllou et al. 2008. S. Triantaphyllou, M.P. Richards, C. Zerner, S. Voutsaki, 'Isotopic Dietary Reconstruction from Middle Bronze Age Lerna, Argolid, Greece', *Journal of Archaeological Science* 35, 3028–34.

Triantaphyllou et al. 2008. S. Triantaphyllou, M.P. Richards, G. Touchais, A. Philippa-Touchais, S. Voutsaki, 'Analyses of Middle Helladic Skeletal Material from Aspis, Argos, 2. Stable Isotope Analysis of Human Remains', *Bulletin de Correspondance Hellénique* 130, 627–637.

Tritsaroli 2006. P. Tritsaroli, *Pratiques funéraires en Grèce centrale à la période byzantine: Analyse à partir des données archéologiques et biologiques*, PhD diss., Université de Paris.

Tritsaroli and Valentin 2008. P. Tritsaroli and F. Valentin, 'Byzantine Burials Practices for Children: Case Studies Based on a Bioarchaeological Approach to Cemeteries from Greece', in F. Gusi Jener, S. Muriel and C. Olària (eds), *Nasciturus, infans, puerulus vobis mater terra: la muerte en la infancia*, Castellón: Diputació de Castelló, Servei d'Investigacions Arqueològiques i Prehistòriques (SIAP), Spain, 93–113. Available online at <http://dialnet.unirioja.es/servlet/articulo?codigo=2794985>.

Trotter 1970. M. Trotter, 'Estimation of Stature from Intact Limb Bones', in T.D. Stewart (ed.), *Personal Identification in Mass Disasters*, Washington DC: Smithsonian Institution, 71–83.

Tsakalos 2005. A. Tsakalos, 2005. *Συλλογή Γεωργίου Τσολοζίδη. Έργα βυζαντινής και μεταβυζαντινής τέχνης*. Κατάλογος έκθεσης, Athens: ΥΠ.ΠΟ.-Βυζαντινό και Χριστιανικό Μουσείο.

Tsougarakis 1988. D. Tsougarakis, *Byzantine Crete from the 5th Century to the Venetian Occupation*, Athens: D. Vasilopoulos.

Tsougarakis 1991. D. Tsougarakis, 'Παρατηρήσεις στό χαρακτήρα τῶν οἰκισμῶν τῆς Βυζαντινῆς Κρήτης', in *Πεπραγμένα του ΣΤ΄Διεθνούς Κρητολογικού Συνεδρίου*, Τόμος Β΄, Chania: Φιλολογικός Σύλλογος 'ο Χρυσόστομος', 591–619.

Tsougarakis 2007. D. Tsougarakis, 'Η Ελιά και το λάδι στα βυζαντινά χρόνια', in *Ωδή στην Ελιά*, Athens: Ακαδημία Αθηνών, Κέντρον Ερεύνης της Ελληνικής Λαογραφίας-ΥΠ.ΠΟ.-Τ.Α.Π.Α., 101–9.

Tyrell et al. 1984. H.F. Tyrrell, G. Pelletier, R. Chevalier, C. Hillaire-Marcel, M. Gagnon, 'Use of Carbon 13 as a Tracer in Metabolism Studies', *Canadian Journal of Animal Science* Supplement 64, 127–9.

Tzifopoulos 2000. Y.Z. Tzifopoulos, 'The Inscriptions', in P. Themelis (ed.), *Πρωτοβυζαντινή Ελεύθερνα Τομέας I*, τόμος Β΄, Rethymno: Πανεπιστήμιο Κρήτης, 237–59.

Ubelaker 1989. D.H. Ubelaker, *Human Skeletal Remains: Excavation, Analysis, Interpretation*, Manuals on Archaeology 2, Washington DC: Taraxacum Press.

Ubelaker, Katzenberg and Doyon 1995. D.H. Ubelaker, M.A. Katzenberg and L.G. Doyon, 'Status and Diet in Precontact Highland Ecuador', *American Journal of Physical Anthropology* 97, 403–11.

Ulijaszek 1990. S.J. Ulijaszek, 'Nutritional Status and Susceptibility to Infectious Disease', in G.A Harrison and J.C. Waterlow (eds), *Diet and Disease in Traditional and Developing Societies*, Cambridge: Cambridge University Press, 137–54.

Vakaloudi 2001. A.D. Vakaloudi, *Η μαγεία ως κοινωνικό φαινόμενο στο πρώϊμο Βυζάντιο (4ος–7ος μ.Χ. αι.)*, Athens: Εκδ. Ενάλιος.

van Klinken, Richards and Hedges 2000. G.J. van Klinken, M.P. Richards and R.E.M. Hedges, 'An Overview of Causes for Stable Isotopic Variations in Past European Human Populations: Environmental, Ecophysiological, and Cultural Effects', in S. Ambrose and A. Katzenberg, (eds), *Biogeochemical Approaches to Paleodietary Analysis*, New York: Kluwer Academic/Plenum Publishers, 39–63.

Velkovska 2001. E. Velkovska, 'Funeral Rites According to the Byzantine Liturgical Sources', *Dumbarton Oaks Papers* 55, 21–51.

Vika 2007. E. Vika, *A Diachronic Bioarchaeological Approach to the Society of Thebes, Greece: Paleopathological Investigations and Paleodietary Reconstruction Using $\delta^{13}C$, $\delta^{15}N$ and $\delta^{32}S$ Isotope Analysis*, PhD diss., University of Bradford.

Vika et al. forthcoming. E. Vika, M.P. Richards, H. Schutkowski, V. Aravantinos, 'Temporal and Spatial Variations in Diet in Prehistoric Thebes: The Case of the Bronze Age Mass Burial', in M.P. Richards and A. Papathanasiou (eds), *Stable Isotope Dietary Studies of Prehistoric and Historic Greek Populations*, OWLS vol. 2, Princeton: American School of Classical Studies in Athens.

Vika, Aravantinos and Richards 2009. E.Vika, V.Aravantinos and M.P. Richards, 'Aristophanes and Stable Isotopes: A Taste for Freshwater Fish in Classical Thebes (Greece)?', *Antiquity* 83, 1076–83.

Vikan 1973. G. Vikan (ed.), *Illuminated Greek Manuscripts from American Collections: An Exhibition in Honor of Kurt Weitzmann*, Princeton: Princeton University Press.

Vikan 1982. G. Vikan, 'Security in Byzantium: Keys', *Jahrbuch der Österreichischen Byzantinistik* 32, 503–11.

Vikan 1984. G. Vikan, 'Art, Medicine, and Magic in Early Byzantium', *Dumbarton Oaks Papers* 38, 65–86.

Virginia and Delwiche 1982. R.A. Virginia and C.C. Delwiche, 'Natural ^{15}N Abundance of Presumed N_2-fixing and Non-N_2-fixing Plants from Selected Ecosystems', *Oecologia* 54, 317–25.

Vogel 1978. J.C. Vogel, 'Isotopic Assessment of the Dietary Habits of Ungulates', *South African Journal of Science* 74, 298–301.

Vogt 1991–93. C. Vogt, 'Πρωτοβυζαντινή κεραμική από την Αγία Γαλήνη', *Κρητική Εστία* 4, 39–75.

Vogt 2000. C. Vogt, 'The Early Byzantine Pottery', in P. Themelis (ed.), *Πρωτοβυζαντινή Ελεύθερνα Τομέας I*, τόμος Β΄, Rethymno: Πανεπιστήμιο Κρήτης, 37–199.

Volanakis 2002. I. Volanakis, '*Βυζαντινά γυάλινα* μυροδοχεία *από* τη Ρόδο', in P. Themelis (ed.), *Το γυαλί από την αρχαιότητα ως σήμερα*, Athens: Εταιρεία Μεσσηνιακών Αρχαιολογικών Σπουδών, 153–70.

Vroom 2007. J. Vroom, 'The Changing Dining Habits at Christ's Table', in L. Brubaker and K. Linardou (eds), *Eat, Drink and Be Merry (Luke 12:19): Food and Wine in Byzantium*, Society for the Promotion of Byzantine Studies 13, Aldershot: Ashgate, 191–222.

Wagner et al. 2000. A.L. Wagner, F.R. Murtagh, J.A. Arrington, D. Stallworth, 'Relationships of Schmorl's Nodes to Vertebral Body Endplate Fractures and Acute Endplate Disk Extrusions', *American Journal of Neuroradiology* 21, 276–81.

Waldron 1992. T. Waldron, 'Osteoarthritis in a Black Death Cemetery in London', *International Journal of Osteoarchaeology* 2, 235–40.

Waldron, Taylor and Rudling 1999. T. Waldron, G. Taylor and D. Rudling, 'Sexing of Romano-British Baby Burials from the Beddingham and Bignor Villas', *Sussex Archaeological Collections* 137, 71–79.

Walker 1986. P.L. Walker, 'Porotic Hyperostosis in a Marine Depending California Indian Population', *American Journal of Physical Anthropology* 69, 345–54.

Walker 1989. P.L. Walker, 'Cranial Injuries as Evidence of Violence in Prehistoric Southern California', *American Journal of Physical Anthropology* 80, 313–23.

Walker 1997. P.L. Walker, 'Skeletal Evidence for Child Abuse: A Physical Anthropological Perspective', *Journal of Forensic Science* 42, 196–207.

Walker 2001. P.L. Walker, 'A Bioarchaeological Perspective on the History of Violence', *Annual Revue of Anthropology* 30, 573–96.

Walker 2003. A. Walker, 'Wife and Husband: "A Golden Team"', in I. Kalavrezou (ed.), *Byzantine Women and Their World*, Cambridge, MA: Harvard University Art Museums, 215–21.

Walker et al. 2009. P.L. Walker, R.R. Bathurst, R. Richman, T. Gjerdrum, V.A. Andrushko, 'The Causes of Porotic Hyperostosis and Cribra Orbitalia: A Reappraisal of the Iron-Deficiency-Anemia Hypothesis', *American Journal of Physical Anthropology* 139, 109–25.

Wapler, Crubézy and Schultz 2004. U. Wapler, E. Crubézy and M. Schultz, 'Is Cribra Orbitalia Synonymous with Anemia? Analysis and Interpretation of Cranial Pathology in Sudan', *American Journal of Physical Anthropology* 123, 333–9.

Weber 1980. T. Weber, 'Essen und Trinken im Konstantinopel des 10. Jahrhunderts nach den Berichten Liutprands von Cremona', in J. Koder and T. Weber (eds), *Liutprand von Cremona in Konstantinopel: Untersuchungen zum griechischen Sprachschatz und zu realenkundlichen Aussagen in seinen Werken*, BV 8, Vienna: Österreichische Akademie der Wissenschaften, 71–99.

Weiss and Jurmain 2007. E. Weiss and R. Jurmain, 'Osteoarthritis Revisited: A Contemporary Review of Aetiology', *International Journal of Osteoarchaeology* 17, 437–450.

Weitzmann 1977. K. Weitzmann, *Late Antique and Early Christian Book Illumination*, New York: Braziller.

Wells 1962. C. Wells, 'Joint Pathology in Ancient Anglo-Saxons', *Journal of Bone and Joint Surgery* 44, 948.

Wells 1963. C. Wells, 'Hip Disease in Ancient Man. Report of Three Cases', *Journal of Bone and Joint Surgery* 45, 790–91.

Wells 1972. C. Wells, 'Ancient Arthritis', *M&B Pharmaceutical Bulletin*, December, 1–4.

Wesolowsky 1973. A. Wesolowsky, 'The Skeletons of Lerna Hollow', *Hesperia* 42, 340–51.

Weston 2006. D.A. Weston, 'Investigating the Specificity of Periosteal Reactions in Pathology Museum Specimens', *American Journal of Physical Anthropology* 137, 48–59.

White, Healy and Schwarcz 1993. C.D. White, P.F. Healy and H.P.Schwarcz, 'Intensive Agriculture, Social Status and Maya Diet at Pacbitum, Belize', *Journal of Anthropological Research* 49, 347–75.

WHO 1999. World Health Organization (WHO), *Scurvy and Its Prevention and Control in Major Emergencies*, Geneva: World Health Organization.

WHO 2006. World Health Organization (WHO), *Neonatal and Perinatal Mortality: Country, Regional and Global Estimates*, Geneva: World Health Organization.

Wiechmann and Grupe 2005. I. Wiechmann and G. Grupe, 'Detection of *Yersinia pestis* DNA in Two Early Medieval Skeletal Finds from Aschheim (Upper Bavaria, 6th century AD)', *American Journal of Physical Anthropology* 126, 48–55.

Wiggins 1991. R. Wiggins, *Porotic Hyperostosis, Cribra Orbitalia, Enamel Hypoplasia, Periosteal Reaction and Metopism: A Correlation of Their Prevalence and an Assessment of the Nature of Porotic Hyperostosis in Three British Archaeological Populations*, MSc thesis, University of Bradford.

Wileman 2005. J. Wileman, *Hide and Seek: The Archaeology of Childhood*, Stroud: Tempus.

Williams, White and Longstaffe 2005. J.S. Williams, C.D. White and F.J. Longstaffe, 'Trophic Level and Macronutrient Shift Effects Associated with the Weaning Process in the Post-Classic Maya', *American Journal of Physical Anthropology* 128, 781–90.

Wilson, MacLeod and Humphrey 2008. L.A. Wilson, N. MacLeod and L.T. Humphrey, 'Morphometric Criteria for Sexing Juvenile Human Skeletons Using the Ilium', *Journal of Forensic Science* 53, 269–78.

Wood 1996. L. Wood, 'Frequency and Chronological Distribution of Linear Enamel Hypoplasia in a North American Colonical Skeletal Sample', *American Journal of Physical Anthropology* 100, 247–59.

Wood et al. 1992. J.W. Wood, G.R Milner, H.C. Harpending, K.M. Weiss, 'The Osteological Paradox: Problems of Inferring Prehistoric Health from Skeletal Samples', *Current Anthropology* 33, 343–70.

Wood-Jones 1910. F. Wood-Jones, 'Fractured Bones and Dislocations', in G.E. Smith and F. Wood-Jones (eds), *The Archaeological Survey of Nubia Report for 1907–1908*, Cairo: National Printing Department, 1910, 293–342.

Wright and Schwarcz 1998. L.E. Wright and H.P. Schwarcz, 'Stable Carbon and Oxygen Isotopes in Human Tooth Enamel: Identifying Breast-Feeding in Prehistory', *American Journal of Physical Anthropology* 106, 1–18.

Wright and Schwarcz 1999. L.E. Wright and H.P. Schwarcz, 'Correspondence between Stable Carbon, Oxygen and Nitrogen Isotopes in Human Tooth Enamel and Dentine: Infant Diets at Kaminaljuyu', *Journal of Archaeological Science* 26, 1159–70.

Wright and Yoder 2003. L.E. Wright and C.J. Yoder, 'Recent Progress in Bioarchaeology: Approaches to the Osteological Paradox', *Journal of Archaeological Research* 11, 43–70.

Yangaki 2004a. A. Yangaki, 'Οι τάφοι', in P. Themelis (ed.), *Πρωτοβυζαντινή Ελεύθερνα, Τομέας I*, τόμος Α', Athens: Πανεπιστήμιο Κρήτης, 115–83.

Yangaki 2004b. A. Yangaki, 'Τα χρυσά φυλακτά', in P. Themelis (ed.), *Πρωτοβυζαντινή Ελεύθερνα, Τομέας I*, τόμος Α', Athens: Πανεπιστήμιο Κρήτης, 187–204.

Yangaki 2005. A. Yangaki, *La céramique des IVe–VIIe siècles ap. J.-C. d'Eleutherna*, Athens: Université de Crète.

Zanini 2003. E. Zanini, 'Indagini nell'area del "quartiere byzantino" di Gortina: seconda relazione preliminare (campagna 2003)', *Annuario della Scuola Archeologica di Atene*, LXXXI, 913–30.

Zanini 2004. E. Zanini, 'Indagini archeologiche nell'area del "quartiere byzantino" del Pythion di Gortina: terza relazione preliminare (campagna 2004)', *Annuario della Scuola Archeologica di Atene*, LXXXII, 751–768.

Zygouri 2005. V. Zygouri, *Human Skeletal Remains from Kefali of Kastelli Pediados, Central Crete: A Study and Comparative Analysis of Health Status*, MSc thesis, University of Durham.

Index